Cartilage and Osteoarthritis

METHODS IN MOLECULAR MEDICINE™

John M. Walker, SERIES EDITOR

METHODS IN MOLECULAR MEDICINE™

Cartilage
and
Osteoarthritis

VOLUME 1

Cellular and Molecular Tools

Edited by

Massimo Sabatini

Philippe Pastoureau

Frédéric De Ceuninck

Division de Rhumatologie
Institut de Recherches Servier
Suresnes, France

HUMANA PRESS ✳ TOTOWA, NEW JERSEY

© 2004 Humana Press Inc.
999 Riverview Drive, Suite 208
Totowa, New Jersey 07512

www.humanapress.com

This publication is printed on acid-free paper. ∞
ANSI Z39.48-1984 (American Standards Institute)

Permanence of Paper for Printed Library Materials.

Cover design by Patricia F. Cleary.
Cover illustrations: Stained sections of normal (background) and osteoarthritic cartilage (foreground). Artwork courtesy of Massimo Sabatini, Philippe Pastoureau, and Frédéric De Ceuninck.

For additional copies, pricing for bulk purchases, and/or information about other Humana titles, contact Humana at the above address or at any of the following numbers: Tel.: 973-256-1699; Fax: 973-256-8341; E-mail: humana@humanapr.com; or visit our Website: www.humanapress.com

Printed in the United States of America. 10 9 8 7 6 5 4 3 2 1

eISBN 1-59259-810-2
ISSN 1543-1894

Library of Congress Cataloging-in-Publication Data

Cartilage and osteoarthritis.
        p. ; cm. — (Methods in molecular medicine ; 100, etc.)
    Contents: v. 1. Cellular and molecular tools / edited by Massimo Sabatini, Philippe Pastoureau, Frédéric De Ceuninck.
    Includes bibliographical references and index.
    ISBN 1-58829-247-9 (v. 1 : alk. paper)
    1. Cartilage cells—Laboratory manuals. 2. Osteoarthritis—Laboratory manuals. I. Sabatini, Massimo. II. Pastoureau, Philippe. III. De Ceuninck, Frédéric. IV. Series.
    [DNLM: 1. Chondrocytes—pathology. 2. Osteoarthritis. 3. Chondrocytes—metabolism. WE 348 C3268 2004]
    QP88.23.C36 2004
    616.7'223—dc22

                                                                                                200302809

Preface

Osteoarthritis (OA), the most common form of arthritis, is generally characterized by a slowly progressive degeneration of articular cartilage, particularly in the weight-bearing joints. It has a stronger prevalence in women, and its incidence increases with age. OA is a major and growing health concern in developed countries, owing to steadily increasing life expectancy and the demand for better quality of life. Because of its chronic nature and nonfatal outcome, OA affects the growing population of the elderly over an increasing time span. Moreover, despite its relatively benign character, OA is one of the most disabling diseases; it is responsible for increasing financial and social burdens in terms of medical treatments, forced inactivity, loss of mobility, and dependence.

Despite a growing awareness of OA as a medical problem that has yet to reach its maximum impact on society, there is a surprising absence of effective medical treatments beyond pain control and surgery. So far, only symptom-modifying drugs are available, while there remains a major demand for disease-modifying treatments of proven clinical efficacy. This demand will hopefully be met in the future by some of the drugs that have been pressed into development and are now at different stages of clinical investigation. Nevertheless, the current lack of effective treatments reflects a still insufficient knowledge of cartilage with respect to its metabolism, interactions with other joint tissues, and causes and mechanisms (possibly of very different nature) leading to failure of its turnover. As is seen in other therapeutic fields, the future availability of better drugs will depend on a deeper knowledge of OA physiopathology, allowing rational definition of new molecular targets for pharmacological intervention. This new interest in OA is fostering an intense research effort both in academic institutions and in the pharmaceutical industry.

In this context, two volumes of the *Methods in Molecular Medicine*™ series are dedicated to research protocols on cartilage and osteoarthritis. *Cartilage and Osteoarthritis*, Volume 1, *Cellular and Molecular Tools* combines classical but still evolving techniques with emerging methods that promise to add critical knowledge to our understanding of cartilage metabolism in health and disease. Authors with hands-on expertise have described protocols for the in vitro study of normal and osteoarthritic cartilage through biochemical, biomolecular, immunological, and physical approaches. Volume 2: *Structure and In Vivo Analysis* is dedicated to procedures for study at the tissue level of turnover, structure, and functioning of normal and diseased articular cartilage, through invasive and noninvasive means.

v

539 7/8 58

We hope and expect that the two volumes of *Cartilage and Osteoarthritis* will constitute a welcome addition to the literature of research protocols, as well as a helpful and trusted laboratory companion.

Massimo Sabatini
Philippe Pastoureau
Frédéric De Ceuninck

Acknowledgments

We would like to thank Corinne Morlat, Research Assistant, Institut de Recherches Servier, for her invaluable secretarial help in editing this book.

Contents of Volume 1

Cellular and Molecular Tools

vii

CONTENTS OF COMPANION VOLUME

Volume 2: *Structure and In Vivo Analysis*

Contributors

THOMAS AIGNER • *Cartilage Research, Department of Pathology, University of Erlangen-Nürnberg, Erlangen, Germany*

WON C. BAE • *Department of Bioengineering and Whitaker Institute of Biomedical Engineering, University of California, San Diego, San Diego, CA*

BRIGITTE BAU • *Cartilage Research, Department of Pathology, University of Erlangen-Nürnberg, Erlangen, Germany*

MICHEL BECCHI • *UMR 5086 CNRS, Institut de Biologie et Chimie des Protéines, Université Lyon I et IFR 128-Biosciences Lyon-Gerland, Lyon, France*

FRANCIS BERENBAUM • *UPRES-A CNRS 7079, Université Pierre et Marie Curie, Paris, France*

R. CLARK BILLINGHURST • *Department of Health Sciences, St. Lawrence College, Kingston, Ontario, Canada*

AUDREY CALIEZ • *Division de Rhumatologie, Institut de Recherches Servier, Suresnes, France*

ARNOLD I. CAPLAN • *Skeletal Research Center, Department of Biology, Case Western Reserve University, Cleveland, OH*

KANIKA CHAWLA • *Department of Bioengineering and Whitaker Institute of Biomedical Engineering, University of California, San Diego, San Diego, CA*

JANG-SOO CHUN • *Department of Life Science, Kwangju Institute of Science and Technology, Gwangju, Korea*

FRÉDÉRIC DE CEUNINCK • *Division de Rhumatologie, Institut de Recherches Servier, Suresnes, France*

DARRYL D. D'LIMA • *Director, Orthopaedic Research Laboratories, Scripps Clinic Center for Orthopaedic Research and Education, La Jolla, CA*

DIRK ELEWAUT • *Department of Rhumatology, Ghent University Hospital, Ghent University, Ghent, Belgium*

CHRISTOPHER H. EVANS • *Center for Molecular Orthopaedics, Harvard Medical School, Boston, MA*

ANNE-MARIE FREYRIA • *UMR 5086 CNRS, Institut de Biologie et Chimie des Protéines, Université Lyon I et IFR 128-Biosciences Lyon-Gerland, Lyon, France*

PIA M. GEBHARD • *Cartilage Research, Department of Pathology, University of Erlangen-Nürnberg, Erlangen, Germany*

STEVEN C. GHIVIZZANI • *Center for Molecular Orthopedics, Harvard Medical School, Boston, MA*

MARY B. GOLDRING • *Beth Israel Deaconess Medical Center, Division of Rheumatology, New England Baptist Bone and Joint Institute, Harvard Institutes of Medicine, Boston, MA*

JÉRÔME GOUTTENOIRE • *Laboratory of Biology and Engineering of Cartilage, CNRS UMR 5086, Institut de Biologie et Chimie des Protéines, Lyon, France*

ELVIRE GOUZE • *Center for Molecular Orthopaedics, Harvard Medical School, Boston, MA*

JEAN-NOEL GOUZE • *Center for Molecular Orthopaedics, Harvard Medical School, Boston, and Center for Biomedical Engineering, Massachusetts Institute of Technology, Cambridge, MA*

ALAN J. GRODZINSKY • *Center for Biomedical Engineering, Massachusetts Institute of Technology, Cambridge, MA*

JOCHEN HAAG • *Cartilage Research, Department of Pathology, University of Erlangen-Nürnberg, Erlangen, Germany*

ANTHONY HOLLANDER • *University of Bristol Academic Rheumatology, AMBI, Avon Orthopaedic Centre, Southmead Hospital, Bristol, United Kingdom*

MIRELA IONESCU • *Joint Diseases Laboratory, Shriners Hospital for Children, Montreal, Quebec, Canada*

TRAVIS J. KLEIN • *Department of Bioengineering and Whitaker Institute of Biomedical Engineering, University of California, San Diego, San Diego, CA*

MARTIN M. KNIGHT • *Department of Engineering, Queen Mary College, University of London, London, United Kingdom*

THOMAS KNORR • *Cartilage Research, Department of Pathology, University of Erlangen–Nürnberg, Erlangen, Germany*

KLAUS KUHN • *Division of Arthritis Research, The Scripps Research Institute, La Jolla, CA*

DAVID A. LEE • *IRC in Biomedical Materials and Medical Engineering Division, Department of Engineering, Queen Mary College, University of London, London, United Kingdom*

DONALD P. LENNON • *Skeletal Research Center, Department of Biology, Case Western Reserve University, Cleveland, OH*

CHRISTOPHE LESUR • *Division de Rhumatologie, Institut de Recherches Servier, Suresnes, France*

KELVIN W. LI • *Department of Bioengineering and Whitaker Institute of Biomedical Engineering, University of California, San Diego, San Diego, CA*

MARTIN K. LOTZ • *Division of Arthritis Research, The Scripps Research Institute, La Jolla, CA*

FRÉDÉRIC MALLEIN-GERIN • *Laboratory of Biology and Engineering of Cartilage, CNRS UMR 5086, Institut de Biologie et Chimie des Protéines, Lyon, France*

AUDREY MCALINDEN • *Department of Orthopaedic Surgery, School of Medicine, Washington University in St. Louis, St. Louis, MO*

JOHN S. MORT • *Joint Diseases Laboratory, Shriners Hospital for Children, and Departments of Surgery and Medicine, McGill University, Montreal, Canada*

FACKSON MWALE • *The Sir Mortimer B. Davis-Jewish General Hospital, Montreal, Quebec, Canada*

GAYLE E. NUGENT • *Department of Bioengineering and Whitaker Institute of Biomedical Engineering, University of California, San Diego, San Diego, CA*

GLYN D. PALMER • *Center for Molecular Orthopaedics, Brigham and Women's Hospital, Harvard Medical School, Boston, MA*

PHILIPPE PASTOUREAU • *Division de Rhumatologie, Institut de Recherches Servier, Suresnes, France*

A. ROBIN POOLE • *Joint Diseases Laboratory, Shriners Hospital for Children; McGill University, Montreal, Quebec, Canada*

GAËLLE ROLLAND-VALOGNES • *Division de Rhumatologie, Institut de Recherches Servier, Suresnes, France*

PETER J. ROUGHLEY • *Genetics Unit, Shriners Hospital for Children, and Departments of Surgery and Human Genetics, McGill University, Montreal, Canada*

JOACHIM SAAS • *Disease Group Osteoarthritis, Aventis Pharma GmbH, Frankfurt, Germany*

MASSIMO SABATINI • *Division de Rhumatologie, Institut de Recherches Servier, Suresnes, France*

ROBERT L. SAH • *Department of Bioengineering and Whitaker Institute of Biomedical Engineering, University of California, San Diego, San Diego, CA*

LUIS A. SOLCHAGA • *Department of Orthopaedics, Case Western Reserve University and University Hospitals of Cleveland, Cleveland, OH*

MATTHEW C. STEWART • *Department of Veterinary Clinical Medicine, University of Illinois at Urbana–Champaign, Urbana, IL*

MARTIN J. STODDART • *Center for Molecular Orthopaedics, Harvard Medical School, Boston, MA, and Laboratory for Experimental Cartilage Research, Center for Rheumatology and Bone Disease, Zürich, Switzerland*

SYLVIE THIRION • *UMR CNRS 6544, Laboratoire Interactions Cellulaires Neuroendocriennes, Institut Fédératif de Recherche Jean Roche, Faculté de Médecine Nord, Université Aix–Marseille II, Marseille, France*

GUST VERBRUGGEN • *Department of Rhumatology, Ghent University Hospital, Ghent University, Ghent, Belgium*

ERIC M. VEYS • *Department of Rhumatology, Ghent University Hospital, Ghent University, Ghent, Belgium*

JUN WANG • *Department of Rhumatology, Ghent University Hospital, Ghent University, Ghent, Belgium*

LAI WANG • *Department of Rhumatology, Ghent University Hospital, Ghent University, Ghent, Belgium*

JEAN F. WELTER • *Department of Orthopaedics, Case Western Reserve University and University Hospitals of Cleveland, Cleveland, OH*

ALEXANDER ZIEN • *Cartilage Research, Department of Pathology, University of Erlangen–Nürnberg, Erlangen, Germany*

RALF ZIMMER • *Cartilage Research, Department of Pathology, University of Erlangen–Nürnberg, Erlangen, Germany*

1

Culture and Phenotyping of Chondrocytes in Primary Culture

Sylvie Thirion and Francis Berenbaum

Summary

The culture of chondrocytes is one of the most powerful tool for exploring the intracellular and molecular features of chondrocyte differentiation and activation. However, chondrocytes tend to dedifferentiate to fibroblasts when they are subcultured, which is a major problem. This chapter describes several protocols for culturing chondrocytes of different anatomical origins (articular and costal chondrocytes) from various species (humans, mice, rabbits, and cattle). All these protocols involve primary cultures in order to limit dedifferentiation. This chapter also describes a new protocol for culturing mouse articular chondrocytes.

Key Words: Primary cell culture; isolation; cartilage; articular chondrocytes; costal chondrocytes; human; mice; rabbit; cattle.

1. Introduction

Normal cartilage has two main components: the collagen- and proteoglycan-rich extracellular matrix and a population of isolated chondrocytes lying within this matrix. From the outermost cartilage layer to the growth plate zone, these chondrocytes show phenotypic variations that reflect their progress through a cascade of differentiating events triggered by environmental signals that either stimulate or suppress the conversion from articular chondrocytes to hypertrophic chondrocytes (also called epiphyseal chondrocytes) *(1–3)*. Articular chondrocytes produce a matrix that confers tensile strength and flexibility to articular surfaces, whereas growth plate chondrocytes produce a matrix capable of undergoing mineralization *(4)*. These functional differences explain the specific phenotype of articular and hypertrophic chondrocytes *(2)*. Articular chondrocytes mainly express collagen types II, IX, and XI, as well as aggrecan *(1,5)*. Hypertrophic chondrocytes reach more advanced stages of differentia-

From: *Methods in Molecular Medicine, Vol. 100: Cartilage and Osteoarthritis, Vol. 1: Cellular and Molecular Tools*
Edited by: M. Sabatini, P. Pastoureau, and F. De Ceuninck © Humana Press Inc., Totowa, NJ

tion and express collagen type X and alkaline phosphatase, along with collagen types II and IX and aggrecan *(6–8)*.

Chondrocyte cultures remain one of the most powerful tools for investigating intracellular and molecular events associated with chondrocyte differentiation and activation *(9,10)*. However, culturing can produce artifacts that bias results *(1,2)*. The main problem is that cultured chondrocytes tend to dedifferentiate into fibroblasts. Factors associated with an increased tendency toward dedifferentiation include the following:

1. Low-density plating *(11)*.
2. Monolayer culturing *(3,12)*.
3. Treatment with proinflammatory cytokines, such as interleukin-1 (IL-1) *(13–15)*.
4. Extraction from human adult cartilage.
5. Extraction from chondrosarcoma or immortalization *(16–18)*.

Conversion from the chondrocyte to the fibroblast phenotype can be detected based on a switch from collagen type II (articular chondrocytes) or type X (epiphyseal chondrocytes) to collagen types I and III, and from high-molecular-weight proteoglycans (aggrecan) to low-molecular-weight proteoglycans (biglycan and decorin) *(13–15)*. To minimize conversion to fibroblasts, studies of nonsubcultured chondrocytes in monolayers have made extensive use of cells from young animals such as rabbits, cattle, or rats, which are more stable than human adult chondrocytes.

Over the last 20 yr, efforts to obtain a better phenotype than that of 2D cultured chondrocytes have involved embedding the cells in an artificial matrix made of alginate (*see* Chapter 2), agarose, or collagens *(3,12,16)*. However, although this approach improves the chondrocyte phenotype, it slows cell growth, so that less material is available for study. In addition, extracting the cells from the matrix is technically challenging. Cell lines from chondrosarcoma produce larger numbers of cells but have tumorigenic properties that may fail to replicate physiological processes *(12,17,18)*. Recently, immortalized chondrocytes have been developed to overcome this problem *(14,19)*. Several immortalized chondrocyte cell lines have been shown to express a chondrocyte-specific phenotype with a high proliferation rate. However, phenotypic stability is lost more quickly during expansion in serial monolayer cultures, compared with primary cultures of cells from juvenile animals.

Finally, many genetically modified animal models have been developed recently, providing new powerful tools for understanding cartilage differentiation or degradation. However, attempts to culture mouse articular chondrocytes have been frustrated by the small size of the joints, which limits the feasibility of extracting chondrocytes from the cartilage matrix. In addition to the method for culturing chondrocytes from numerous species, a new method for culturing articular chondrocytes from newborn mice is detailed.

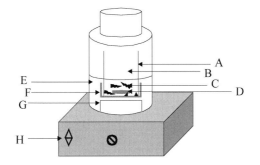

Fig. 1. Cartilage digestion chamber. Bottle used for isolating chondrocytes. A nylon mesh forms a barrier between the inner and outer chambers. The filter is fastened to a glass tube with a glass ring (not shown here) and placed on a glass-rod triangle, in order to leave a narrow space between the filter and the bottom of the vessel. The chondrocytes released into this space are withdrawn with a pipet. A magnetic bar is placed in the inner chamber. A, glass cylinder; B, inner chamber; C, cartilage pieces; D, magnetic bar; E, outer chamber; F, nylon mesh (48-µm pore size); G, platform; H, battery-powered magnetic stirrer.

2. Materials

2.1. Human Primary Articular Chondrocytes

1. Cell culture medium: Dulbecco's modified Eagle's medium (DMEM high glucose, Sigma, France), supplemented with 4 mM L-glutamine, 100 U/mL penicillin, and 0.1 mg/mL streptomycin.
2. Complete culture medium consists of DMEM high glucose supplemented with antibiotics as above and with 10% (v/v) fetal calf serum (FCS). Store FCS aliquots at –20°C and do not refreeze after thawing (*see* **Note 1**).
3. Sterile Dulbecco's phosphate-buffered Ca^{2+}- and Mg^{2+}-free saline (PBS).
4. Enzymes (Roche Diagnostics, Meylan, France): hyaluronidase 0.05% (w/v) in PBS; trypsin, 0.2% (w/v) in PBS; collagenase A from *Clostridium histolyticum*, 0.2% (w/v) in PBS (*see* **Note 2**). Enzyme solutions are freshly prepared and filtered through a sterile 0.22-µm filter.
5. Scalpels.
6. 30-mL Flat-bottomed glass vial, glass ring, glass cylinder, and glass triangle (custom glassware prepared by a local glassblower and adapted as shown in **Fig. 1**).
7. Magnetic stirrer (battery-powered).
8. Nylon mesh, 48 µm (WWR for Sefar AG, Rüschlikon, Switzerland).
9. Tissue culture plastic: sterile pipets, culture flasks, and Petri dishes.
10. CO_2 incubator.
11. Centrifuge.
12. Inverted light microscope.
13. Hemocytometer.

2.2. Isolation and Culture of Rabbit
Primary Articular Chondrocytes

The following was adapted from **ref. *20***.

1. Cell culture medium: Ham's F-12 medium (Sigma, France) supplemented with 4 m*M* L-glutamine, 100 U/mL penicillin, and 0.1 mg/mL streptomycin.
2. Complete culture medium consists of Ham's F-12 medium supplemented with antibiotics as above and with 10% (v/v) FCS.
3. Animal shaver.
4. 15-mL Custom glassware as shown in **Fig. 1**.
5. All other materials and equipment as in **Subheading 2.1.** (For enzymes, *see* **Note 3**.)

2.3. Isolation and Culture of Rat
and Bovine Primary Articular Chondrocytes

The following was adapted from **ref. *21***.

1. Cell culture medium: DMEM/Ham's F-12 medium supplemented with 2 m*M* L-glutamine, 50 µg/mL gentamicin, and 0.25 µg/mL amphotericin B.
2. Complete culture medium consists of DMEM/Ham's F-12 medium supplemented as above with, in addition, 10% (v/v) FCS.
3. Enzymes (Roche Diagnostics): pronase 1% (w/v) in cell culture medium containing 5% FCS; bacterial collagenase 0.4% (w/v) in cell culture medium containing 5% FCS. Enzyme solutions are freshly prepared and filtered through a sterile 0.22-µm filter.
4. 15-mL Custom glassware as shown in **Fig. 1**.
5. All other materials and equipments as in **Subheading 2.1.**

2.4. Isolation and Culture of Newborn Mouse Rib Chondrocytes

The following was adapted from **ref. *22***.

1. Cell culture medium: DMEM (Sigma, France) supplemented with 2 m*M* L-glutamine, 50 U/mL penicillin, and 0.05 mg/mL streptomycin.
2. Complete culture medium consists of DMEM supplemented as above with, in addition, 10% (v/v) FCS.
3. Enzyme (Roche Diagnostics): collagenase D from *Clostridium histolyticum*, 3 mg/mL in cell culture medium (*see* **Note 2**). The enzyme solution is freshly prepared and filtered through a sterile 0.22-µm filter.
4. 70% Ethanol.
5. All other materials and equipment as in **Subheading 2.1.**

2.5. Isolation and Culture of Mouse Primary Articular Chondrocytes

1. All solutions, materials, and equipment as in **Subheading 2.4.** plus 0.5 mg/mL collagenase D in cell culture medium.

3. Methods

3.1. Human Primary Articular Chondrocytes (see Note 4)

3.1.1. Collection of Articular Specimens

As soon as possible after surgery, place the knees or hips in cold collection medium and store at 4°C. Specimens collected and stored in this way can be used for chondrocyte isolation up to 48 h after surgery.

Osteoarthritic cartilage specimens can be obtained from the tibial plateaus and femoral condyles of adults undergoing total knee replacement. They are excised from the superficial and middle layers, avoiding the calcified layer. Nonarthritic human articular cartilage can be isolated from femoral heads of patients with displaced femoral neck fractures or at autopsy of individuals with no history of joint disease and with normal cartilage by gross examination and microscopy. Each culture is run with chondrocytes from a single patient (*see* **Note 5**).

3.1.2. Isolation and Culture of Human Chondrocytes

1. Under a laminar flow hood, place the joints in a dish containing complete culture medium. When necessary, remove mesenchymal repair tissue with scissors and scalpels to clear the cartilaginous layer completely. Cut across the surface to obtain full-thickness strips of cartilage, excluding subchondral bone, and tip the strips of cartilage into 10-cm dishes containing 0.05% hyaluronidase in PBS.
2. Finely mince all collected cartilage slices into about $1–3$-mm^3 pieces, using scalpels.
3. Remove the hyaluronidase solution and rinse the cartilage once with PBS.
4. Transfer the pieces of cartilage from the Petri dish to the inner chamber of the sterile mounted glass vial (**Fig. 1**) and carefully add to the inner chamber 10 mL of 0.2% trypsin solution.
5. Transfer the vial to the CO_2 incubator previously equipped with a battery-powered shaker and subject the mixture to magnetic stirring at low speed at 37°C for 45 min.
6. Discard the trypsin solution from the outer chamber and resuspend the cartilage slices in 10 mL of 0.2% collagenase solution.
7. Incubate the vial in a CO_2 incubator at 37°C for 90 min while shaking.
8. Aspirate the suspension from the outer chamber of the vial and use a pipet to transfer it to a new sterile 50-mL polypropylene tube.
9. Add 10 mL fresh 0.2% collagenase solution to the inner chamber and incubate for 45 min at 37°C in a CO_2 incubator while shaking.
10. During **step 9**, centrifuge the 50-mL polypropylene tube for 5 min at 200g and discard the supernatant.
11. Resuspend the pellet in 10 mL of complete culture medium.
12. At the end of the second collagenase digestion, aspirate the suspension from the outer chamber of the vial and add to the 50-mL tube containing the first suspended cells (*see* **step 11**).

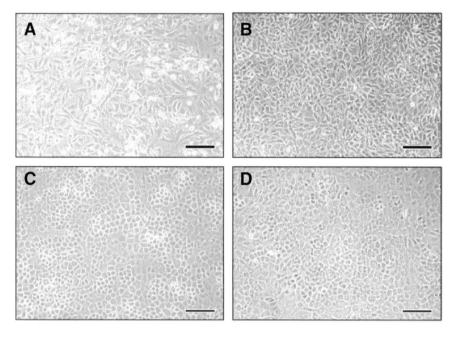

Fig. 2. Micrographs of different species of primary cultured chondrocytes. (**A**) Human articular chondrocytes. (**B**) Rabbit articular chondrocytes. (**C**) Mouse rib chondrocytes. (**D**) Mouse articular chondrocytes. Phase-contrast micrograph. Original magnification ×120; scale bars, 100 μm.

13. Wash the remaining cartilage pieces in adding 10 mL serum-free culture medium to the inner chamber of the vial. Incubate for 90 min at 37°C in a CO_2 incubator while shaking. During this step, centrifuge the 50-mL polypropylene tube for 5 min at 200g and discard the supernatant.
14. Resuspend the pellet in 10 mL of complete culture medium.
15. Pipet the cell suspension from the outer chamber of the vial and add to the 50-mL tube containing the suspended cells.
16. Centrifuge for 5 min at 200g and discard the supernatant.
17. Resuspend the pellet in 10 mL of complete culture medium and count the cells in a hemocytometer. Bring up to volume with complete culture medium and seed the suspended chondrocytes onto tissue culture plates or dishes at a density of 1×10^5 cells/cm^2.
18. Incubate the culture plates or dishes for 2 d undisturbed at 37°C under humidified conditions and 5% CO_2/95% air to ensure strong attachment.
19. Change the medium on the day before harvest. To avoid dedifferentiation, we use human primary chondrocytes between 3 and 6 d after seeding. (Their morphological appearance is shown in **Fig. 2A**.)

3.2. Isolation and Culture of Rabbit Primary Articular Chondrocytes

1. Sacrifice 3-wk-old female Fauve-de-Bourgogne rabbits under general anesthesia (*see* **Note 6**). Shave each limb of the animal and clean with a disinfectant; use sterile equipment to remove the joints.
2. Dissected out the shoulders, knees, and femoral heads of the rabbit and transfer to 50-mL sterile polypropylene tubes containing complete culture medium.
3. Under a laminar flow hood, place the joints in a dish containing complete culture medium. Remove extraneous tissue with scissors and scalpels to clear the cartilaginous layer completely.
4. Cut the cartilage into longitudinal slices, and tip the slices into 10-cm dishes containing 0.05% hyaluronidase in PBS.
5. Repeat **steps 2–15** of **Subheading 3.1.2.**, but add only 5 mL of enzyme in **steps 4, 6,** and **9** and 5 mL of complete culture medium in **steps 11–17**. Incubate for 60 min in **steps 7** and **13** and for 30 min in **step 9**. Use a 15-mL polypropylene tube instead of a 50-mL tube.
6. Transfer the cell suspension to a new sterile 50-mL polypropylene tube, centrifuge for 5 min at 200g, and discard the supernatant.
7. Resuspend the pellet in 20 mL complete culture medium and count the cells in a hemocytometer. Bring up to volume with complete culture medium and seed the suspended chondrocytes onto tissue culture plates or dishes at a density of 8 × 10^3 cells/cm^2 (*see* **Note 7**).
8. Incubate the culture plates or dishes for 4 d undisturbed at 37°C under humidified conditions and 5% CO_2/95% air to ensure strong attachment.
9. After 4 d, replace the medium with fresh complete culture medium every 2–3 d and monitor the progress of the cultures by observing them under a phase-contrast inverted microscope. The chondrocytes expand and may grow to confluence within 6–8 d (*see* **Fig. 2B**).

3.3. Isolation and Culture of Rat and Bovine Primary Articular Chondrocytes

3.3.1. Tissue Samples

1. Bovine.
   a. Harvest bovine articular cartilage from various joints of young calves (about 2–4 wk old) or adult steers (18–24 mo old), obtained from the local slaughterhouse.
   b. Depending on the studies, aseptically collect full-thickness articular cartilage slices from the metatarsophalangeal *(23)*, metacarpophalangeal *(21)*, humeroscapular *(24)*, or femoropatellar *(22)* joints.
   c. Immediately place the articular cartilage slices in culture medium.
2. Rats
   a. Male Wistar rats (130–150 g) are housed under controlled temperature and lighting conditions, with food and water *ad libitum*.

  b. Sacrifice the rats under general anesthesia (ketamine and acepromazine), and cut into slices joint cartilage taken surgically from the knees and hips (*see* **Note 6**).

3.3.2. Isolation and Culture of Chondrocytes

1. Tip slices of cartilage into 10-cm dishes containing 1% pronase (w/v) in culture medium containing 5% FCS (*see* **Note 8**).
2. Finely mince all collected cartilage slices into about 1-mm³ pieces, using scalpels.
3. Incubate the cartilage fragments in a CO_2 incubator at 37°C, for 90 min.
4. Remove the pronase solution and rinse the cartilage once with PBS.
5. Transfer the pieces of cartilage from the Petri dish to the inner chamber of the digestion sterile glass vial and carefully add 5 mL of 0.4% collagenase solution to the inner chamber (*see* **Note 9**).
6. Transfer the vial to the CO_2 incubator previously equipped with a battery-powered shaker and subject the mixture to magnetic stirring at low speed at 37°C for 180 min.
7. Aspirate the suspension from the outer chamber of the vial and use a pipet to transfer it to a new sterile 15-mL polypropylene tube.
8. Centrifuge the 15-mL polypropylene tube for 5 min at 200*g* and discard the supernatant.
9. Resuspend the pellet in 10 mL PBS.
10. Centrifuge the 15-mL polypropylene tube for 5 min at 200*g* and discard the supernatant.
11. Repeat **steps 9** and **10**.
12. Resuspend the pellet in 5 mL complete culture medium.
13. Count the cells in a hemocytometer. Bring up to volume with complete culture medium and *seed* the suspended chondrocytes onto tissue culture plates or dishes at a density of 1.5×10^5 cells/cm².
14. Incubate the culture plates or dishes for 4 d undisturbed at 37°C under humidified conditions and 5% CO_2/95% air to ensure strong attachment.
15. After 4 d, replace the medium with fresh complete culture medium every 2–3 d and monitor the progress of the cultures by observing them under a phase-contrast inverted microscope. The chondrocytes expand and may grow to confluence within 6–8 d.

3.4. Isolation and Culture of Newborn Mouse Rib Chondrocytes

1. Sacrifice newborn mice (0–4 d old) under general anesthesia (*see* **Note 6**).
2. After washing with 70% ethanol, place the mouse on its back and keep in position by pinning the mouse to a paper-covered corkplate.
3. Make a longitudinal incision through the skin of the abdomen and rib cage, pull the skin to the sides, and open the front of the rib cage longitudinally along the midline.
4. Dissect the ventral part of the rib cage and place in a sterile 50-mL polypropylene tube containing cold PBS.

5. Under a laminar flow hood, wash the rib cages two or three times with sterile PBS.
6. Incubate the rib cages in collagenase D (about 1 mL/rib cage) in the CO_2 incubator at 37°C for 90 min.
7. Check that all the soft tissues are digested or can be detached from the cartilages with a few pipetings. If not, incubate longer.
8. Transfer the pieces into a 50-mL sterile polypropylene tube.
9. Fill with PBS; allow the rib cartilages (and bones) to settle for just a few minutes and immediately remove the supernatant.
10. Fill again with PBS, mix gently, allow the cartilages to settle, and remove the supernatant.
11. Repeat **steps 9** and **10** until the cartilages seem clean. These washes must eliminate most of the soft tissues contaminating the cartilages.
12. Resuspend the cartilages in collagenase D (about 1 mL/cage) and transfer to a 10-cm Petri dish. (Do not leave in the tube, as this would cause the cells to die.)
13. Leave in the incubator for 5–6 h or until the cartilages are completely digested. (Withdraw and expel in the pipet a few times to check digestion.) At the end of the incubation, only the bony parts of the ribs are left undigested (*see* **Note 10**).
14. Transfer the supernatant, which contains the chondrocytes, to a new 50-mL sterile polypropylene tube (avoid all bony particles).
15. Fill the tube with PBS
16. Centrifuge at 200*g* for 10 min to pellet the cells.
17. Remove the supernatant.
18. Repeat **steps 15–17**.
19. Fill the tube with complete medium.
20. Centrifuge at 200*g* for 10 min to pellet the cells.
21. Remove the supernatant.
22. Resuspend the cells in 8 mL of complete medium and count them.
23. Plate the chondrocytes at high density, 1–2 million cells per 10-cm^2 dish in 8 mL of complete medium (*see* **Note 11** and **Fig. 2C**).

3.5. Isolation and Culture of Mouse Primary Articular Chondrocytes

1. Sacrifice newborn mice (5 d old) under general anesthesia (*see* **Notes 6** and **12**)
2. After washing with 70% ethanol, place the mouse on its abdomen and keep in position by pinning the mouse to a paper-covered corkplate.
3. Remove the skin and soft tissue from the hind legs using scissors and one pair of sterile curved forceps.
4. Dislocate the femur from the hip using scissors and remove the soft tissues surrounding the femoral head.
5. Block the femoral head (which resembles the head of a pin) between the curved tips of forceps, and clamp hard to cut it off. Pick up the femoral head carefully and place it in a 50-mL sterile polypropylene tube containing complete culture medium.
6. Incise the knee joint capsules to expose the femoral condyles and the tibial plateau.

7. Crack the bone open to isolate the femoral condyles and the tibial plateau and place in the 50-mL tube containing the femoral heads.
8. Transfer the pieces of tissue from the tube to a sterile 100-mm Petri dish containing 12 mL collagenase D, 3 mg/mL, in cell culture medium.
9. Incubate for 45 min at 37°C in the incubator.
10. Use a sterile plastic 25-mL pipet to agitate the tissue fragments for 30 s and transfer the pieces to a new sterile 100-mm Petri dish containing fresh collagenase D solution (3 mg/mL).
11. Incubate typically for 45 min at 37°C in the incubator and check that all the soft tissues have then been removed.
12. Use a sterile plastic 25-mL pipet to agitate the tissue fragments for 30 s and transfer the pieces to a new sterile 100-mm Petri dish containing 20 mL collagenase D, 0.5 mg/mL, overnight at 37°C.
13. Dislodge the smaller sheets of cells from the bone heads by vigorous agitation, first with a sterile plastic 5-mL pipet and then with a plastic 2-mL pipet. The cell suspension should be well mixed to disperse any cell aggregates in order to obtain a suspension of single cells.
14. Allow the Petri dish to stand for 2 min to let the bone fragments to settle to the bottom of the dish. Then draw off the cell suspension.
15. Pass the cell suspension through sterile 48-µm nylon mesh into a fresh 50-mL polypropylene tube in order to remove any sheets of dead cells.
16. Centrifuge for 10 min at 200g and discard the supernatant.
17. Resuspend the pellet in 10 mL complete culture medium and count the cells in a hemocytometer. Bring up to volume with complete culture medium and seed the suspended chondrocytes onto tissue culture plates or dishes at a density of 8×10^3 cells/cm^2. A 6-d-old culture is shown in **Fig. 2D**.

4. Notes

1. Batches of serum vary in their ability to support the proliferation and differentiated phenotype expression of chondrocytes in primary culture. It is advisable to screen the batches and to keep a large reserve of serum once a suitable batch has been identified. We used serum from Gibco-BRL (Cergy Pontoise, France).
2. The collagenase most commonly used for tissue dissociation is a crude preparation from *C. histolyticum* containing clostridiopeptidase A in addition to a number of other proteases, polysaccharidases, and lipases. Crude collagenase is apparently ideal for tissue dissociation since it contains the enzyme required to attack native collagen, in addition to the enzymes that hydrolyze the other proteins, polysaccharides, and lipids in the extracellular matrix of tissues. Collagenases A, B, and D are prepared from extracellular *C. histolyticum* culture filtrate. These crude preparations contain collagenase and other proteases, including clostripain, trypsin-like activity, and a neutral protease. This mixture of enzyme activities makes crude collagenases ideal for gentle tissue dissociation to generate single cells. Collagenases A, B, and D contain different ratios of the various proteolytic activities. This allows for selection of the preparation best suited for

disaggregation of a particular tissue. In our hands, the best results were obtained using collagenase A for rabbit and human chondrocyte dissociation and collagenase D for mouse chondrocyte dissociation.

3. An alternative method for rabbit articular chondrocyte dissociation uses pronase E (2 mg/g cartilage, 30 min, 37°C) instead of trypsin *(25)*.

4. Many protocols have been described for isolating chondrocytes from adult human joints *(26–28)*. Some studies have used fetal human chondrocytes *(29,30)*, and in general the fetal human joint has been found to be superior to the adult human joint in terms of cell numbers. However, the qualitative differences between fetal and adult cells cannot be disregarded, as fetal tissues consist mainly of epiphyseal cartilage. Based on the various published modifications of isolation techniques, we describe here a protocol that, in our laboratory, provides both high yields and good preservation of phenotypic properties.

5. Some authors divided the cartilage specimens of each donor into more severely degraded and less severely degraded samples *(31)*.

6. Ethical guidelines for experimental investigations in animals must be followed. In particular, the experimental procedure for euthanasia must be discussed and accepted by the local ethics committee for animal experimentation.

7. To ensure plating at a uniform density, repeatedly aspirate and expel the cell suspension during its distribution among the dishes. After completion of the full digestion procedure, this usually provides 20×10^6 cells per rabbit.

8. A method that has been used successfully for isolating bovine chondrocytes is digestion with trypsin 0.25% in Hanks' solution for 20 min followed by collagenase 0.25% in culture medium for 40 min *(32)* . This protocol has also been adapted for rat chondrocyte isolation *(33)*, with minor changes such as a longer collagenase incubation (180 min) *(34)*.

9. A commonly used alternative involves digestion with 1.5% (w/v) bacterial collagenase B in culture medium without serum, overnight at 37°C *(35,36)*.

10. Alternatively, digestion can be performed overnight by diluting the collagenase six-fold in complete culture medium.

11. In our hands, one mouse yields about 2 million chondrocytes.

12. Younger mouse pups have tiny joints that are very difficult to handle and easy to tear. Older mice provide fewer chondrocytes per joint, probably because their cells divide more slowly. The instruments used are autoclaved before the procedure. An entire litter of mouse pups is usually handled at one sitting, and the instruments are resterilized between pups by dipping in 70% ethanol before each use.

Acknowledgments

We are grateful to Colette Salvat for her outstanding technical expertise in the development and optimization of cultured mouse articular chondrocytes and to Lydie Humbert and Audrey Pigenet for their high-quality technical assistance. We thank Claire Jacques for her expertise and detailed information about cultured mouse rib chondrocytes. We are indebted to Professor C. Sautet (Saint Antoine UFR, Paris) for providing human articular cartilage.

References

1. Aydelotte, M. B., and Kuettner, K. E. (1988) Differences between sub-populations of cultured bovine articular chondrocytes. I. Morphology and cartilage matrix production. *Connect. Tissue Res.* **18,** 205–222
2. von der Mark, K. and Conrad, G. (1979) Cartilage cell differentiation. *Clin. Orthop.* **139,** 185–205
3. Stokes, D. G., Liu, G., Coimbra, I. B., Piera-Velazquez, S., Crowl, R. M., and Jimenez, S. A. (2002) Assessment of the gene expression profile of differentiated and dedifferentiated human fetal chondrocytes by microarray analysis. *Arthritis Rheum.* **46,** 404–419.
4. Kergosien, N., Sautier, J., and Forest, N. (1998) Gene and protein expression during differentiation and matrix mineralization in a chondrocyte cell culture system. *Calcif. Tissue Int.* **62,** 114–121.
5. Hauselmann, H. J., Aydelotte, M. B., Schumacher, B. L., Kuettner, K. E., Gitelis, S. H., and Thonar, E. J. (1992) Synthesis and turnover of proteoglycans by human and bovine adult articular chondrocytes cultured in alginate beads. *Matrix* **12,** 116–129.
6. Karsenty, G. (2001) Chondrogenesis just ain't what it used to be. *J. Clin. Invest.* **107,** 405–407.
7. Corvol, M. T., Dumontier, M. F., and Rappaport, R. (1975) Culture of chondrocytes from the proliferative zone of epiphyseal growth plate cartilage from prepubertal rabbits. *Biomedicine* **23,** 103–107.
8. Mwale, F., Billinghurst, C., Wu, W., et al. (2000) Selective assembly and remodelling of collagens II and IX associated with expression of the chondrocyte hypertrophic phenotype. *Dev. Dyn.* **218,** 648–662.
9. Goldring, M. B. (2000) The role of the chondrocyte in osteoarthritis. *Arthritis Rheum.* **43,** 1916–1926.
10. Goldring, M. B. and Berenbaum, F. (1999) Human chondrocyte culture models for studying cyclooxygenase expression and prostaglandin regulation of collagen gene expression. *Osteoarthritis Cartilage* **7,** 386–388.
11. Watt, F. M. (1988) Effect of seeding density on stability of the differentiated phenotype of pig articular chondrocytes in culture. *J. Cell. Sci.* **89,** 373–378.
12. Stokes, D. G., Liu, G., Dharmavaram, R., Hawkins, D., Piera-Velazquez, S., and Jimenez, S. A. (2001) Regulation of type-II collagen gene expression during human chondrocyte de-differentiation and recovery of chondrocyte-specific phenotype in culture involves Sry-type high-mobility-group box (SOX) transcription factors. *Biochem. J.* **360,** 461–470.
13. Goldring, M. B., Birkhead, J., Sandell, L. J., Kimura, T., and Krane, S. M. (1988) Interleukin 1 suppresses expression of cartilage-specific types II and IX collagens and increases types I and III collagens in human chondrocytes. *J. Clin. Invest.* **82,** 2026–2037.
14. Goldring, M. B., Birkhead, J. R., Suen, L. F., et al. (1994) Interleukin-1 beta-modulated gene expression in immortalized human chondrocytes. *J. Clin. Invest.* **94,** 2307–2316.

15. Demoor-Fossard, M., Redini, F., Boittin, M., and Pujol, J. P. (1998) Expression of decorin and biglycan by rabbit articular chondrocytes. Effects of cytokines and phenotypic modulation. *Biochim. Biophys. Acta* **1398,** 179–191.

16. Gibson, G. J., Schor, S. L., and Grant, M. E. (1982) Effects of matrix macromolecules on chondrocyte gene expression: synthesis of a low molecular weight collagen species by cells cultured within collagen gels. *J. Cell Biol.* **93,** 767–774.

17. Takigawa, M., Pan, H. O., Kinoshita, A., Tajima, K., and Takano, Y. (1991) Establishment from a human chondrosarcoma of a new immortal cell line with high tumorigenicity in vivo, which is able to form proteoglycan- rich cartilage-like nodules and to respond to insulin in vitro. *Int. J. Cancer* **48,** 717–725.

18. Mallein-Gerin, F., and Olsen, B. R. (1993) Expression of simian virus 40 large T (tumor) oncogene in mouse chondrocytes induces cell proliferation without loss of the differentiated phenotype. *Proc. Natl. Acad. Sci. USA* **90,** 3289–3293.

19. Robbins, J. R., Thomas, B., Tan, L., et al. (2000) Immortalized human adult articular chondrocytes maintain cartilage- specific phenotype and responses to interleukin-1β. *Arthritis Rheum.* **43,** 2189–2201.

20. Adolphe, M., Froger, B., Ronot, X., Corvol, M. T., and Forest, N. (1984) Cell multiplication and type II collagen production by rabbit articular chondrocytes cultivated in a defined medium. *Exp. Cell Res.* **155,** 527–536.

22. Martin, I., Vunjak-Novakovic, G., Yang, J., Langer, R., and Freed, L. E. (1999) Mammalian chondrocytes expanded in the presence of fibroblast growth factor 2 maintain the ability to differentiate and regenerate three-dimensional cartilaginous tissue. *Exp. Cell Res.* **253,** 681–688.

21. Kuettner, K. E., Memoli, V. A., Pauli, B. U., Wrobel, N. C., Thonar, E. J., and Daniel, J. C. (1982) Synthesis of cartilage matrix by mammalian chondrocytes in vitro. II. Maintenance of collagen and proteoglycan phenotype. *J. Cell Biol.* **93,** 751–757.

23. Domm, C., Schunke, M., Christesen, K., and Kurz, B. (2002) Redifferentiation of dedifferentiated bovine articular chondrocytes in alginate culture under low oxygen tension. *Osteoarthritis Cartilage* **10,** 13–22.

24. Zaucke, F., Dinser, R., Maurer, P., and Paulsson, M. (2001) Cartilage oligomeric matrix protein (COMP) and collagen IX are sensitive markers for the differentiation state of articular primary chondrocytes. *Biochem. J.* **358,** 17–24.

25. Rahfoth, B., Weisser, J., Sternkopf, F., Aigner, T., von der Mark, K., and Brauer, R. (1998) Transplantation of allograft chondrocytes embedded in agarose gel into cartilage defects of rabbits. *Osteoarthritis Cartilage* **6,** 50–65.

26. Robbins, J. R. and Goldring, M. B. (1998) Preparation of immortalized human chondrocyte cell lines, in *Tissue Engineering*, Vol. 18 (Morgan, J. R., and Yarmush, M. L., eds.), Humana, Totowa, NJ, pp. 173–192.

27. Goldring, M. B. (1996) Human chondrocyte cultures as models of cartilage-specific gene regulation, in *Human Cell Culture Protocols*, Vol. 2 (Gareth, E. J., ed.), Humana, Totowa, NJ, pp. 217–232.

28. Aulthouse, A. L., Beck, M., Griffey, E., et al. (1989) Expression of the human chondrocyte phenotype in vitro. *In Vitro Cell Dev. Biol.* **25,** 659–668.

29. Carrascosa, A., Audi, L., and Ballabriga, A. (1985) Morphologic and metabolic development of human fetal epiphyseal chondrocytes in primary culture. *Pediatr. Res.* **19,** 720–727.

30. Reginato, A. M., Iozzo, R. V., and Jimenez, S. A. (1994) Formation of nodular structures resembling mature articular cartilage in long-term primary cultures of human fetal epiphyseal chondrocytes on a hydrogel substrate. *Arthritis Rheum.* **37,** 1338–1349.

31. Stove, J., Gerlach, C., Huch, K., et al. (2001) Gene expression of stromelysin and aggrecan in osteoarthritic cartilage. *Pathobiology* **69,** 333–338.

32. Kawiak, J., Moskalewski, S., and Darzynkiewicz, Z. (1965) Isolation of chondrocytes from calf cartilage. *Exp. Cell Res.* **39,** 59–68.

33. Nedelec, E., Abid, A., Cipolletta, C., et al. (2001) Stimulation of cyclooxygenase-2-activity by nitric oxide-derived species in rat chondrocyte: lack of contribution to loss of cartilage anabolism. *Biochem. Pharmacol.* **61,** 965–978.

34. Okazaki, M., Higuchi, Y., and Kitamura, H. (2003) AG-041R stimulates cartilage matrix synthesis without promoting terminal differentiation in rat articular chondrocytes. *Osteoarthritis Cartilage* **11,** 122–132.

35. Gouze, J. N., Bordji, K., Gulberti, S., et al. (2001) Interleukin-1beta down-regulates the expression of glucuronosyltransferase I, a key enzyme priming glycosaminogly-can biosynthesis: influence of glucosamine on interleukin-1β-mediated effects in rat chondrocytes. *Arthritis Rheum.* **44,** 351–360.

36. Gouze, J. N., Bianchi, A., Becuwe, P., et al. (2002) Glucosamine modulates IL-1-induced activation of rat chondrocytes at a receptor level, and by inhibiting the NF-k B pathway. *FEBS Lett.* **510,** 166–170.

2

Culture of Chondrocytes in Alginate Beads

**Frédéric De Ceuninck, Christophe Lesur,
Philippe Pastoureau, Audrey Caliez, and Massimo Sabatini**

Summary

A classic method for the encapsulation and culture of chondrocytes in alginate beads is described. Chondrocytes are released from cartilage matrix by collagenase/dispase digestion and mixed with a solution of 1.25% alginic acid until a homogenous suspension is obtained. The suspension is drawn into a syringe and pushed gently through a needle, so that drops fall into a solution of calcium chloride. Beads form instantaneously and further polymerize after 5 min in the calcium chloride solution. Chondrocytes from any species, including human osteoarthritic chondrocytes, can be cultured with this technique. Under these conditions, chondrocytes maintain a high degree of differentiation. Beads can be dissolved by chelation of calcium with EDTA. In this way, chondrocytes can be recovered and further separated from the matrix by centrifugation. Almost all molecular and biochemical techniques, as well as a number of biological assays, are compatible with the culture of chondrocytes in alginate.

Key Words: Chondrocyte; cartilage; alginate; differentiation; cell culture.

1. Introduction

After being released from their cartilaginous matrix by enzyme digestion, chondrocytes have a tendency to dedifferentiate, especially if they are cultured at a low density in monolayer culture. The round cells rapidly lose their cartilage phenotype and transform into flattened fibroblast-like cells. Under these conditions, certain specific markers of the chondrocytic phenotype are downregulated, and some nonchondrocytic proteins such as type I collagen are synthesized (*1*). To prevent dedifferentation, culture at a high density (more than 5×10^4 cells/cm^2) is recommended and passage culture must be avoided. These are important constraints, especially when working on human osteoarthritic chondrocytes, which are often obtained in low amounts from a single cartilage specimen.

From: *Methods in Molecular Medicine, Vol. 100: Cartilage and Osteoarthritis, Vol. 1: Cellular and Molecular Tools*
Edited by: M. Sabatini, P. Pastoureau, and F. De Ceuninck © Humana Press Inc., Totowa, NJ

To maintain chondrocytes in their original phenotype, various methods have been developed, including culture in scaffolding materials, such as collagen sponges, agarose, or alginate. Among these techniques, culture in alginate is often used, as it offers many advantages over the others. Chondrocytes can be homogeneously dispersed and encapsulated in alginate beads and cultured for more than 8 mo without any apparent phenotype loss *(2)*. Alginate beads allow the reconstitution of a tridimensional scaffold closely resembling that of the cartilage matrix *(3)*. Chondrocytes express proteoglycans, especially aggrecan, and also type II, but not type I collagen *(2–8)*. Encapsulated chondrocytes are still able to respond to growth factors and cytokines usually known to affect chondrocyte metabolism *(9–11)*. Beads are easy to handle, and many molecular, biochemical, and biological applications are compatible with this mode of culture *(2–18)*. Cells can be recovered from beads by simple chelation of divalent ions with ethylenediamine tetraacetic acid (EDTA) followed by centrifugation. Culture in alginate beads is also useful to redifferentiate chondrocytes that have dedifferentiated because of expansion in bidimensional culture *(16–18)*. The original method of culture of chondrocytes in alginate beads was developed in the late eighties by Guo et al. *(19)* and was then employed and improved by many researchers. We describe here the method routinely used in our laboratory.

2. Materials

1. Articular cartilage explants from guinea pigs, rabbits, or rats or from human normal or osteoarthritic cartilage.
2. Hanks' balanced salt solution (HBSS; Gibco-BRL)
3. Ham's F-12 culture medium with Glutamax (Ham F-12; Gibco-BRL).
4. Fetal calf serum (FCS).
5. 10,000 U/mL Penicillin /10,000 µg/mL streptomycin stock solution (PS; Gibco-BRL).
6. Dispase/collagenase solution for guinea pig, rabbit, or rat cartilage: 2 mg/mL dispase (from *Bacillus polymixa*; Gibco-BRL) and 3 mg/mL collagenase type I (Worthington) in HBSS. Sterilize through a 0.22 µm filter.
7. Dispase/collagenase solution for human cartilage: 2 mg/mL dispase (from *B. polymixa*; Gibco-BRL) and 3 mg/mL collagenase type I (Worthington) in Ham F-12 supplemented with 10% FCS. Sterilize through a 0.22 µm filter.
8. Cell culture equipment, including 10-mm-diameter Petri dishes, pipets, multipipets, and appropriate tips or combitips.
9. 50-mL Capacity beaker sterilized by autoclaving.
10. Cell strainer, 40 µm nylon (Falcon, cat. no. 2340).
11. Blue max 50-mL sterile tubes (Falcon, cat. no. 2070).
12. 21-Gage needle (Terumo, cat. no. NN-2125R) with syringe of 2, 5, or 10 mL (Terumo).
13. Sterile 0.9% NaCl solution.

14. Alginate solution: 1.25% alginic acid (Fluka, cat. no. 71238), 20 mM HEPES, 150 mM NaCl, pH 7.4. First dissolve HEPES and NaCl powders in deionized water. Warm up the mixture at 60°C and add the alginate powder with constant stirring until the solution is homogeneous. It may take more than 1 h to achieve complete dissolution. Let the solution cool down to room temperature and adjust to pH 7.4 (*see* **Note 1**) . Adjust the final volume of the solution with deionized water. Autoclave.
15. Polymerization solution: 102 mM CaCl$_2$, 10 mM HEPES, pH 7.4. Pass through a 0.22 μm-filter.
16. Dissolution solution: 55 mM EDTA, 10 mM HEPES, pH 7.4. Pass through a 0.22 μm-filter.
17. Tissue culture incubator, set at 37°C, with water-saturated, 5% CO$_2$ air.

3. Methods

3.1. Chondrocyte Isolation

Chondrocytes from any species may be used with this technique.

1. Guinea pig, rat, or rabbit cartilage explants: finely mince articular cartilage down to fragments of around 1 mm^3. Transfer the fragments (0.25–0.5 g) into a Petri dish containing 20 mL of dispase/collagenase solution in HBSS. Incubate at 37°C for 5 h, or until the explants are digested.
2. Human cartilage: finely mince articular cartilage down to fragments of around 1 mm^3 . Transfer the fragments (0.25–0.5 g) into a Petri dish containing 20 mL of dispase/collagenase solution in Ham F-12 with 10% FCS. Incubate at 37°C for 16 h or until the explants are digested (*see* **Notes 2 and 3**).
3. Pellet cells by 3-min centrifugation at 900g.
4. Resuspend cell pellet in Ham F-12 medium supplemented with 10% FCS and 1% PS. Count the cells on a hemacytometer, and centrifuge the suspension for 3 min at 900g. Discard the supernatant and keep the cell pellet.

3.2. Encapsulation of Chondrocytes in Alginate Beads

The overall method is depicted in **Fig. 1** and described here in detail. All steps should be performed under a sterile hood.

1. Resuspend the cell pellet obtained in **Subheading 3.1., step 4** by adding a volume of alginate solution **(Fig. 1A),** so as to have 2 million cells/mL of alginate solution (*see* **Note 4).**
2. Aspirate the suspension into a syringe and cap with a 21-gage needle.
3. Gently push the piston of the syringe so that the solution is released dropwise into 30 mL of polymerization solution, maintained under gentle stirring by a magnet, in a 50 mL sterile beaker **(Fig. 1B)**.
4. Beads instantly polymerize when falling into the solution, entrapping the chondrocytes. Let beads polymerize completely under gentle agitation for an additional 10 min.

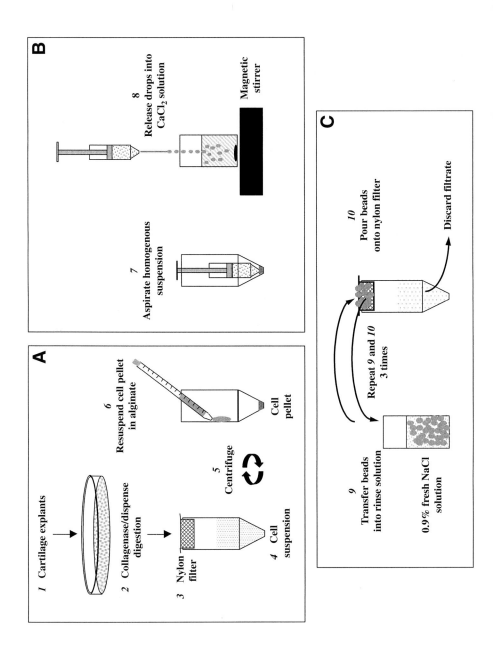

18

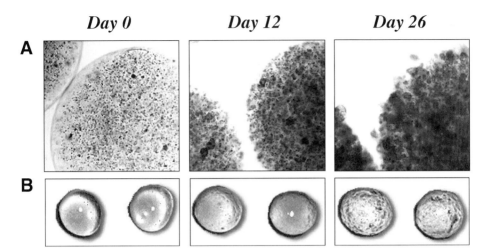

Fig 2. (A) Morphological appearance of alginate beads with encapsulated rabbit chondrocytes. Beads were cultured in medium containing 10% FCS. The increase of cell density was evident at d 12. Cell density was further increased at d 26. **(B)** Macroscopic view of beads as a function of time. The volume of beads increased by about 40% at d 26.

5. Pour the solution containing the beads on the cell strainer laid on top of a 50-mL Falcon tube. Discard the filtered polymerization solution and carefully pick up the beads with a spatula.

6. Transfer the beads into 30 mL of a sterile 0.9% NaCl solution (*see* **Note 5**) in a 50-mL capacity beaker and wash beads by gentle stirring for 1–2 min.

7. Repeat **step 6** three times (**Fig. 1C**) and finally rinse beads with complete culture medium.

8. The gross appearance of alginate beads with entrapped rabbit chondrocytes cultured in FCS-containing medium is shown in **Fig. 2**. The granular aspect and increase of density of beads at d 26 postencapsulation accounts for the proliferation of chondrocytes and the synthesis of matrix components. By contrast, human osteoarthritic chondrocytes do not proliferate in alginate beads (**Fig. 3**). However, they are still capable of synthetic activities.

Fig 1. *(opposite page)* Schematic representation of the encapsulation of chondrocytes in alginate beads. **(A)** Isolated cells are suspended at 2 million/mL of 1.25% alginic acid solution. **(B)** The mixture is aspirated in a syringe, and then released dropwise into a calcium chloride solution by passage through a 21-gage needle. Beads form instantly and completely polymerize by 10 min in this solution. **(C)** Beads undergo three washes in a 0.9% sterile NaCl solution and are then ready for culture.

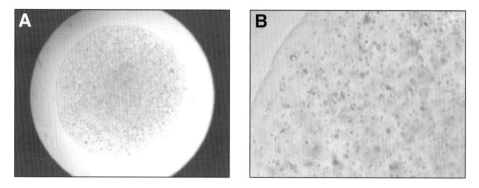

Fig. 3. (**A**) Morphological appearance of an alginate bead with encapsulated human osteoarthritic chondrocytes 12 wk after encapsulation. Unlike the rabbit chondrocytes in Fig. 2, human osteoarthritic chondrocytes do not proliferate in alginate beads cultured in serum-containing medium. (**B**) Magnification (×5) of the bead shown in **A**.

9. Culture beads as long as required in Petri dishes in Ham F-12 medium containing Glutamax plus 10% FCS and 1% PS. Replace medium every 2 d. In our hands, chondrocytes need about 3 wk to reestablish a consistent pericellular and territorial extracellular matrix.

3.3. Experimental Procedures: Recommendations

1. Perform experiments in serum-free medium if required, after a prior 24-h washing-out period to ensure that all interfering serum constituents have been removed from the beads.
2. For certain experimental procedures, it may be necessary to separate cells from the alginate matrix: for this, incubate beads in dissolution solution (at a ratio of about 200 µL/bead) for 5 min. Centrifuge. Recover cells in the pellet and the matrix in the supernatant.
3. Depending on the experiments, the results can be normalized relative to the weight of beads, the number of chondrocytes, or the DNA content within each bead.

4. Notes

1. Care must be taken not to exceed the pH 7.4 limit since any attempt to bring back pH to 7.4 with HCl may lead to precipitation.
2. Digestion of human cartilage is slower than that of cartilage from rat, rabbit, or guinea pig, even when the same digestion volume/cartilage weight is used. To ensure chondrocyte viability, the digestion is performed in culture medium supplemented with FCS, even if the presence of endogenous collagenase inhibitors in FCS may somewhat slow down the digestion. For reproducible digestion conditions, it is recommended to maintain the same enzyme/tissue ratio and to distribute the explants, if necessary, across several Petri dishes.

3. For a similar weight of explants before digestion, the number of cells obtained from human cartilage will not be more than half that obtained from cartilage of rat, rabbit, or guinea pig and will be highly dependent on the age of the donor and stage of osteoarthritis.
4. Expect about 200–300 drops, i.e., 200–300 beads starting from a 5-mL homogenous suspension. This means that each bead will contain about 33–50 × 10³ cells.
5. Using other solutions (such as phosphate-buffered saline) to wash the beads may lead to precipitation.

References

1. Benya, P. D. and Shaffer, J. D. (1982) Dedifferentiated chondrocytes reexpress the differentiated collagen phenotype when cultured in agarose gels. *Cell* **30**, 215–224.
2. Hauselmann, H. J., Fernandes, R. J., Mok, S. S., et al. (1994) Phenotypic stability of bovine articular chondrocytes after long-term culture in alginate beads. *J. Cell Sci.* **107**, 17–27.
3. Hauselmann, H. J., Masuda, K., Hunziker, E. B., et al. (1996) Adult human chondrocytes cultured in alginate form a matrix similar to native human articular cartilage. *Am. J. Physiol.* **271**, C742–C752.
4. Tamponnet, C., Ramdi, H., Guyot, J. B., and Lievremont, M. (1992) Rabbit articular chondrocytes in alginate gel: characterization of immobilized preparations and potential applications. *Appl. Microbiol. Biotechnol.* **37**, 311–315.
5. Hauselmann, H. J., Aydelotte, M. B., Schumacher, B. L., Kuettner, K. E., Gitelis, S. H., and Thonar, E., J. (1992) Synthesis and turnover of proteoglycans by human and bovine adult articular chondrocytes cultured in alginate beads. *Matrix* **12**, 116–129.
6. Mok, S. S., Masuda, K., Hauselmann, H. J., Aydelotte, M. B., and Thonar, E. J. (1994) Aggrecan synthesized by mature bovine chondrocytes suspended in alginate; identification of two distinct metabolic matrix pools. *J. Biol. Chem.* **269**, 33021–33027.
7. Petit, B., Masuda, K., D'Souza, A. L., et al. (1996) Characterization of crosslinked collagens synthesized by mature articular chondrocytes cultured in alginate beads: comparison of two distinct matrix compartments. *Exp. Cell Res.* **225**, 151–161.
8. Beekman, B., Verzijl, N., Bank, R. A., von der Mark, K., and TeKoppele, J. M. (1997) Synthesis of collagen by bovine chondrocytes cultured in alginate; posttranslational modifications and cell-matrix interaction. *Exp. Cell Res.* **237**, 135–141.
9. Redini, F., Min, W., Demoor-Fossard, M., Boittin, M., and Pujol, J. P. (1997) Differential expression of membrane-anchored proteoglycans in rabbit articular chondrocytes cultured in monolayers and in alginate beads. Effect of transforming growth factor-beta 1. *Biochim. Biophys. Acta* **1355**, 20–32.
10. Beekman, B., Verzijl, N., de Roos, J. A., and TeKoppele, J. M. (1998) Matrix degradation by chondrocytes cultured in alginate: IL-1β induces proteoglycan degradation and proMMP synthesis but does not result in collagen degradation. *Osteoarthritis Cartilage* **6**, 330–340.

11. Loeser, R. F., Todd, M. D., and Seely, B. L. (2003) Prolonged treatment of human osteoarthritic chondrocytes with insulin-like growth factor-I stimulates proteoglycan synthesis but not proteoglycan matrix accumulation in alginate cultures. *J. Rheumatol.* **30**, 1565–1570.

12. Chubinskaya, S., Huch, K., Schulze, M., Otten, L., Aydelotte, M. B., and Cole, A. A. (2001) Gene expression by human articular chondrocytes cultured in alginate beads. *J. Histochem. Cytochem.* **49**, 1211–1219.

13. Stove, J., Fiedler, J., Huch, K., Gunther, K. P., Puhl, W., and Brenner, R. (2002) Lipofection of rabbit chondrocytes and long lasting expression of a lacZ reporter system in alginate beads. *Osteoarthritis Cartilage* **10**, 212–217.

14. Knight, M. M., van de Breevaart Bravenboer, J., Lee, D. A., van Osch, G. J., Weinans, H., and Bader, D. L. (2002) Cell and nucleus deformation in compressed chondrocyte-alginate constructs: temporal changes and calculation of cell modulus. *Biochim. Biophys. Acta* **1570**, 1–8.

15. Enobakhare, B. O., Bader, D. L., and Lee, D. A. (1996) Quantification of sulfated glycosaminoglycans in chondrocyte/alginate cultures, by use of 1,9-dimethyl-methylene blue. *Anal. Biochem.* **243**, 189–191.

16. Bonaventure, J., Kadhom, N., Cohen-Solal, L., et al. (1994) Reexpression of cartilage-specific genes by dedifferentiated human chondrocytes cultured in alginate beads. *Exp. Cell Res.* **212**, 97–104.

17. Lemare, F., Steimberg, N., Le Griel, C., Demignot, S., and Adolphe, M. (1998) Dedifferentiated chondrocytes cultured in alginate beads: restoration of the differentiated phenotype and of the metabolic responses to interleukin-1β. *J. Cell. Physiol.* **176**, 303–313.

18. Liu, H., Lee, Y. W., and Dean, M. F. (1998) Re-expression of differentiated proteoglycan phenotype by dedifferentiated human chondrocytes during culture in alginate beads. *Biochim. Biophys. Acta* **1425**, 505–515.

19. Guo, J. F., Jourdian, G. W., and MacCallum, D. K. (1989) Culture and growth characteristics of chondrocytes encapsulated in alginate beads. *Connect. Tissue Res.* **19**, 277–297.

3

Immortalization of Human Articular Chondrocytes for Generation of Stable, Differentiated Cell Lines

Mary B. Goldring

Summary

Immortalized chondrocytes of human origin have been developed to serve as reproducible models for studying chondrocyte function. In this chapter, methods for immortalization of primary human chondrocytes with SV40-TAg, HPV-16 E6/E7, and telomerase by retrovirally mediated transduction and selection for neomycin resistance are described. However, stable integration of an immortalizing gene stabilizes proliferative capacity, but not the differentiated chondrocyte phenotype. Thus, strategies for selection of chondrocyte cell lines, involving the maintenance of high cell density and moderation of cell proliferation, are also described. The methods for immortalization and selection are applicable to the development of chondrocyte cell lines using any immortalizing agent. Although immortalized chondrocytes should not be considered as substitutes for primary chondrocytes, they may be useful tools for evaluating and further validating mechanisms relevant to cartilage biology.

Key Words: Immortalized chondrocytes; type II collagen; aggrecan; retrovirus production; viral titer; retroviral infection; simian virus 40 large T antigen (SV40-TAg); human papillomavirus type 16 early function genes E6 and E7 (HPV-16 E6/E7); telomerase; chondrocyte morphology; chondrocyte proliferation; G418; hyaluronidase; polybrene; Nutridoma.

1. Introduction

Successful development of therapeutic strategies that prevent degradation of cartilage matrix in patients with osteoarthritis and permit cartilage regeneration and repair depends on the availability of reproducible cell culture models of human origin. Primary cultures of articular chondrocytes isolated from various animal and human sources have served as useful models for studying the mechanisms controlling responses to growth factors and cytokines (*1*). The use of chondrocytes of human origin has been problematical, because the source of the cartilage cannot be controlled, sufficient numbers of cells are not readily

From: *Methods in Molecular Medicine, Vol. 100: Cartilage and Osteoarthritis, Vol. 1: Cellular and Molecular Tools*
Edited by: M. Sabatini, P. Pastoureau, and F. De Ceuninck © Humana Press Inc., Totowa, NJ

obtained from random operative procedures, and the phenotypic stability and proliferative capacity in adult human chondrocytes is quickly lost upon expansion in serial monolayer cultures *(2)*. Thus, a reproducible source of chondrocytes of human origin would be most desirable for studying cartilage function relevant to human osteoarthritis. Furthermore, the availability of phenotypically stable culture systems employing immortalized human chondrocytes would permit prior testing in vitro of strategies for improving autologous chondrocyte transplantation, implantation of chondrocyte-laden biomaterials, and gene transfer *(3)*.

Several different approaches have been used in the attempt to develop cell lines that maintain the chondrocyte phenotype. Chondrocyte cell lines that display high proliferative capacities and retain at least some features of the differentiated phenotype have been derived from nonhuman sources using viral oncogenes *(4–8)*. Chondrocyte cell lines have also arisen spontaneously from fetal rat calvaria *(9,10)* or have been derived from transgenic mice harboring the temperature-sensitive mutant of simian virus 40 (SV40) large T antigen (TAg) *(11,12)*.

Recent studies have focused on adult human articular chondrocytes as target cells for immortalization, since articular cartilage is the primary joint tissue requiring replacement or reconstruction after it is damaged in osteoarthritis. Stable expression of SV40-TAg using plasmid or retroviral vectors has been used as a popular method for immortalizing human chondrocytes *(13–16)*. Articular chondrocyte cell lines have also been established using the human papilloma virus type 16 (HPV-16) early function genes E6 and E7 *(17)* and telomerase *(18)*. A common finding, however, is that stable integration of immortalizing genes disrupts normal cell-cycle control but does not stabilize expression of the type II collagen gene (*COL2A1*), the most sensitive marker of the differentiated chondrocyte phenotype. This is true even when a chondrocyte-specific promoter is used to drive TAg expression *(14)*. Indeed, the expression of the differentiated phenotype in chondrocyte cell lines appears to be inversely related to the proliferative capacity of the cell line. Thus, strategies that maintain high cell density and decrease cell proliferation have been used to develop cell lines that express chondrocyte-specific phenotype *(15–17)*.

This chapter will focus on strategies for immortalization and selection that may be applied to the development of a chondrocyte cell line using any immortalizing agent. Immortalized chondrocytes cannot be considered as substitutes for primary cultures but are useful for validation and further elucidation of mechanisms uncovered in nonimmortalized chondrocytes. Furthermore, immortalization of osteoarthritic chondrocytes will not necessarily stabilize characteristics observed in primary cultures of these cells, unless they are hereditary features of the original chondrocytes *in situ*. However, immortalized cell lines may be useful as reproducible culture systems for evaluating chondrocyte functions, and additional approaches are described in Chapter 4.

2. Materials
2.1. Culture Reagents

1. Growth medium for packaging cell lines: Dulbecco's modified Eagle's medium (DMEM) with high glucose (4.5 g/L), L-glutamine and sodium pyruvate, and without HEPES, containing 10% fetal calf serum (FCS).
2. Growth medium for chondrocytes: DMEM/Ham's F-12, 1:1 (v/v). Mix equal volumes of DMEM, high glucose, with L-glutamine and Ham's F-1, with L-glutamine (Cambrex, Walkersville, MD), both without HEPES, to give final concentrations of 3.151 g/L glucose, L-glutamine (365 mg/L)/L-glutamic acid (7.36 mg/L), and sodium pyruvate (110 mg/L). Add 10% FCS immediately before use.
3. Dulbecco's phosphate-buffered Ca^{2+}- and Mg^{2+}-free saline (PBS).
4. Trypsin-EDTA solution: 0.05% trypsin and 0.02% ethylenediamine tetraacetic acid (EDTA) in Hanks' balanced salt solution without Ca^{2+} and Mg^{2+} (Life Technologies, Gaithersburg, MD).
5. Serum substitutes for experimental incubations of immortalized chondrocytes: Nutridoma-SP (Roche Applied Science) is provided as sterile concentrate (100X, pH 7.4; storage at 15–25°C protected from light). Dilute 1:100 (v/v) with sterile DMEM/Ham's F-12, without FCS, and use immediately. ITS+ (BD Biosciences) is an alternative serum substitute.
6. Hyaluronidase (type I-S, Sigma, St. Louis, MO): Reconstituted in 50 mM sodium acetate, pH 6.0, at 1000X stock concentration and added freshly to medium at 4 U/mL.

Except where specified, cell culture reagents can be obtained from a number of different suppliers, including Life Technologies, Cambrex, Sigma, or Intergen (Purchase, NY). Reserve serum testing, which is offered by these suppliers, is recommended for selection of lots of FCS that maintain chondrocyte phenotype (*see* **Note 1**). Cell culture reagents have shelf lives as recommended by the suppliers. FCS and trypsin-EDTA are stored at –20°C but should not be refrozen after thawing for use.

2.2. Packaging Cell Lines

The retrovirus packaging cell lines (*see* **Note 2**) that are amphotropic, producing virus particles that infect human cells with high titer, include PA317 (ATTC, CRL-9078) *(19)*, PT67 (BD Biosciences Clontech), or 293GPG (Phoenix cell line from Gary Nolan, Stanford University) *(20)*. They may be obtained commercially or derived by stable transfection with the plasmid form of the retroviral vector containing a selectable marker, such as Neo^{R}. Replication-defective mutants of SV40-TAg, inserted in the pZipNeoSV(X) shuttle vector, including the U19 mutant that does not bind the SV40 origin *(21)* and tsA58-3 that encodes a temperature-sensitive (ts) mutant of SV40-TAg *(22)*, may be packaged in PA317 or 293GPG. SV40-TAg-containing vectors are generally available by request from the investigators who have developed them. However, other immortalizing vectors may be the agents of choice. PA317-LXSN-16E6E7 (ATTC, CRL2203) is a packaging cell line that produces HPV-16 E6/E7. The telomerase reverse transcriptase (hTERT) expression plasmid (C. Harley *[23]*, Geron Corporation, Menlo Park, CA), inserted in the pLNCX vector (BD Biosciences Clontech), is packaged in the PT67 cell line. Since the current technology is advancing rapidly, advice should be sought from collaborators in the field or institutional experts.

2.3. Retrovirus Production and Infection of Chondrocytes

1. Polybrene (Sigma): 8 mg/mL in PBS (1000X stock), sterile filtered, and stored at –20°C. Add to freshly thawed virus-containing medium to a final concentration of 8 µg/mL.
2. G418 sulfate (neomycin analog, also known as Geneticin; Sigma or Life Technologies): 30 mg/mL in PBS (100X stock), sterile filtered, freshly prepared or stored in aliquots at –20°C. (Avoid freeze/thawing.) Add to culture medium at a final concentration of 300–400 µg/mL for selection and 200 µg/mL for maintenance (*see* **Note 3**). For production of virus in the 293GPG packaging cell line, also prepare 1000X stocks of puromycin (Sigma) and tetracycline (Sigma) to give final concentrations of 2 and 1 µg/mL, respectively.
3. Antibodies for detection of immortalizing antigens, including SV40-TAg. HPV16-E6, HPV16-E7, and hTERT are available from Santa Cruz Biotechnology. The TRAPeze kit used to detect telomerase activity is available from Intergen. The telomeric probe $(TTAGGG)_3$ is from Genset (LaJolla, CA).

3. Methods

The methods describe immortalization strategies using retroviral vectors containing Neo^R as the selectable marker, although the approaches for selection and subsequent expansion are generally applicable when other types of immortalization vectors are used. The methods for isolation and primary culture of chondrocytes and phenotypic characterization are described in Chapters 1 and 14. The methods described below outline: (1) retrovirus production, (2) retroviral infection of chondrocytes, (3) selection and establishment of immortalized chondrocytes, and (4) characterization of established cell lines.

3.1. Retrovirus Production

3.1.1. Production of Stably Transfected Packaging Cell Line *(24)*

1. One day before transfection, plate packaging cells at a density of 4×10^5 per 6-cm dish or 25-cm^2 flask.
2. Transfect cells 16–24 h later with 10–15 µg of plasmid DNA encoding the immortalizing retrovirus by the calcium-phosphate technique, using one of several commercially available kits.

3. Before the cells reach confluence, 24–48 h after the transfection, split the cells from each dish into two 10-cm dishes containing 400 μg/mL of G418 (*see* **Note 3**). Change medium containing fresh G418 every 2–3 d. Once cell death is evident, the G418 concentration can be changed to 200 μg/mL until G418-resistant colonies are visible. Colonies may then be isolated, expanded, and selected for high viral titer, or the entire G418-selected population may be expanded if the viral titer is sufficiently high.

4. Liquid nitrogen storage of packaging cell line: expand the cell line in several 10-cm dishes. When the cultures are nearly confluent, trypsinize and wash the cells in PBS and count with a hemocytometer. Pellet the cells and resuspend at a concentration of 2×10^6 cells/mL in DMEM containing 10% FCS and 10% dimethylsulfoxide (DMSO) with gentle swirling. Pipet 1.5 mL aliquots of cell suspension into 1.8-mL cryovials. Freeze the vials at –70°C for 24 h in a styrofoam rack with a lid or a Cryo 1°C Freezing Chamber (Nalgene). Transfer the vials to liquid nitrogen for long-term storage. Subsequent experiments should be carried out with cultures derived from freshly thawed cells.

3.1.2. Production of Retrovirus (24)

1. Culture the packaging cell line in DMEM containing 10% FCS at 37°C in 25-cm^2 flasks. Passage the cultures twice weekly with a split ratio of 1:15 (*see* **Note 4**).

2. Collect virus-containing conditioned medium in 15-mL centrifuge tubes from subconfluent, actively dividing cultures. Filter through a 0.45-μm filter and use immediately, or quick-freeze on dry ice and store at –70°C in 5-mL aliquots until needed.

3. To determine viral titer in the culture supernatants:

   a. Split the producer cell line at 1:10 or 1:20 into several 6-cm dishes the day before the infection.

   b. Remove medium and add 1–2 mL of fresh medium containing different dilutions of virus stock ranging from 0.01 μL to 0.1 mL (volume of viral stock added per mL = "replication factor"). Use at least two dilutions that differ by 10-fold and will give a countable number of colonies after selection. Add polybrene to a final concentration of 8 μg/mL and incubate cells at 37°C for 1–3 h.

   c. Add medium to dilute the polybrene to 2 μg/mL and incubate at least 2–3 d.

   d. Split the infected cells at 1:10 and 1:20 (1/10 or 1/20 = "fraction of infected cells plated") into selection medium containing 400 μg/mL of G418 and incubate for 3 d. Change to fresh medium containing G418 and incubate until colonies are obvious (7–10 d). Count colonies before they spread and calculate titer as:

$$\text{G418–resistant CFU/mL} = \frac{\text{no. of colonies}}{\text{virus vol.} \times \text{replication factor} \times \text{fraction of infected cells plated}}$$

in which CFU = colony-forming units.

3.2. Retroviral Infection of Chondrocytes

1. Plate freshly isolated chondrocytes at a density of 2.5×10^4 per cm^2 in flasks or dishes. Culture at 37°C for 3–4 d, with medium changes every 2 d, or until the cells begin to divide rapidly and have covered more than 50% of the plate (*see* **Note 5**).

2. At 24 and 3 h prior to infection, remove the spent medium from chondrocyte cultures and add fresh growth medium to stimulate cell division. Hyaluronidase may be added during these medium changes to facilitate the infection efficiency (*see* **Note 6**).

3. Begin infection by removing the medium and adding 5 mL of freshly thawed virus-containing medium supplemented with polybrene at 8 μg/mL to promote the binding of virus to the cells. Replace the dishes in the 37°C incubator and incubate for 4–6 h or overnight (*see* **Note 7**).

4. Remove the polybrene-containing medium and replace with fresh growth medium. Incubate for at least 24 h, until the cultures become confluent, or for at least one cell division cycle.

3.3. Selection and Establishment of Immortalized Chondrocytes

1. Passage confluent cultures with a split ratio of 1:2, and begin selection with G418 the following day. Cultures infected with tsSV40-TAg may be transferred to a 32°C incubator at this point.

2. Remove the medium and add fresh growth medium containing G418 at 300 μg/mL (*see* **Note 3**). Continue selection for 3–4 wk, feeding the cultures three times per week with fresh growth medium supplemented with G418. During selection a percentage of the cells will die, substantially reducing the culture density. After 4–8 wk, however, G418-resistant cells should repopulate the dishes, and when the cultures become confluent, they should be passaged and maintained in fresh growth medium containing G418 at 200 μg/mL.

3. Establish cultures by passaging more than 50 times in growth medium without G418, ensuring that the cultures are allowed only to reach "confluence" and not overgrow, with the appearance of floating cells (*see* **Note 8**). Cultures are maintained as nonclonal populations or cloned by limiting dilution after "crisis" (*see* **Note 9**). After stable growth for approx 25 or more population doublings (same as passage number in cultures split from one to two dishes), a gradual decline in growth rate is observed with a progressive failure of the cells to grow to confluence. This crisis period is marked by morphological changes in a portion of the cells that are destined to die and the accumulation of cellular debris. Some cultures undergo a latency period of a few weeks, after which the rate of cell division returns to that prior to crisis.

4. Verify the presence of the immortalizing antigen in established, G418-resistant chondrocyte cell lines by immunocytochemistry and/or by Western blotting using specific antibodies against the immortalizing antigen, i.e., SV40-TAg, HPV16-E6, HPV16-E7, or hTERT. The mRNAs encoding these antigens may also be analyzed by reverse transcriptase polymerase chain reaction (RT-PCR).

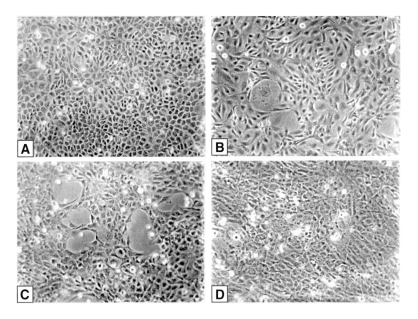

Fig. 1. Morphologies of immortalized human chondrocytes in monolayer culture. **(A)** T/C-28a4, **(B)** C-28/I2, **(C)** C-20/A4, and **(D)** tsT/AC62 cells were cultured to confluency and photographed using phase-contrast microscopy. The T/C-28a4, C-28/ I2, and C-20/A4 cell lines were derived from primary cultures of juvenile human costal chondrocytes by immortalization with a retroviral or plasmid vector encoding SV40-TAg *(15)*. The tsT/AC62 cell line was derived from primary cultures of adult human articular chondrocytes by immortalization with a temperature-sensitive mutant of SV40-TAg *(16)*. Note that the T/C-28 cells are small and rounded. The tsT/AC62 cells become more fibroblastic during passage and may be "redifferentiated" about every 12 passages by culture in alginate or in suspension for 1–2 wk. (Reproduced with permission from ref. *30*.)

Telomerase activity in hTERT-immortalized cells is analyzed by the telomerase repeat amplification protocol (TRAP). Telomeric length, which decreases with senescence and increases in hTERT-immortalized cells, is detected by Southern blotting using genomic DNA digested with the restriction enzymes *Rsa*I and *Msp*I or *Hin*fI and the ^{32}P end-labeled telomeric probe (TTAGGG)$_3$ *(25)*. Mean telomeric length is determined by densitometric analysis of autoradiographs of the Southern blots *(26)*.

3.4. Characterization of Established Chondrocyte Cell Lines

1. Morphology: if cultures are passaged at confluence at split ratios that permit appropriate densities (*see* **Note 8**), chondrocyte cell lines will maintain the typical rounded to polygonal morphology in monolayer culture, although the size and volume may vary, as shown in **Fig. 1**.

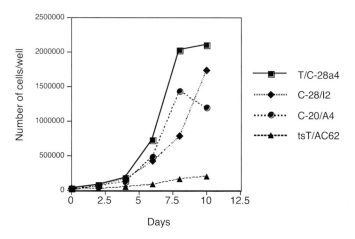

Fig. 2. Representative growth curves from established immortalized chondrocyte cell lines expressing different forms of SV40-TAg. Cells were seeded into multiwell plates at a density of 2.5×10^4 cells/cm^2 and cultured in DMEM/F-12 supplemented with 10% FCS for the indicated time periods with medium changes every 3 d. The T/C-28a4, C-28/I2, and C-20/A4 cell lines are grown at 37°C. The tsT/AC62 cell line is grown at 32°C, the permissive temperature for expression of tsTAg. (Reproduced with permission from ref. *30*.)

2. Growth kinetics: trypsinize the cells from a 10-cm dish and wash with PBS. Plate cells in 12-well plates at a concentration of 50,000 cells/well in 2 mL of growth medium. At intervals of 48 h, trypsinize duplicate wells from each plate and determine the cell counts using a hemocytometer or Coulter counter. Cell counts should be obtained until the cultures reach confluence. The proliferative capacity may also vary from one cell line to another, depending on the source of cartilage and the technique of immortalization (**Fig. 2**).

3. Phenotypic characterization (*see* **Note 10**): it is necessary to verify the presence of the definitive markers of the phenotype in chondrocyte cell lines after selection and to screen frequently once they are established. Phenotype can be monitored conveniently by the analysis of mRNAs encoding *COL2A1* and aggrecan using sensitive RT-PCR methods (*see* **Note 11**), as described previously *(27–30)* and in Chapters 6 and 7, in this volume. As shown in **Fig. 3**, the expression of *COL2A1* mRNA is lower in proliferating chondrocyte cell lines, where it is suppressed by 10% FCS, and can be enhanced in the presence of an insulin-containing serum substitute, such as Nutridoma-SP or ITS+. The expression of aggrecan mRNA is not coordinately regulated with *COL2A1* mRNA and is less susceptible to changes in the culture conditions (*see* **Note 12**). Experimental incubations are performed as follows:

   a. Passage cells into 6-well culture plates at $2.5–5 \times 10^5$ cells/well in DMEM/F-12 containing 10% FCS and allow the cells to grow to 50–95% confluence.

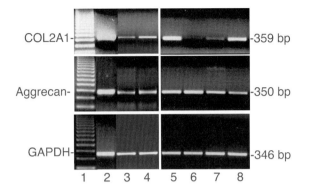

Fig. 3. Matrix gene expression in immortalized chondrocyte cell lines. Total RNA was isolated and analyzed by RT-PCR for expression of *COL2A1*, aggrecan, and GAPDH mRNAs. Lane 1, DNA ladder; lane 2, primary adult articular chondrocytes; lane 3, T/C-28a4 cultured in medium with 10% FCS; lane 4, T/C28a4 in serum-free medium with 1% Nutridoma-SP; lane 5, C-28/I2 in 1% Nutridoma-SP; lane 6, C-28/I2 in 10% FCS; lane 7, C-20/A4 in 10% FCS; lane 8, tsT/AC62 in 10% FCS at 32°C. Note that some cell lines are susceptible to a loss of the *COL2A1* phenotype in serum-containing growth medium. (Reproduced with permission from ref. *30*.)

   b. Remove culture medium, wash with PBS, and replace with DMEM/F-12 containing 1% Nutridoma-SP or 1% ITS+.

   c. Incubate overnight for up to 24 h, add treatments in a small volume without medium change, and continue incubations for the times desired.

4. Notes

1. Batches of serum should be tested and selected on the basis of the capacity to support expression of chondrocyte-specific matrix gene expression. High capacity to induce cell proliferation is not necessarily associated with the ability to maintain phenotype.

2. Human chondrocytes, similar to other human cell types, are not as easily immortalized with retroviruses as their mouse counterparts. Amphotropic packaging cell lines that have a broad host range are used for the production of helper virus-free stocks that will infect human cells *(24)*.

3. The appropriate G418 concentration should be determined empirically for each cell line prior to transfection. For most packaging cell lines, 300–400 µg/mL is optimal for death of nontransfected cells. The neomycin-sensitive cells should stop growing within 24 h, and cell death should be evident within 1 wk. Since multiplying cells are susceptible to G418, frequent changes of medium containing fresh G418 should be applied. Once cell death is evident, the G418 concentration can be changed to 200 µg/mL.

4. Safety considerations in handling viral stocks: Special care should be taken to prevent skin contamination and aerosol of virus particles. Spent medium, pipets, vacuum flasks, and any other materials in contact with virus-containing media should be treated with a 10% solution of bleach or handled as recommended by institutional standards.

5. After initial plating of the primary cultures, the chondrocytes require 2–3 d before they have settled down and spread out completely. Although the cultures may continue to express chondrocyte phenotype (e.g., type II collagen and aggrecan mRNAs) for several weeks, expression of nonspecific collagens I and III may begin as early as d 7 after isolation. Thus, it is recommended that infection with the immortalizing retrovirus be carried out between d 4 and 7 after isolation. Since cells must be actively dividing in order to be infected efficiently with retroviruses, the culture medium should be changed 24 and 3 h prior to addition of the retroviral supernatants.

6. Hyaluronidase added before and/or during transfections has been shown to increase transfection efficiencies in chondrocytes *(31–33)* and also to facilitate retroviral gene transfer in other cell types by degrading hyaluronan and GAGs in the pericellular coat and cell surface *(34)*.

7. Since viral activity is depleted after 4–6 h of incubation at 37°C, it is not necessary to leave the viral supernatants on the chondrocytes overnight except as a convenience.

8. The expansion of immortalized chondrocytes in monolayer culture in medium containing 10% FCS favors a loss of phenotype. Established cultures should not be plated at densities lower than those resulting from a split ratio of 1:2 for adult articular chondrocytes and 1:5–1:10 for more rapidly growing chondrocytes, such as juvenile costal chondrocytes. They should be passaged immediately upon reaching confluence, but not more than twice weekly. Since prolonged passaging of immortalized cell lines will select for rapidly growing cells, the cell lines should be expanded as soon as they are established and frozen down in liquid nitrogen.

9. Cultures are maintained as nonclonal populations, at least until they are established, in order to preserve potential cellular interactions among clonal cell types that might aid in survival and the preservation of phenotype. If the cells are cloned immediately after G418 selection, when immortalized cells have not completely repopulated the dish, survival is poor compared with other cell types. Greater success can be achieved if cloning by limiting dilution is performed on established cultures after crisis.

10. A note of caution is that immortalized human chondrocyte cell lines should not serve as a replacement for primary cultures. Because of the stable proliferative capacities of established cell lines, the cultures may be expanded to produce sufficient numbers of cells for selected types of experiments (*see* Chapter 4).

11. *COL2A1* mRNA, detected by RT-PCR, is the most sensitive marker of the chondrocyte phenotype, since it is lost more easily than aggrecan mRNA.

12. Further notes on culture of human chondrocytes and on chondrocyte immortalization may be found in previous volumes of *Methods in Molecular Medicine (27,28)*.

Acknowledgments

This work was supported in part by NIH grants AR45378 and AG22021 and a Biomedical Science Grant from the Arthritis Foundation.

References

1. Goldring, M. B. (2000) The role of the chondrocyte in osteoarthritis. *Arthritis Rheum.* **4**, 1916–1926.
2. Goldring, M. B., Sandell, L. J., Stephenson, M. L., and Krane, S. M. (1986) Immune interferon suppresses levels of procollagen mRNA and type II collagen synthesis in cultured human articular and costal chondrocytes. *J. Biol. Chem.* **261**, 9049–9056.
3. Brittberg, M., Lindahl, A., Nilsson, A., Ohlsson, C., Isaksson, O., and Peterson, L. (1994) Treatment of deep cartilage defects in the knee with autologous chondrocyte transplantation. *N. Engl. J. Med.* **331**, 889–895.
4. Alema, S., Tato, F., and Boettiger, D. (1985) Myc and src oncogenes have complementary effects on cell proliferation and expression of specific extracellular matrix components in definitive chondroblasts. *Mol. Cell. Biol.* **5**, 538–544.
5. Gionti, E., Pontarelli, G., and Cancedda, R. (1985) Avian myelocytomatosis virus immortalizes differentiated quail chondrocytes. *Proc. Natl. Acad. Sci. USA* **82**, 2756–2760.
6. Horton, W. E., Jr, Cleveland, J., Rapp, U., et al. (1988) An established rat cell line expressing chondrocyte properties. *Exp. Cell Res.* **178**, 457–468.
7. Thenet, S., Benya, P. D., Demignot, S., Feunteun, J., and Adolphe, M. (1992) SV40-immortalization of rabbit articular chondrocytes: alteration of differentiated functions. *J. Cell. Physiol.* **150**, 158–167.
8. Mallein-Gerin, F. and Olsen, B. R. (1993) Expression of simian virus 40 large T (tumor) oncogene in chondrocytes induces cell proliferation without loss of the differentiated phenotype. *Proc. Natl. Acad. Sci. USA* **90**, 3289–3293.
9. Grigoriadis, A. E., Heersche, J. N. M., and Aubin, J. E. (1988) Differentiation of muscle, fat, cartilage, and bone from progenitor cells present in a bone-derived clonal cell population: effect of dexamethasone. *J. Cell Biol.* **106**, 2139–2151.
10. Bernier, S. M. and Goltzman, D. (1993) Regulation of expression of the chondrogenic phenotype in a skeletal cell line (CFK2) in vitro. *J. Bone Miner. Res.* **8**, 475–484.
11. Lefebvre, V., Garofalo, S., and deCrombrugghe, B. (1995) Type X collagen gene expression in mouse chondrocytes immortalized by a temperature-sensitive simian virus 40 large tumor antigen. *J. Cell Biol.* **128**, 239–245.
12. Mataga, N., Tamura, M., Yanai, N., et al. (1996) Establishment of a novel chondrocyte-like cell line derived from transgenic mice harboring the temperature-sensitive simian virus 40 large T-antigen. *J. Bone Miner. Res.* **11**, 1646–1654.
13. Benoit, B., Thenet-Gauci, S., Hoffschir, F., Penformis, P., Demignot, S., and Adolphe, M. (1995) SV40 large T antigen immortalization of human articular chondrocytes. *In Vitro Cell. Dev. Biol.* **31**, 174–177.
14. Steimberg, N., Viengchareun, S., Biehlmann, F., et al. (1999) SV40 large T antigen expression driven by col2a1 regulatory sequences immortalizes articular

chondrocytes but does not allow stabilization of type II collagen expression. *Exp. Cell Res.* **249,** 248–259.

15. Goldring, M. B., Birkhead, J. R., Suen, L.-F., et al. (1994) Interleukin-1β-modulated gene expression in immortalized human chondrocytes. *J. Clin. Invest.* **94,** 2307–2316.

16. Robbins, J. R., Thomas, B., Tan, L., et al. (2000) Immortalized human adult articular chondrocytes maintain cartilage-specific phenotype and responses to interleukin-1β. *Arthritis Rheum.* **43,** 2189–2201.

17. Grigolo, B., Roseti, L., Neri, S., et al. (2002) Human articular chondrocytes immortalized by HPV-16 E6 and E7 genes: maintenance of differentiated phenotype under defined culture conditions. *Osteoarthritis Cartilage* **10,** 879–889.

18. Piera-Velazquez, S., Jimenez, S. A., and Stokes, D. (2002) Increased life span of human osteoarthritic chondrocytes by exogenous expression of telomerase. *Arthritis Rheum.* **46,** 683–693.

19. Miller, A. D. and Buttimore, C. (1986) Redesign of retrovirus packaging cell lines to avoid recombination leading to helper virus production. *Mol. Cell Biol.* **6,** 2895–2902.

20. Ory, D. S., Neugeboren, B. A., and Mulligan, R. C. (1996) A stable human-derived packaging cell line for production of high titer retrovirus/vesicular stomatitis virus G pseudotypes. *Proc. Natl. Acad. Sci. USA* **93,** 11,400–11,406.

21. Jat, P. S., Cepko, C. L., Mulligan, R. C., and Sharp, P. A. (1986) Recombinant retroviruses encoding simian virus 40 large T antigen and polyomavirus large and middle T antigens. *Mol. Cell Biol.* **6,** 1204–1217.

22. Jat, P. S. and Sharp, P. A. (1989) Cell lines established by a temperature-sensitive simian virus 40 large-T-antigen gene are growth restricted at the nonpermissive temperature. *Mol. Cell. Biol.* **9,** 1672–1681.

23. Harley, C. B. (2002) Telomerase is not an oncogene. *Oncogene* **21,** 494–502.

24. Cepko, C. L. and Pear, W. (2002) Introduction of DNA into mammalian cells, in *Short Protocols in Molecular Biology*, 5th Ed., Vol. 1, (Ausebel, F. M., Brent, R., Kingston, R. E., et al., eds.), John Wiley, New York, NY, pp. 9-1–9-77.

25. Bodnar, A. G., Ouellette, M., Frolkis, M., et al. (1998) Extension of life-span by introduction of telomerase into normal human cells. *Science* **279,** 349–352.

26. Harley, C. B., Futcher, A. B., and Greider, C. W. (1990) Telomeres shorten during ageing of human fibroblasts. *Nature* **345,** 458–460.

27. Goldring, M. B. (1996) Human chondrocyte cultures as models of cartilage-specific gene regulation, in *Methods in Molecular Biology: Human Cell Culture Protocols* (Jones, G. E., ed.), Humana, Totowa, NJ, pp. 217–231.

28. Robbins, J. R. and Goldring, M. B. (1998) Methods for preparation of immortalized human chondrocyte cell lines, in *Methods in Molecular Medicine: Tissue Engineering Methods and Protocols* (Morgan, J. R. and Yarmush, M. L., eds.), Humana, Totowa, NJ, pp. 173–192.

29. Kokenyesi, R., Tan, L., Robbins, J. R., and Goldring, M. B. (2000) Proteoglycan production by immortalized human chondrocyte cell lines cultured under conditions that promote expression of the differentiated phenotype. *Arch. Biochem. Biophys.* **383,** 79–90.

30. Loeser, R. F., Sadiev, S., Tan, L., and Goldring, M. B. (2000) Integrin expression by primary and immortalized human chondrocytes: evidence of a differential role for $\alpha1\beta1$ and $\alpha2\beta1$ integrins in mediating chondrocyte adhesion to types II and VI collagen. *Osteoarthritis Cartilage* **8,** 96–105.
31. Lu Valle, P., Iwamoto, M., Fanning, P., Pacifici, M., and Olsen, B. R. (1993) Multiple negative elements in a gene that codes for an extracellular matrix protein, collagen X, restrict expression to hypertrophic chondrocytes. *J. Cell Biol.* **121,** 1173–1179.
32. Viengchareun, S., Thenet-Gauci, S., Steimberg, N., Blancher, C., Crisanti, P., and Adolphe, M. (1997) The transfection of rabbit articular chondrocytes is independent of their differentiation state. *In Vitro Cell Dev. Biol. Anim.* **33,** 15–17.
33. Madry, H. and Trippel, S. B. (2000) Efficient lipid-mediated gene transfer to articular chondrocytes. *Gene Ther.* **7,** 286–291.
34. Batra, R. K., Olsen, J. C., Hoganson, D. K., Caterson, B., and Boucher, R. C. (1997) Retroviral gene transfer is inhibited by chondroitin sulfate proteoglycans/glycosaminoglycans in malignant pleural effusions. *J. Biol. Chem.* **272,** 11,736–11,743.

4

Culture of Immortalized Chondrocytes and Their Use As Models of Chondrocyte Function

Mary B. Goldring

Summary

Immortalization of chondrocytes increases life span and proliferative capacity but does not necessarily stabilize the differentiated phenotype. Expansion of chondrocyte cell lines in continuous monolayer culture may result in the loss of phenotype, particularly if high cell density is not maintained. This chapter describes strategies for maintaining or restoring differentiated phenotype in established chondrocyte cell lines involving culture in serum-free defined culture medium, in suspension over agarose or polyHEMA, or within alginate or collagen scaffolds. Chondrocyte cell lines have been used successfully to develop reproducible models for studying the regulation of gene expression in experiments requiring large numbers of cells. Thus, approaches for studying transcriptional regulation by transfection of promoter-driven reporter genes and cotransfection of expression vectors for wild-type or mutant proteins are also described.

Key Words: Immortalized chondrocytes; type II collagen; aggrecan; monolayer culture; suspension culture; alginate; agarose; polyHEMA; three-dimensional (3D) scaffolds; collagen scaffolds; ascorbate; Nutridoma; transfections; luciferase reporter plasmids; green fluorescent protein (GFP) reporter plasmids; adenoviral-mediated expression; luciferase assay.

1. Introduction

Simian virus 40 large T antigen (SV40-TAg), human papillomavirus type 16 early function genes E6 and E7 (HPV-16 E6/E7), and telomerase have been used with varying degrees of success for immortalizing human chondrocytes, as described in Chapter 3. However, a general observation is that phenotypic stability is lost during serial subculture of immortalized chondrocytes in monolayer culture. Clonal expansion usually results in type II collagen-negative cell lines that express type I and type III collagens in monolayer culture (*1,2*). The loss of phenotype may be reversible if established monolayer cultures are

From: *Methods in Molecular Medicine, Vol. 100: Cartilage and Osteoarthritis, Vol. 1: Cellular and Molecular Tools*
Edited by: M. Sabatini, P. Pastoureau, and F. De Ceuninck © Humana Press Inc., Totowa, NJ

maintained as nonclonal populations and selected by passaging through suspension cultures *(3,4)*. Furthermore, phenotype can be restored by transfer to three-dimensional (3D) culture in alginate *(4)* or hyaluronan *(5)* or to suspension culture on poly-2-hydroxyethyl-methacrylate (polyHEMA)-coated dishes *(6)*. Interestingly, long-term pellet culture of a clonal cell line of tsTAg-immortalized human articular chondrocytes at 37°C, the nonpermissive temperature for proliferation, induced expression of type X collagen, a hypertrophic chondrocyte marker not found in normal articular cartilage *(7)*.

Success in establishing immortalized human chondrocyte cell lines that can be used as models for studying cartilage breakdown and repair depends not only on the source and developmental state of the tissue from which the cell lines are established, but also more importantly on the ability of the culture system to support the differentiated phenotype. Regardless of the immortalization strategy, however, matrix protein synthesis and secretion in general and chondrocyte-specific phenotype in particular may be reduced after selection and expansion in monolayer culture. Thus, short-term incubation in serum-free defined medium supplemented with an insulin-containing serum substitute has been used as an experimental strategy *(3–5)*. This chapter focuses on strategies for culture and characterization that are applicable to any chondrocyte cell line and also describes approaches for using immortalized chondrocytes as reproducible models for evaluating chondrocyte functions.

2. Materials

2.1. Culture Reagents

1. Growth medium for chondrocytes: Dulbecco's modified Eagle's medium (DMEM)/Ham's F-12, 1:1 (v/v). Mix equal volumes of DMEM, high glucose, with L-glutamine and Ham's F-1, with L-glutamine (Cambrex, Walkersville, MD), both without HEPES, to give final concentrations of 3.151 g/L glucose, L-glutamine (365 mg/L)/L-glutamic acid (7.36 mg/L), and sodium pyruvate (110 mg/L). Add 10% FCS immediately before use.
2. Dulbecco's phosphate-buffered Ca^{2+}- and Mg^{2+}-free saline (PBS).
3. Trypsin-EDTA solution: 0.05% trypsin and 0.02% ethylenediamine tetraacetic acid (EDTA) in Hanks' balanced salt solution without Ca^{2+} and Mg^{2+} (Life Technologies, Gaithersburg, MD).
4. Hanks' balanced salt solution with Ca^{2+} and Mg^{2+} (HBSS; Life Technologies).
5. Serum substitutes for experimental incubations of immortalized chondrocytes: Nutridoma-SP (Roche Applied Science) is provided as sterile concentrate (100X, pH 7.4; storage at 15–25°C protected from light). Dilute 1:100 (v/v) with sterile DMEM/Ham's F-12, without FCS, and use immediately. ITS+ (BD Biosciences) is an alternative serum substitute.

Except where specified, cell culture reagents can be obtained from a number of different suppliers, including Life Technologies, Cambrex, Sigma (St.

Louis, MO), or Intergen (Purchase, NY). Reserve serum testing, which is offered by these suppliers, is recommended for selection of lots of FCS that maintain chondrocyte phenotype (*see* **Note 1**). FCS and trypsin-EDTA are stored at –20°C but should not be refrozen after thawing for use.

2.2. Culture Systems for Immortalized Chondrocytes

1. Agarose-coated dishes *(8)*.
   a. Weigh out 10 mL of high melting point agarose in an autoclavable bottle and add 100 mL of dH$_2$O.
   b. Autoclave with cap tightened loosely, allow to cool to approx 55°C, and pipet quickly into culture dishes (1 mL/3.5-cm well of 6-well plate, 3 mL/6-cm dish, or 9 mL/10-cm dish).
   c. Allow the gel to set at 4°C for 30 min and wash the surface two to three times with PBS.
   d. Plates may be used immediately or wrapped tightly with plastic or foil to prevent evaporation and stored at 4°C.
2. Dishes coated with polyHEMA *(9)*.
   a. Prepare a 10% (w/v) solution by dissolving 5 g of polyHEMA (BD Biosciences) in 50 mL of ethanol in a sterile capped bottle or centrifuge tube.
   b. Leave overnight at 37°C with gentle shaking to dissolve polymer completely.
   c. Centrifuge the viscous solution for 30 min at 2000*g* to remove undissolved particles.
   d. Layer the polyHEMA solution on dishes at 0.3 mL/well of 6-well plate or 0.9 mL/6-cm dish and leave with lids in place to dry overnight in a tissue culture hood.
   e. Expose open dishes to bactericidal ultraviolet light for 30 min to sterilize.
3. Alginate (Keltone LVCR, NF; ISP Alginates, San Diego, CA). Low viscosity (LV) alginate is generally used. Request LVCR for more highly purified preparation.
   a. Prepare 1.2% (w/v) solution of alginate in 0.15 *M* NaCl.
   b. Dissolve alginate in a 0.15 *M* NaCl solution, heating the solution in a microwave oven until it just begins to boil. Swirl and heat again two or three times until the alginate is dissolved completely. (**Caution:** Do not autoclave.) Allow the solution to cool to about 37°C and sterile filter. Filtering when warm permits the viscous solution to pass through the filter.
   c. Prepare 102 m*M* CaCl$_2$ and 0.15 *M* NaCl solutions in tissue culture bottles and autoclave.
   d. Prepare 55 m*M* Na citrate, 0.15 *M* NaCl, pH 6.0, sterile filter, and store at 4°C. Make fresh weekly.
4. 3D scaffolds: several types of scaffolds are available commercially, including the following:
   a. Gelfoam® (Pharmacia & Upjohn, Kalamazoo, MI), sterile absorbable collagen sponge, purchased as size 12–7 (2 cm × 6 cm × 7 mm; cat. no. 09-0315-03, box of 12).

    b. BD™ Three Dimensional Collagen Composite Scaffold (BD Biosciences): contains a mixture of bovine type 1 and type III collagens and is provided as 3D scaffolds with 48-well plates.

    c. BD™ Three Dimensional OPLA® Scaffold (BD Biosciences): contains a synthetic polymer synthesized from D,D,-L,L polylactic acid and is provided as 3D scaffolds with 48-well plates.

5. Recovery of cells from scaffolds:

    a. Cell lysis solution: 0.2% v/v Triton X-100, 10 mM Tris-HCl, pH 7.0, 1 mM EDTA.

    b. Collagenase solution: 0.03% (w/v) collagenase (Worthington, Freehold, NJ) in HBSS.

    c. RNA extraction kits: TRIzol® reagent (Life Technologies) or RNeasy Mini Kit (Qiagen).

2.3. Immortalized Chondrocyte Cell Lines As Models for Studying Chondrocyte Function

1. EndoFree Plasmid Maxi Kit (Qiagen).
2. Lipid-based transfection reagent such as LipofectAMINE PLUS™ Reagent (Life Technologies) or FuGENE 6 (Roche Applied Science, Indianapolis, IN).
3. Serum-free culture medium for transfections: Opti-MEM (Life Technologies) or DMEM/F-12 (test for optimal transfection efficiency).
4. Passive Lysis Buffer (Promega).
5. Coomassie Plus Protein Assay Reagent (Pierce, Rockford, IL).
6. Luciferase Assay System (Promega, Madison, WI).
7. Dual-Luciferase Reporter Assay (Promega) with the pRL-TK Renilla luciferase control vector.
8. Adenovirus producer cell line: 293 (ATTC CRL 1573; transformed primary human embryonic kidney).

3. Methods

Immortalization strategies and approaches for selection and expansion of chondrocyte cell lines are described in Chapter 3. The methods described below outline: (1) culture systems for immortalized chondrocytes, and (2) the use of established cell lines as models for studying chondrocyte function.

3.1. Culture Systems for Immortalized Chondrocytes

Immortalization of a number of human somatic cell types, including dermal fibroblasts, osteoblasts, endothelial cells, and epithelial cells, using SV40-TAg, HPV-16 E6/E7, or hTERT has been shown to increase life span and proliferative capacity, but it does not necessarily preserve the differentiated phenotype. Since proliferating chondrocytes in monolayer culture are particularly susceptible to loss of phenotype during prolonged culture, it is necessary to use culture conditions that maintain differentiated chondrocyte features or that permit redifferentiation (*see* **Note 2**).

3.1.1. Monolayer Cultures

1. Immortalized chondrocytes are cultured routinely in 10-cm dishes and passaged immediately upon reaching confluence. Adult articular chondrocytes are passaged every 7–10 d and more rapidly growing cultures, such as juvenile costal chondrocytes, are passaged every 4–6 d.

2. For passaging, remove culture medium by aspiration with a sterile Pasteur pipet attached to a vacuum flask and wash with PBS (Ca^{2+}- and Mg^{2+}-free). Add trypsin-EDTA solution (*not* trypsin alone) at 1.5 mL/10-cm dish to cover cell layer, and immediately remove 1 mL. Leave at room temperatures with periodic gentle shaking of dish. Check in microscope to ensure that all cells have come off the plate in a single cell suspension (*see* **Note 3**). If significant numbers of cells remain attached, continue the incubation for a longer time (20 min or less) at 37°C and/or gently scrape the cell layer with a sterile plastic scraper, Teflon policeman, or syringe plunger.

3. Bring up cells in 5- or 10-mL pipet containing culture medium, aspirating in and out several times to break up cell clumps. Transfer to a sterile conical 15- or 50-mL polypropylene tube and perform cell counts to determine the split ratio required (usually 1 dish into 2 [1:2] for adult articular chondrocytes, or 1 dish into 5, 8, or 10 for more rapidly growing juvenile chondrocytes). Distribute equal volumes of the cell suspension in dishes or wells that already contain culture medium, rocking plates back and forth (not swirling) immediately after each addition to ensure uniform plating density throughout the plate.

4. For experiments, plate cells in 12-well plates at a concentration of 100,000 cells/well in 2 mL of growth medium or in 6-well plates at 250,000 cells/well in 3 mL of medium. Remove growth medium 1–3 d after passaging, when the cultures are subconfluent. Add serum-free medium containing a serum substitute (*see* **Note 4**), such as Nutridoma-SP, followed immediately or 1–24 h later by the test agent of interest. Continue incubation at 37°C for short-term time courses of 0.25–24 h or longer time-courses of 24–72 h.

3.1.2. Fluid Suspension Cultures on Agarose- or polyHEMA-Coated Dishes

1. Trypsinize monolayer cultures, spin down cells, wash with PBS, centrifuge, and resuspend in culture medium containing 10% FCS at 1×10^6 cells/mL.

2. Transfer chondrocyte suspension to dishes that have been coated with 1% agarose or with 0.9% polyHEMA and culture for 2–4 wk. The cells first form large clumps that begin to break up after 7–10 d and eventually form single-cell suspensions.

3. Change the medium weekly by carefully removing the medium above settled cells while tilting the dish, centrifuging the remaining suspended cells and replacing them in the dish after resuspension in fresh culture medium.

4. To recover cells for direct experimental analysis, for redistribution in agarose- or polyHEMA-coated wells, or for culture in monolayer, transfer the cell suspension to 15- or 50-mL conical tubes, gently washing the agarose surface at least twice with culture medium to recover remaining cells; then spin down and resuspend cells in an appropriate volume of culture medium for plating or in extraction buffer for subsequent experimental analysis.

3.1.3. Alginate Bead Cultures (see **Note 5**)

1. Trypsinize several 10-cm plates and wash the cells with PBS. Determine the cell count with a hemocytometer and pellet the cells. Resuspend the pellet in a 1.2% solution of alginate, 0.15 M NaCl at a concentration of 4×10^6 cells/mL.
2. Express the alginate suspension in a dropwise manner through a 10-mL syringe equipped with a 25-gage needle into a 50-mL centrifuge tube containing 40 mL of 10^2 mM $CaCl_2$. Allow the beads to polymerize in the $CaCl_2$ solution for 10 min and wash twice with 25 mL of 0.15 M NaCl. The alginate beads should *not* be washed in PBS, as they will become cloudy.
3. Resuspend the beads (7–15 beads/mL) in 20 mL of growth medium supplemented with 25 µg/mL Na ascorbate (*see* **Note 6**), and decant the beads to a 10-cm dish. As many as 150 beads (approx 9×10^6 cells) can be cultured in a single dish with medium changes every 3 d.
4. To recover cells from alginate, carefully aspirate the medium from the cultures and wash twice with PBS. Depolymerize the alginate by adding three volumes of a solution of 55 mM Na citrate/0.15 M NaCl and incubate at 37°C for 10 min. Aspirate the solution over the surface of the dish several times to dislodge adherent cells (the cells are sticky) and transfer the suspension to a 50-mL centrifuge tube.
5. Because the solution is quite viscous, centrifuge the cells at 2000g for a minimum of 10 min to pellet the cells completely. Wash the cells twice with PBS before using them for further analysis.

3.1.4. Culture on 3D Scaffolds (see **Note 7**)

1. Gelfoam: use a sterile scalpel blade to cut into pieces of $1 \times 1 \times 0.5$ cm^3 and place in wells of sterile 6-well plates. Inoculate by dropping 50 µL of growth medium containing 10^6 cells on each sponge. Place in incubator for 1.5–2 h, and then add 100 µL medium and culture for an additional 1–3 h. Add medium to cover and continue incubation overnight or longer.
2. BD 3D Collagen Composite or OPLA Scaffolds: place scaffolds (0.5 cm^3) in the 48-well plates provided, in 96-well plates, or in other plates as required. Seed scaffolds by dropping 100 µL of growth medium containing $1–5 \times 10^4$ cells. Incubate for 1 h, add 150 µL of medium to each scaffold, and incubate for 1.5–3 h. Add medium as required for further culture and experimental conditions.
3. Recovery of cells from scaffolds for analysis:
   a. Prepare cell lysates for DNA analysis using 250–500 µL of cell lysis solution (0.2% v/v Triton X-100, 10 mM Tris-HCl, pH 7.0, 1 mM EDTA) per scaffold

in 1.5-mL tube. Freeze samples at –70°C and subject to two freeze/thaw cycles, thawing at room temperature for 45–60 min. Break up scaffolds with pipet tip, centrifuge, and transfer lysates to fresh tubes. The cell lysates may be analyzed using the Picogreen Assay Kit according to the manufacture's protocol (Molecular Probes).

b. Recover cells for RNA extraction and other analyses by treatment of minced scaffolds with 0.03% (w/v) collagenase in HBSS for 10–15 min at 37°C. Collect cells by centrifugation, wash with PBS, and extract total RNA using TRIzol reagent or RNeasy Mini Kit.

3.2. Immortalized Chondrocyte Cell Lines As Models for Studying Chondrocyte Function

Immortalized chondrocyte cell lines serve as reproducible models to study the expression of chondrocyte-specific matrix genes and to examine the effects of cytokines and growth/differentiation factors on chondrocyte phenotypic markers, as shown in **Figs. 1** and **2**. In 3D cultures, it is also useful to characterize the proteoglycans synthesized *(4,10,11)* (*see* also Chapters 14 and 15), stain the matrix components with alcian blue *(4,10)*, toluidine blue, or other dyes, or perform immunohistochemistry using specific antibodies against these proteins *(3)* (*see* Chapters 17 and 18). Other features of the chondrocyte phenotype include the expression of the three members of the SRY-type HMG box (SOX) family of transcription factors, L-Sox5, Sox6, and Sox9 *(12)*, which are required for chondrocyte differentiation during development. The capacity to respond to interleukin-1β (IL-1β) by increasing expression of cyclooxygenase-2 (COX-2) and matrix metalloproteinase-13 (MMP-13) is somewhat dependent on the differentiated phenotype *(13)*. Integrin profiles should be consistent with those expressed on normal chondrocytes but may also reflect the types of integrins found on proliferating cells *(14)*. However, immortalized chondrocytes should not be considered as substitutes for primary chondrocytes, which should be used to validate key findings.

Chondrocyte cell lines have served most beneficially as models to delineate the cytokine- and growth factor-induced signaling pathways and transcription factors involved in the regulation of gene expression. They may be used to study the effects of selective protein kinase inhibitors, as described *(4,13)*, employing techniques described in Chapter 20. Because they can be cultured in sufficient numbers, they are convenient models for examining transiently or stably expressed reporter genes or recombinant wild-type and mutant proteins *(13,15–20)* and for examining specific DNA binding activities in nuclear extracts *(12,21)*. They may also be used to test approaches for gene therapy using viral vectors *(22)* and RNA interference (RNAi) strategies *(23)*.

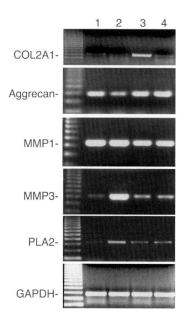

Fig. 1. RT-PCR analysis of mRNAs expressed by immortalized human chondrocytes. The tsT/AC62 cells were passaged into 6-well plates in DMEM/F-12 containing 10% FCS and incubated at 32°C for 4 d, at which time the medium was changed. On d 5, IL-1β (100 pg/mL) or hBMP-2 (100 ng/mL) was added alone or in combination, and incubations were continued until d 7. Total RNA was extracted using TRIzol reagent and mRNAs encoding *COL2A1*, aggrecan, matrix metalloproteinase (MMP)-1, MMP-3, phospholipase A2 (PLA2), and GAPDH were analyzed by RT-PCR as described in Robbins et al. *(4)*. The DNA ladder is shown on the left. Lane 1, untreated control; lane 2, IL-1β; lane 3, BMP-2; and lane 4, IL-1β and BMP-2.

Plasmid vectors, in which the expression of reporter genes such as CAT (3), luciferase (**Fig. 3**) *(4,12,21)*, or green fluorescent protein (GFP) (**Fig. 4**) is driven by gene regulatory sequences, such as those regulating COL2A1 transcription, may be transfected in immortalized cell lines to study chondrocyte-specific responses, as described below. Coexpression of wild-type or dominant-negative mutants of transcription factors, protein kinases, and other regulatory molecules, mediated by plasmid or adenoviral vectors, may be performed to dissect further the mechanisms involved.

3.2.1. Transient Transfections Using Luciferase Reporter Plasmids

1. Prepare plasmids using the EndoFree Plasmid Maxi Kit, according to the manufacturer's instructions (Qiagen), to generate endotoxin-free DNA (*see* **Note 8**).

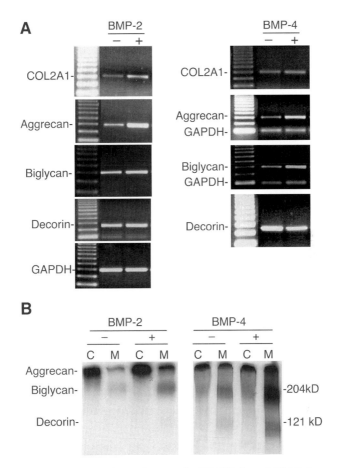

Fig. 2. Effects of bone morphogenic protein (BMP)-2 and BMP-4 on matrix gene expression and proteoglycan synthesis by T/C-28a2 immortalized chondrocytes. The T/C-28 cells were passaged into 6-well plates in DMEM/F-12 containing 10% FCS and incubated at 37°C for 2 d, at which time the medium was changed to serum-free medium containing 1% Nutridoma. On d 3, BMP-2 (100 ng/mL) or BMP-4 (100 ng/mL) was added to wells as indicated, and incubations were continued until d 5. **(A)** Total RNA was extracted using TRIzol reagent and mRNAs encoding *COL2A1*, aggrecan, biglycan, decorin, and reduced glyceraldehyde-phosphate dehydrogenase (GAPDH) were analyzed by RT-PCR, as described *(4)*. DNA ladders are shown in the left lanes of each panel. Note that different GAPDH primers were used in the left and right panels. **(B)** Proteoglycans were biosynthetically labeled with [^{35}S]sulfate in the presence of ascorbate (25 μg/mL) during the final 12 h of incubation. The cell layers (C) and media (M) were extracted separately, as described *(11)*, prior to electrophoresis on SDS-polyacrylamide 4–20% gradient gels and visualization by fluorography. Aggrecan, biglycan, and decorin migrate as indicated on the left of the panel. Molecular weight standards are indicated to the right of the panel.

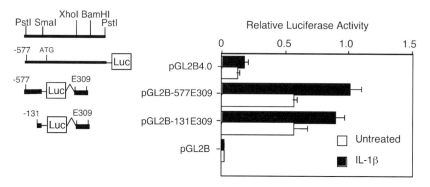

Fig. 3. Regulation of *COL2A1* promoter activity by interleukin-1β (IL-1β) in immortalized human chondrocytes. Luciferase reporter constructs containing *COL2A1* sequences were transfected into C-28/I2 cells using LipofectAMINE+ and treated with IL-1β in DMEM/F-12 containing 1% Nutridoma for 18 h prior to harvest for luciferase assay. The promoter constructs, pGL2B4.0, pGL2B-577/+125, and pGL2B-131/+125 containing the E309 enhancer region (+2388/+2696 bp) from intron 1 were compared. Luciferase activity was normalized to the amount of protein and expressed as relative activity to that of untreated cells transfected with pGL2B-577/+125E309. Each value is calculated as the mean ± SD of the results from three to six wells, and results are representative of at least three experiments. Note that the empty vector, pGL2-Basic, expressed at 1–2% of the levels of the *COL2A1* promoter constructs and did not respond to IL-1β.

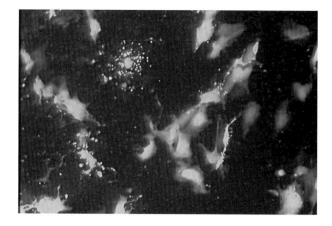

Fig. 4. Transient expression of green fluorescent protein in immortalized human chondrocytes. The C-20/A4 cells were transfected using LipofectAMINE+ with pEGFP-N2 at 1 µg/well in 6-well plates and cultured for 24 h in medium containing 10% FCS. Live cultures were visualized by fluorescence microscopy (Nikon Eclipse TE300). Expression of the green fluorescent protein is driven by the CMV promoter in this vector (BD Biosciences Clontech).

2. On the day before transfection, seed cells in 6-well tissue culture plates at 2.5–5 × 10⁵ cells/well in DMEM/F-12 containing 10% FCS. (Determine optimal cell number to ensure that cultures are 50–95% confluent at the time of transfection.)

3. On the day of the transfection, prepare lipid/DNA complexes in serum-free DMEM/F-12 or Opti-MEM using LipofectAMINE+ or FuGENE 6, according to the manufacturer's protocol. Prepare in bulk for multiple transfections. Do not vortex at any step:

   a. LipofectAMINE+: for each well, add 92 μL of serum-free medium to a small sterile polypropylene tube, add 1 μL of plasmid DNA (maximum of 1 μg; *see* **Note 9**), and tap gently to mix. Add 6 μL of PLUS reagent, mix, and incubate for 15 min at room temperature. Dilute 4 μL of LipofectAMINE+ reagent into 100 μL of serum-free medium, mix, and add to each reaction mixture. Mix and leave at room temperature for an additional 15–30 min at room temperature.

   b. FuGENE 6: for each well, add 96 μL of serum-free medium to a small sterile polypropylene tube, add 3 μL of FuGENE 6 reagent, and tap gently to mix. Add 1 μL plasmid of DNA (maximum of 1 μg) to the prediluted FuGENE 6 reagent and incubate for 15 min at room temperature.

4. While the lipid/DNA complexes are forming, replace culture medium on cells with serum-free medium to give a final volume of 1 mL. Add the lipid/DNA complex mixture dropwise to the well and incubate for 4 h at 37°C.

5. Dilute the transfection medium by adding to the wells an equal volume of DMEM/F-12 containing 2% Nutridoma-SP (or 20% FCS) and incubate 2 h to overnight. Add test agent without medium change and incubate for a further 18 h (up to 48 h) (*see* **Note 10**).

3.2.2. Cotransfections Using Plasmid Vectors for Expression of Recombinant Proteins

1. Prepare plasmids as described above in **Subheading 3.2.1.**

2. Titrate each expression vector and its corresponding empty vector, at amounts ranging from 10 to 200 ng per well, against a fixed amount of reporter vector. Equalize the total amount of reporter plus expression plasmid in each well (<1 μg/well) by adding empty vector and maintain equal volumes (*see* **Note 9**).

3. After cotransfection, incubate the cells for 18–24 h to permit expression of recombinant protein prior to treatment with test reagents.

3.2.3. Adenovirally Mediated Expression of Recombinant Proteins

1. Infect the 293 producer cell line with adenoviral vector containing the cDNA encoding the wild-type or mutant protein to be coexpressed and determine the titer (multiplicity of infection [MOI]) by standard techniques.

2. Incubate immortalized chondrocytes in DMEM/F-12 containing 10% FCS for 18 h following transfection of the reporter construct.

3. Remove medium and wash cells with PBS.

4. Add 1 mL of serum-free medium containing adenovirus at 1:125 MOI. Incubate at 37°C for 90 min.
5. Add 1 mL of DMEM/F-12 containing 20% FCS and continue incubation for 18 h.
6. Change medium to fresh DMEM/F-12 containing 10% FCS or 1% Nutridoma-SP, incubate for 1 h, and treat with test agent for 18 h.

3.2.4. Luciferase Assay

1. Prepare cell lysates by extraction with 200 μL of Passive Lysis Buffer, which will passively lyse cells without the requirement of a freeze-thaw cycle. Scrape cells with a policeman and transfer solubilized cells to a 1.5-mL microcentrifuge tube. Microcentrifuge for 5 min at maximum speed at 4°C, transfer supernatant to a clean microcentrifuge tube, and store on ice.
2. Determine the protein content using the Coomassie Plus Protein Assay Reagent.
3. Determine luciferase activities using the Luciferase Assay System or equivalent, according to the manufacturer's protocol. Mix, manually or automatically, 20 μL of cell lysate with 100 μL of Luciferase Assay Reagent and read in a luminometer. Normalize to the amount of protein (or internal control such as β-galactosidase) and express as relative activity against the empty vector or untreated control. Perform each treatment in triplicate wells and each experiment at least three times to ensure reproducibility and significance.
4. The Dual-Luciferase Reporter Assay, in which 20 ng of the pRL-TK Renilla luciferase control vector is included in the transfections, may be used routinely or when it is necessary to check the purity of new plasmid preparations or relative activities of mutant and wild-type constructs.

4. Notes

1. Batches of serum should be tested and selected on the basis of the capacity to support expression of chondrocyte-specific matrix expression. High capacity to induce cell proliferation is not necessarily associated with the ability to maintain phenotype.
2. After prolonged passaging in a monolayer, immortalized chondrocytes may be redifferentiated by 1–2 wk of culture in alginate beads or in suspension over agarose or polyHEMA. Note that culture of chondrocytes embedded in agarose is not discussed here because it is difficult to recover cells for further culture or other manipulations.
3. Since chondrocytes are strongly adherent to tissue culture plastic, possibly because of calcium ion-binding glycosaminoglycans in the pericellular matrix, a trypsin-EDTA solution rather than trypsin alone is used for full release of chondrocytes from tissue culture plastic during passaging. Immortalized adult articular chondrocytes adhere more strongly to the culture dish than the more rapidly proliferating immortalized juvenile chondrocytes.
4. The synthetic activities of immortalized chondrocytes in monolayer culture are inversely related to proliferative activities. Thus, the expression of genes encoding matrix proteins and their deposition into the extracellular matrix decrease

compared with housekeeping and cell growth-associated genes. For experiments, the growth medium is removed 1–3 d after passaging, when the cultures are subconfluent, and serum-free medium supplemented with an insulin-containing serum substitute such as Nutridoma-SP or ITS+ is added, followed immediately 1–24 h later by the addition (without medium change) of the test agent of interest. Confluent cultures may tolerate serum-free medium containing 0.3% bovine serum albumin for up to 48 h or longer.

5. The method for culture of chondrocytes in alginate beads has been adapted from previously published methods *(24,25)*. This method was developed for nonimmortalized articular chondrocytes that do not proliferate when cultured in fluid or gel suspension. Immortalized chondrocytes continue to proliferate in alginate, and rapidly proliferating cell lines cannot be kept in alginate longer than 1 or 2 wk. Since the alginate does not remodel, the clonal growth forms bundles of cells that cannot expand into the matrix, the cytoplasmic volume is reduced, and cell death may occur in the middle of the cell mass. Immortalized adult articular chondrocytes, which tend to grow more slowly, can be kept in alginate culture for longer periods, as described *(4,13)*.

6. Ascorbate, which is required for synthesis and secretion of proteoglycans and collagens, is added daily to alginate or other 3D cultures to permit secretion and deposition of extracellular matrix, particularly when staining techniques are to be used. Add 25 µg/mL of ascorbate during the final 24–72 h of incubation when radiolabeling proteoglycans with [^{35}S] sulfate or collagens with [^{3}H]proline for characterization by sodium dodecyl sulfate polyacrylamide gel electrophoresis. Do not use ascorbate, which inhibits *COL2A1* transcription (M. B. Goldring, unpublished observation), if analysis of type II collagen mRNA is the endpoint.

7. Culture of immortalized chondrocytes in 3D scaffolds is a useful approach for tissue engineering applications. The commercially available methods are recommended because of their ease of use. Published methods are available for fabricating collagen sponges *(26)* and other 3D scaffolds, in which the composition may be manipulated, for example, by using type II collagen and/or adding glycosaminoglycans and other cartilage-specific matrix components. The biodegradable scaffolds are particularly useful if the cell-seeded scaffolds are to be implanted in animals. For studies entirely in vitro, in which incubation periods of more than a few days are required, it is recommended that cultures be performed in wells that fit the size of the scaffolds. Otherwise, the culture surface of the well or dish should be coated with a nonadherent substrate or treated in such a way as to prevent attachment of cells that may migrate out from the sponges. Additional analytical methods have been described using Gelfoam *(27)* and BD 3D scaffolds (*see* Website: http://www.bdbiosciences.com/discovery_Labware/Products/tissue_engineering/).

8. Although chondrocytes are generally less susceptible than monocyte/macrophages and other immune cells to endotoxin, it is possible that the transfection conditions, the proliferative state of the cell lines, or other factors may sensitize the cells to low concentrations of endotoxin *(28)*. Endotoxin itself induces and

activates transcription factors that are common to inflammatory responses and may thus up- or downregulate the promoter of interest, thereby masking the response to a cytokine or growth factor.

9. The total amount of plasmid to be transfected, including reporter, expression, and internal control plasmids, should not exceed 1 μg, and the optimal amount for the culture system should be tested empirically. If variable amounts of expression vector, for example, are included, the total amount of plasmid in each well should be equalized by the addition of the empty vector. Wells transfected with appropriate empty vector controls, without and with treatment with test agent, should also be included. Of the luciferase reporter vectors available, pXP2 and pGL2 provide reproducible results in immortalized chondrocyte cell lines. Results using pGL3 as the reporter vector are variable depending on the promoter and treatment, and stable transfection may be required when using highly proliferative immortalized chondrocyte cell lines or transformed cells such as the chondrosarcoma cell line SW-1351 *(29)*.

10. The times of incubation following transfection before addition of the test agent may vary according to the cell line and treatment and should be tested empirically. Nutridoma-SP or another serum substitute may be used for experiments with highly proliferative immortalized chondrocyte cell lines for the reasons indicated in **Note 4**. Note also that test agents should be added without medium change to avoid induction of pathways by serum growth factors or other medium constituents.

Acknowledgments

We thank Dr. Elisabeth Morris (Wyeth Research, Cambridge, MA) for providing recombinant BMP-2 and BMP-4. This work was supported in part by NIH grants AR45378 and AG22021 and a Biomedical Science Grant from the Arthritis Foundation.

References

1. Benoit, B., Thenet-Gauci, S., Hoffschir, F., Penformis, P., Demignot, S., and Adolphe, M. (1995) SV40 large T antigen immortalization of human articular chondrocytes. *In Vitro Cell. Dev. Biol.* **31,** 174–177.
2. Steimberg, N., Viengchareun, S., Biehlmann, F., et al. (1999) SV40 large T antigen expression driven by col2a1 regulatory sequences immortalizes articular chondrocytes but does not allow stabilization of type II collagen expression. *Exp. Cell. Res.* **249,** 248–259.
3. Goldring, M. B., Birkhead, J. R., Suen, L.-F., et al. (1994) Interleukin-1β-modulated gene expression in immortalized human chondrocytes. *J. Clin. Invest.* **94,** 2307–2316.
4. Robbins, J. R., Thomas, B., Tan, L., et al. (2000) Immortalized human adult articular chondrocytes maintain cartilage-specific phenotype and responses to interleukin-1β. *Arthritis Rheum.* **43,** 2189–2201.

5. Grigolo, B., Roseti, L., Neri, S., et al. (2002) Human articular chondrocytes immortalized by HPV-16 E6 and E7 genes: maintenance of differentiated phenotype under defined culture conditions. *Osteoarthritis Cartilage* **10**, 879–889.

6. Piera-Velazquez, S., Jimenez, S. A., and Stokes, D. (2002) Increased life span of human osteoarthritic chondrocytes by exogenous expression of telomerase. *Arthritis Rheum.* **46**, 683–693.

7. Oyajobi, B. O., Frazer, A., Hollander, A. P., et al. (1998) Expression of type X collagen and matrix calcification in three-dimensional cultures of immortalized temperature-sensitive chondrocytes derived from adult human articular cartilage. *J. Bone Miner. Res.* **13**, 432–442.

8. Castagnola, P., Moro, G., Descalzi-Cancedda, F., and Cancedda, R. (1986) Type X collagen synthesis during in vitro development of chick embryo tibial chondrocytes. *J. Cell Biol.* **102**, 2310–2317.

9. Reginato, A. M., Iozzo, R. V., and Jimenez, S. A. (1994) Formation of nodular structures resembling mature articular cartilage in long-term primary cultures of human fetal epiphyseal chondrocytes on hydrogel substrate. *Arthritis Rheum.* **37**, 1338–1349.

10. Robbins, J. R. and Goldring, M. B. (1998) Methods for preparation of immortalized human chondrocyte cell lines, in *Methods in Molecular Medicine: Tissue Engineering Methods and Protocols* (Morgan, J. R. and Yarmush, M. L., eds.), Humana, Totowa, NJ, pp. 173–192.

11. Kokenyesi, R., Tan, L., Robbins, J. R., and Goldring, M. B. (2000) Proteoglycan production by immortalized human chondrocyte cell lines cultured under conditions that promote expression of the differentiated phenotype. *Arch. Biochem. Biophys.* **383**, 79–90.

12. Osaki, M., Tan, L., Choy, B. K., et al. (2003) The TATA-containing core promoter of the type II collagen gene (COL2A1) is the target of interferon-γ-mediated inhibition in human chondrocytes: requirement for Stat1α, Jak1, and Jak2. *Biochem. J.* **369**, 103–115.

13. Thomas, B., Thirion, S., Humbert, L., et al. (2002) Differentiation regulates interleukin-1β-induced cyclo-oxygenase-2 in human articular chondrocytes: role of p38 mitogen-activated kinase. *Biochem. J.* **362**, 367–373.

14. Loeser, R. F., Sadiev, S., Tan, L., and Goldring, M. B. (2000) Integrin expression by primary and immortalized human chondrocytes: evidence of a differential role for α1β1 and α2β1 integrins in mediating chondrocyte adhesion to types II and VI collagen. *Osteoarthritis Cartilage* **8**, 96–105.

15. Attur, M. G., Dave, M., Cipolletta, C., et al. (2000) Reversal of autocrine and paracrine effects of interleukin 1 (IL-1) in human arthritis by type II IL-1 decoy receptor. Potential for pharmacological intervention. *J. Biol. Chem.* **275**, 40,307–40,315.

16. Nuttall, M. E., Nadeau, D. P., Fisher, P. W., et al. (2000) Inhibition of caspase-3-like activity prevents apoptosis while retaining functionality of human chondrocytes in vitro. *J. Orthop. Res.* **18**, 356–363.

17. Johnson, K., Vaingankar, S., Chen, Y., et al. (1999) Differential mechanisms of inorganic pyrophosphate production by plasma cell membrane glycoprotein-1 and B10 in chondrocytes. *Arthritis Rheum.* **42**, 1986–1997.

18. Palmer, G., Guerne, P. A., Mezin, F., et al. (2002) Production of interleukin-1 receptor antagonist by human articular chondrocytes. *Arthritis Res.* **4**, 226–231.

19. Laflamme, C., Filion, C., Bridge, J. A., Ladanyi, M., Goldring, M. B., and Labelle, Y. (2003) The homeotic protein Six3 is a coactivator of the nuclear receptor NOR-1 and a corepressor of the fusion protein EWS/NOR-1 in human extraskeletal myxoid chondrosarcomas. *Cancer Res.* **63**, 449–454.

20. Grall, F., Gu, X., Tan, L., et al. (2003) Responses to the pro-inflammatory cytokines interleukin-1 and tumor necrosis factor-α in cells derived from rheumatoid synovium and other joint tissues involve NF-κB-mediated induction of the Ets transcription factor ESE-1. *Arthritis Rheum.* **48**, 1249–1260.

21. Tan, L., Peng, H., Osaki, M., et al. (2003) Egr-1 mediates transcriptional repression of COL2A1 promoter activity by interleukin-1β. *J. Biol. Chem.* **278**, 17,688–17,770.

22. Ulrich-Vinther, M., Maloney, M. D., Goater, J. J., et al. (2002) Light-activated gene transduction enhances adeno-associated virus vector-mediated gene expression in human articular chondrocytes. *Arthritis Rheum.* **46**, 2095–2104.

23. Zwicky, R., Muntener, K., Goldring, M. B., and Baici, A. (2002) Cathepsin B expression and down-regulation by gene silencing and antisense DNA in human chondrocytes. *Biochem. J.* **367**, 209–217.

24. Guo, J., Jourdian, G. W., and MacCallum, D. K. (1989) Culture and growth characteristics of chondrocytes encapsulated in alginate beads. *Connect. Tiss. Res.* **19**, 277–297.

25. Hauselmann, H. J., Fernandes, R. J., Mok, S. S., et al. (1994) Phenotypic stability of bovine articular chondrocytes after long-term culture in alginate beads. *J. Cell Sci.* **107**, 17–27.

26. Mizuno, S., Allemann, F., and Glowacki, J. (2001) Effects of medium perfusion on matrix production by bovine chondrocytes in three-dimensional collagen sponges. *J. Biomed. Mater. Res.* **56**, 368–375.

27. Wu, Q. Q. and Chen, Q. (2000) Mechanoregulation of chondrocyte proliferation, maturation, and hypertrophy: ion-channel dependent transduction of matrix deformation signals. *Exp. Cell Res.* **256**, 383–391.

28. Cotten, M., Baker, A., Saltik, M., Wagner, E., and Buschle, M. (1994) Lipopolysaccharide is a frequent contaminant of plasmid DNA preparations and can be toxic to primary human cells in the presence of adenovirus. *Gene Ther.* **1**, 239–246.

29. Mengshol, J. A., Vincenti, M. P., and Brinckerhoff, C. E. (2001) IL-1 induces collagenase-3 (MMP-13) promoter activity in stably transfected chondrocytic cells: requirement for Runx-2 and activation by p38 MAPK and JNK pathways. *Nucleic Acids Res.* **29**, 4361–4372.

5

Generation of Pluripotent Stem Cells and Their Differentiation to the Chondrocytic Phenotype

Luis A. Solchaga, Jean F. Welter,
Donald P. Lennon, and Arnold I. Caplan

Summary

It is well documented that adult cartilage has minimal self-repair ability. Current methods for treatment of cartilage injury focus on the relief of pain and inflammation and have met with limited long-term success. In the forefront of new therapeutic approaches, autologous chondrocyte transplantation is still only applied to a very small percentage of the patient population.

Our laboratory has focused on cartilage repair using progenitor cells and studied their differentiation into cartilage. Adult mesenchymal stem cells are an attractive candidate as progenitor cells for cartilage repair because of their documented osteogenic and chondrogenic potential, ease of harvest, and ease of expansion in culture; furthermore, their use will obviate the need for harvesting precious healthy cartilage from a patient to obtain autologous chondrocytes for transplantation. However, the need to induce chondrogenic differentiation in the mesenchymal stem cells is superposed on other technical issues associated with cartilage repair; this adds a level of complexity over using mature chondrocytes.

This chapter focuses on the methods involved in the isolation of human mesenchymal stem cells and their differentiation along the chondrogenic lineage. Although we have the technology to accomplish chondrogenic differentiation of stem cells, much is still to be learned regarding the regulatory mechanisms controlling the lineage transitions and maturation of the cartilaginous tissue.

Key Words: Mesenchymal stem cell; chondrogenesis; differentiation; tissue culture; transforming growth factor-β; cartilage; chondrocyte; aggregate culture.

1. Introduction

Tissue Engineering has recently emerged as a discipline that combines the fields of cell biology, engineering, material sciences, and surgery to provide new functional tissues using living cells, biomatrices, and signaling molecules

From: *Methods in Molecular Medicine, Vol. 100: Cartilage and Osteoarthritis, Vol. 1: Cellular and Molecular Tools*
Edited by: M. Sabatini, P. Pastoureau, and F. De Ceuninck © Humana Press Inc., Totowa, NJ

(1–3). In the past decade, this relatively new discipline has greatly expanded, with numerous research groups focused on the development of strategies for the repair and regeneration of a variety of tissues *(4,5)*.

Many of these tissue-engineered approaches have targeted the musculoskeletal system in general, with special emphasis on articular cartilage *(6–14)*. Articular cartilage is especially attractive as a target for tissue engineering strategies because it has been well documented that injuries of the articular cartilage, an avascular tissue without direct access to a significant source of reparative cells, do not heal spontaneously *(15–20)*. The vast majority of approaches to the repair or regeneration of articular cartilage are cell-based, aiming to provide a population of reparative cells to the injured site. Cells used to develop these strategies can be either differentiated chondrocytes, isolated from unaffected areas of the joint surface *(12,21–32)*, or progenitor cells, capable of differentiating into chondrocytes, which can be isolated from a variety of tissues *(33–46)*. Harvesting a tissue biopsy from valuable healthy articular cartilage that cannot repair itself does not seem to be a good choice; therefore a number of research efforts are directed to the isolation of progenitor cells and the understanding of the mechanisms involved in their chondrogenic differentiation.

The isolation and mitotic expansion of adult human bone marrow-derived mesenchymal stem cells *(47–50)*, and the specific culture conditions developed for their chondrogenic differentiation *(51–54)* are described in this chapter.

2. Materials

1. Scalpel blade (Fisher).
2. 20-, 10-, and 5-mL Syringes (Becton Dickinson).
3. Lidocaine (Henry Schein).
4. 11-Gage Jamshidi needle (Henry Schein).
5. Sterile gauze (Henry Schein).
6. Heparin (400 U/mL; Henry Schein).
7. Tissue culture vessels:

    a. 15- and 50-mL Centrifuge tubes (Falcon).
    b. 50-mL Polycarbonate capped centrifuge tubes (Fisher).
    c. 15-mL Polypropylene centrifuge tubes (Falcon).
    d. Pipets and tissue culture dishes and flasks (Falcon).

8. Tissue culture media:

    a. Dulbecco's modified Eagle's medium, low glucose (1.5 g/L; DMEM-LG; Sigma).
    b. DMEM, high glucose (4.5 g/L; DMEM-HG; Sigma).

9. Culture media supplements:

    a. Fetal bovine serum (FBS; best available).
    b. Bovine calf serum (BCS) (Hyclone).

   c. ITS+ Premix Tissue Culture Supplement (Becton Dickinson).
   d. Stock solution of 10^{-5} M dexamethasone in DMEM-HG (100X). Dexamethasone (Sigma) is dissolved at 10^{-3} M in absolute ethanol and diluted 1:100 with DMEM-HG to the 10^{-5} M stock solution.
   e. Stock solution of 100 μM ascorbate-2-phosphate (Wako USA) in H_2O (100X).
   f. MEM sodium pyruvate (100X; Gibco).
   g. Stock solution of 1 $\mu g/mL$ transforming growth factor-β1 (TGF-β1; R&D systems) in 4 mM hydrochloric acid (HCl) and 1% bovine serum albumin (100X).

10. 4% Acetic acid (Fisher) in H_2O.
11. 70% Ethanol in H_2O.
12. 15% Sodium hypochlorite (bleach) in H_2O.
13. Tyrode's salt solution (Sigma).
14. 0.25% Trypsin 53 mM ethylenediamine tetraacetic acid (EDTA) (Gibco-BRL).
15. Percoll gradient: 22.05 mL Percoll (Sigma), 2.45 mL 1.5 M NaCl, 10.5 mL Tyrode's salt solution.

   a. Prepare the Percoll solution in any convenient multiples of these volumes and mix thoroughly.
   b. Add 35 mL of Percoll solution per 50-mL polycarbonate capped sterile centrifuge tubes.
   c. Spin at 21,200g for 15 min in an SS-34 fixed-angle rotor using a Sorvall centrifuge. The resulting density gradient equals 1.03–1.12 g/L.
   d. Percoll can be stored for short periods at 4°C.

16. Benchtop centrifuge.
17. Class II biological safety cabinet.

3. Methods

3.1. Bone Marrow Aspiration

In our Institution, bone marrow is harvested from the posterior superior iliac crest by physicians of the Department of Hematology-Oncology at University Hospitals of Cleveland, affiliated with Case Western Reserve University. The bone marrow sample arrives at our laboratory in a 20-mL syringe and is processed as described in the following steps. The details of the bone marrow aspiration were provided by Dr. Omer Koc of the Department of Hematology-Oncology and are presented here for the reader's information. Research protocols involving human bone marrow must be approved by the Institutional Review Board of the hospital, and donors must give informed consent.

1. Marrow donors who have given informed consent lie in a lateral decubitus position.
2. Locate the posterior superior iliac crest.
3. Wipe the donor's skin over the superior iliac crest with Betadine.
4. Anesthetize with lidocaine (1%) the skin and subcutaneous tissue superficial to the iliac crest.

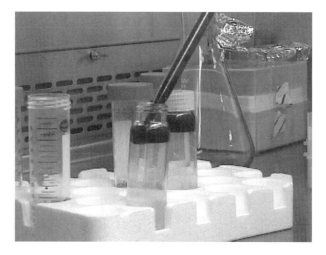

Fig. 3. Bone marrow sample being layered over the preformed Percoll gradient.

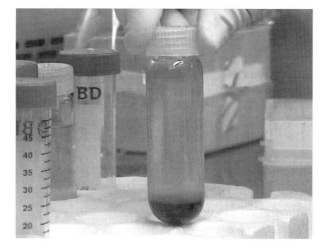

Fig. 4. Sample after gradient fractionation; note the red blood cells at the bottom of the tube and a band of nucleated cells at the top of the gradient.

9. Return the sample (**Fig. 4**) to the biological safety cabinet, carefully pipet off the top layer or layers of cells (about 10–14 mL); (**Fig. 5**), and transfer this volume to another sterile 50-mL centrifuge tube (*see* **Note 2**).
10. Add serum-containing medium to a volume of 50 mL.
11. Spin in a benchtop centrifuge at 500*g* for 5 min.
12. Remove and discard supernatant and resuspend the cell pellet in 10 mL of complete medium.

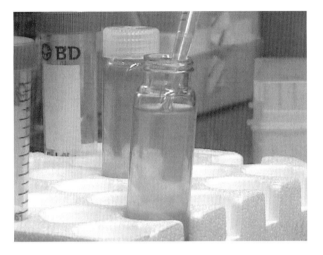

Fig. 5. Recovery of cells from the top fraction of the gradient.

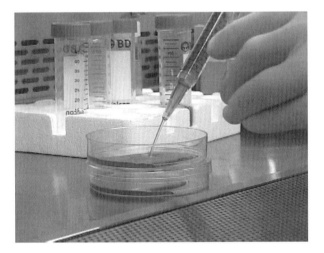

Fig. 6. Inoculation of tissue culture dishes with the cell suspension.

13. Use a 1-mL pipet to take a small sample (about 100 µL) for determination of cell number as described in **step 4**.
14. Plate cells at 1.7×10^6 per cm^2 in tissue culture dishes or flasks in complete medium (*see* **Note 3** and **Fig. 6**).

3.3. Mesenchymal Stem Cell Culture

MSCs are cultured at 37°C in a humidified atmosphere of 95% air and 5% CO_2. Only a small percentage of the cells in the original cell suspension attach

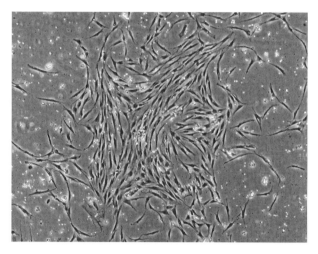

Fig. 7. Microscopic appearance of a colony in a primary culture of MSCs. Original magnification ×4.

to the tissue culture surface. These fibroblast-like cells proliferate and form loose colonies of spindle-shaped cells that are usually visible under the microscope between d 4 and 6 of culture. These colonies increase in size over the next 7–10 d, and should be subcultured before the cells become confluent. (It is important to note that proliferation of these cells is not contact-inhibited.) No efforts are made to remove nonadherent cells. Medium is pipeted or aspirated from the dish without vigorous swirling or rinsing; it is hypothesized that these cells provide cytokines and other factors needed for the growth of the attached cells. Change the medium twice a week.

1. Aspirate spent medium from plates.
2. Add fresh complete medium.

3.4. Mesenchymal Stem Cell Subculture

MSCs must be subcultured before they reach confluence. In primary cultures, the main consideration to determine when the cells should be subcultured is cell density within single colonies rather than the overall level of confluence of the plate, which in the case of primary culture may be low, depending on the colony-forming efficiency of the population. Typically, MSCs are passaged when colonies are 80–90% confluent (**Fig. 7**).

Primary cultures are usually subcultured around d 14 of culture (± 3 d).

1. Aspirate expired medium from plates.
2. Rinse the cell layer with the appropriate volume (5 mL for a 56-cm² tissue culture dish) of Tyrode's salt solution to wash cells.

3. Repeat rinse.
4. Add the appropriate volume of trypsin-EDTA (4 mL for a 56-cm^2 tissue culture dish).
5. Return to the incubator for 5–7 min. Keep the time of exposure as brief as possible.
6. When most of the cells have become well rounded or have detached from the tissue culture surface, stop the reaction by adding bovine calf serum (BCS) equal to half the volume of trypsin-EDTA.
7. Draw up the cell suspension with a pipet and, with the same pipet, use the suspension to wash the remaining cells gently from the dish. It is not necessary (or desirable) to remove all the cells from the dish, as most of the nonfibroblastoid cells (which are not likely to be MSCs) in these cultures are more trypsin-resistant than the spindle-shaped fibroblast-like cells. Thus, trypsinization represents, after attachment of fibroblastic cells to plastic, the second component of the process of selection of MSCs from the total marrow cell population.
8. Transfer the cell suspension from all the cultures to an appropriate size centrifuge tube or tubes.
9. Spin in benchtop centrifuge at 500*g* for 5 min.
10. Resuspend pellet in 5–10 mL of complete medium.
11. Determine cell number with a hemocytometer.
12. Plate cells at $3.5–4.0 \times 10^3$ per cm^2.

Further subculturing is conducted according to the above protocol except for the following considerations:

1. Subcultured hMSCs are evenly distributed on the tissue culture vessel surface (**Fig. 8**) and are not in colonies as for primary cultures. Therefore, the degree of confluence determines when the cells should be trypsinized; as a general rule, hMSCs should be trypsinized before they become confluent.
2. Passaged hMSCs are more easily trypsinized than are primary cultures, so exposure of these cells to trypsin is usually limited to 5 min.

MSCs have a high proliferative capacity and may be subcultured multiple times. During the process of cell expansion, MSCs maintained in complete medium remain in an undifferentiated state *(56)*.

Subcultured MSCs remain spindle-shaped fibroblastic cells, distributed evenly over the culture dish. They are also slightly larger than primary cells, a feature that becomes more pronounced with additional subcultivation.

3.5. Chondrogenic Induction

Bone marrow-derived MSCs can be induced to differentiate into chondrocytes under specific culture conditions. These conditions include 3D conformation of the cells in aggregates in which high cell density and cell–cell interaction play an important role in the mechanism of chondrogenesis. Together with these physical culture conditions, a defined culture medium is required to achieve chondrogenic differentiation *(51,52,57)*.

forming efficiency, and proliferation rate of the cells grown under the different conditions are recorded through primary, first, and second passage cultures. At the end of the second passage, once the sufficient cell number has been obtained, the cells are assayed for their multipotentiality both in vitro (osteogenesis, chondrogenesis, and adipogenesis) and in vivo (osteogenesis and chondrogenesis) *(58)*.

The selection of a particular serum lot is based on the results of this battery of different assays and is, therefore, complicated. Detailed protocols for these assays and for the measurement of the outcome parameters that define the mulipotentiality of MSCs can be found in the chapter "Mesenchymal stem cells" by Lennon and Caplan in the book *Culture of Cells for Tissue Engineering* edited by Freshney and Vunjak currently in preparation.

4. Once the cells are introduced into chondrogenic conditions, it is very important to ensure that the caps of the tubes are loose, so that the air in the tubes can equilibrate with the 5% CO_2, humidified air of the incubator. If the caps are too tight there will be no air exchange, and the cells will probably die owing to lack of oxygen and/or reduced pH.

References

1. Langer, R. and Vacanti, J. P. (1993) Tissue engineering. *Science* **260,** 920–926.
2. Vacanti, C. A. and Vacanti, J. P. (2000) The science of tissue engineering. *Orthop. Clin. North Am.* **31,** 351–356.
3. Vacanti, J. and Langer, R. (1999) Tissue engineering: the design and fabrication of living replacement devices for surgical re-construction and transplantation. *Lancet* **354(Suppl. 1),** SI32–SI34.
4. Bonassar, L. J. and Vacanti, C. A. (1998) Tissue engineering: the first decade and beyond. *J. Cell Biochem. Suppl.* **30–31,** 297–303.
5. Pearson, R. G., Bhandari, R., Quirk, R. A., and Shakesheff, K. M. (2002) Recent advances in tissue engineering: an invited review. *J. Long Term Eff. Med. Implants* **12,** 1–33.
6. Temenoff, J. S. and Mikos, A. G. (2000) Review: tissue engineering for regeneration of articular cartilage. *Biomaterials* **21,** 431–440.
7. O'Driscoll, S. W. (2001) Preclinical cartilage repair: current status and future perspectives. *Clin. Orthop.* **391(Suppl.),** S397–S401.
8. Luyten, F. P., Dell'Accio, F., and De Bari, C. (2001) Skeletal tissue engineering: opportunities and challenges. *Best Pract. Res. Clin. Rheumatol.* **15,** 759–769.
9. Musgrave, D. S., Fu, F. H., and Huard, J. (2002) Gene therapy and tissue engineering in orthopaedic surgery. *J. Am. Acad. Orthop. Surg.* **10,** 6–15.
10. Risbud, M. (2001) Tissue engineering: implications in the treatment of organ and tissue defects. *Biogerontology* **2,** 117–125.
11. Guilak, F., Butler, D. L., and Goldstein, S. A. (2001) Functional tissue engineering: the role of biomechanics in articular cartilage repair. *Clin. Orthop.* **391(Suppl.),** S295–S305.
12. Risbud, M. V. and Sittinger, M. (2002) Tissue engineering: advances in in vitro cartilage generation. *Trends Biotechnol.* **20,** 351–356.

13. Caplan, A. I. and Goldberg, V. M. (1999) Principles of tissue engineered regeneration of skeletal tissues. *Clin. Orthop.* **367(Suppl.),** S12–S16.
14. Caplan, A. I., Elyaderani, M., Mochizuki, Y., Wakitani, S., and Goldberg, V. M. (1997) Principles of cartilage repair and regeneration. *Clin. Orthop. Rel. Res.* **342,** 254–269.
15. Buckwalter, J. (1998) Articular cartilage: injuries and potential for healing. *J. Orthop. Sports Phys. Ther.* **28,** 192–202.
16. Buckwalter, J. and Mankin, H. (1998) Articular cartilage repair and transplantation. *Arthritis Rheum.* **41,** 1331–1342.
17. Buckwalter, J. A. and Mankin, H. J. (1998) Articular cartilage: degeneration and osteoarthritis, repair, regeneration, and transplantation. *Instr. Course Lect.* **47,** 487–504.
18. Mankin, H. J. (1974) The reaction of articular cartilage to injury and osteoarthritis (first of two parts) *N. Engl. J. Med.* **291,** 1285–1292.
19. Mankin, H. J. (1974) The reaction of articular cartilage to injury and osteoarthritis (second of two parts) *N. Engl. J. Med.* **291,** 1335–1340.
20. Mankin, H. J. and Buckwalter, J. A. (1996) Restoration of the osteoarthrotic joint [editorial]. *J. Bone Joint Surg. Am.* **78,** 1–2.
21. Chesterman, P. J. and Smith, A. U. (1968) Homotransplantation of articular cartilage and isolated chondrocytes. An experimental study in rabbits. *J. Bone Joint Surg. Br.* **50,** 184–197.
22. Bentley, G. and Greer, R. B. d. (1971) Homotransplantation of isolated epiphyseal and articular cartilage chondrocytes into joint surfaces of rabbits. Nature 230, 385–388.
23. Wakitani, S., Kimura, T., Hirooka, A., et al. (1989) Repair of rabbit articular surfaces with allograft chondrocytes embedded in collagen gel. *J. Bone Joint Surg. Br.* **71,** 74–80.
24. Vacanti, C. A., Kim, W., Schloo, B., Upton, J., and Vacanti, J. P. (1994) Joint resurfacing with cartilage grown in situ from cell-polymer structures. *Am. J. Sports Med.* **22,** 485–488.
25. Freed, L. E., Grande, D. A., Lingbin, Z., Emmanual, J., Marquis, J. C., and Langer, R. (1994) Joint resurfacing using allograft chondrocytes and synthetic biodegradable polymer scaffolds. *J. Biomed. Mater. Res.* **28,** 891–899.
26. Frenkel, S. R., Toolan, B., Menche, D., Pitman, M. I., and Pachence, J. M. (1997) Chondrocyte transplantation using a collagen bilayer matrix for cartilage repair. *J. Bone Joint Surg. Br.* **79,** 831–836.
27. Nehrer, S., Breinan, H. A., Ramappa, A., et al. (1997) Canine chondrocytes seeded in type I and type II collagen implants investigated in vitro. [erratum appears in (1997) *J. Biomed. Mater. Res.* **38(4),** 288]. *J. Biomed. Mater. Res.* **38,** 95–104.
28. Breinan, H. A., Minas, T., Hsu, H. P., Nehrer, S., Sledge, C. B., and Spector, M. (1997) Effect of cultured autologous chondrocytes on repair of chondral defects in a canine model. *J. Bone Joint Surg. Am.* **79,** 1439–1451.
29. Minas, T. (1998) Chondrocyte implantation in the repair of chondral lesions of the knee: economics and quality of life. *Am. J. Orthop.* **27,** 739–744.

30. Giannini, S., Buda, R., Grigolo, B., and Vannini, F. (2001) Autologous chondrocyte transplantation in osteochondral lesions of the ankle joint. *Foot Ankle Int.* **2,** 513–517.

31. Breinan, H. A., Minas, T., Hsu, H. P., Nehrer, S., Shortkroff, S., and Spector, M. (2001) Autologous chondrocyte implantation in a canine model: change in composition of reparative tissue with time. *J. Orthop. Res.* **19,** 482–492.

32. Brittberg, M., Lindahl, A., Nilsson, A., Ohlsson, C., Isaksson, O., and Peterson, L. (1994) Treatment of deep cartilage defects in the knee with autologous chondrocyte transplantation. *N. Engl. J. Med.* **331,** 889–895.

33. Amiel, D., Coutts, R. D., Abel, M., Stewart, W., Harwood, F., and Akeson, W. H. (1985) Rib perichondrial grafts for the repair of full-thickness articular-cartilage defects. A morphological and biochemical study in rabbits. *J. Bone Joint Surg. Am.* **67,** 911–920.

34. O'Driscoll, S. W., Keeley, F. W., and Salter, R. B. (1986) The chondrogenic potential of free autogenous periosteal grafts for biological resurfacing of major full-thickness defects in joint surfaces under the influence of continuous passive motion. An experimental investigation in the rabbit. *J. Bone Joint Surg. Am.* **68,** 1017–1035.

35. Amiel, D., Coutts, R. D., Harwood, F. L., Ishizue, K. K., and Kleiner, J. B. (1988) The chondrogenesis of rib perichondrial grafts for repair of full thickness articular cartilage defects in a rabbit model: a one year postoperative assessment. *Connect. Tissue Res.* **18,** 27–39.

36. Shahgaldi, B. F., Amis, A. A., Heatley, F. W., McDowell, J., and Bentley, G. (1991) Repair of cartilage lesions using biological implants. A comparative histological and biomechanical study in goats. *J. Bone Joint Surg. Br.* **73,** 57–64.

37. Wakitani, S., Goto, T., Pineda, S. J., et al. (1994) Mesenchymal cell-based repair of large, full-thickness defects of articular cartilage. *J. Bone Joint Surg. Am.* **76,** 579–592.

38. Wakitani, S., Goto, T., Pined, S. J., et al. (1994) Mesenchymal cell-based repair of large, full-thickness defects of articular cartilage. *J. Bone Joint Surg. Am.* **76,** 579–592.

39. Chu, C. R., Coutts, R. D., Yoshioka, M., Harwood, F. L., Monosov, A. Z., and Amiel, D. (1995) Articular cartilage repair using allogeneic perichondrocyte-seeded biodegradable porous polylactic acid (PLA): a tissue-engineering study. *J. Biomed. Mater. Res.* **29,** 1147–1154.

40. Butnariu-Ephrat, M., Robinson, D., Mendes, D. G., Halperin, N., and Nevo, Z. (1996) Resurfacing of goat articular cartilage by chondrocytes derived from bone marrow. *Clin. Orthop.* **330,** 234–243.

41. Hunziker, E. B. and Rosenberg, L. C. (1996) Repair of partial-thickness defects in articular cartilage: cell recruitment from the synovial membrane. *J. Bone Joint Surg. Am.* **78,** 721–733.

42. Chu, C. R., Dounchis, J. S., Yoshioka, M., Sah, R. L., Coutts, R. D., and Amiel, D. (1997) Osteochondral repair using perichondrial cells. A 1-year study in rabbits. *Clin. Orthop.* **340,** 220–229.

43. Goldberg, V. M., Solchaga, L. A., Lundberg, M., et al. (1999) Mesenchymal stem cell repair of osteochondral defects of articular cartilage. *Semin. Arthroplasty* **10,** 30–36.
44. Johnstone, B. and Yoo, J. U. (1999) Autologous mesenchymal progenitor cells in articular cartilage repair. *Clin. Orthop.* **367(Suppl.),** S156–S162.
45. Dounchis, J. S., Bae, W. C., Chen, A. C., Sah, R. L., Coutts, R. D., and Amiel, D. (2000) Cartilage repair with autogenic perichondrium cell and polylactic acid grafts. *Clin. Orthop.* **377,** 248–264.
46. Solchaga, L. A., Gao, J., Dennis, J. E., et al. (2002) Treatment of osteochondral defects with autologous bone marrow in a hyaluronan-based delivery vehicle. *Tissue Eng.* **8,** 333–347..
47. Friedenstein, A. J. (1976) Precursor cells of mechanocytes. *Int. Rev. Cytol.* **47,** 327–359.
48. Caplan, A. I. (1991) Mesenchymal stem cells. *J. Orthop. Res.* **9,** 641–650.
49. Haynesworth, S. E., Goshima, J., Goldberg, V. M., and Caplan, A. I. (1992) Characterization of cells with osteogenic potential from human bone marrow. *Bone* **13,** 81–88.
50. Ashton, B. A., Allen, T. D., Howlett, C. R., Eaglesom, C. C., Hattori, A., and Owen, M. (1980) Formation of bone and cartilage by marrow stromal cells in diffusion chambers in vivo. *Clin. Orthop.* **151,** 294–307.
51. Johnstone, B., Hering, T. M., Caplan, A. I., Goldberg, V. M., and Yoo, J. U. (1998) In vitro chondrogenesis of bone marrow-derived mesenchymal progenitor cells. *Exp. Cell Res.* **238,** 265–272.
52. Yoo, J. U., Barthel, T. S., Nishimura, K., et al. (1998) The chondrogenic potential of human bone-marrow-derived mesenchymal progenitor cells. *J. Bone Joint Surg. Am.* **80,** 1745–1757.
53. Angele, P., Yoo, J. U. Smith, C., et al. (2000) Cyclic hydrostatic pressure enhances the chondrogenic phenotype of human mesenchymal progenitor cells differentiated in vitro. *J. Orthop. Res.* **21,** 451–457.
54. Hanada, K., Solchaga, L. A., Caplan, A. I., et al. (2001) BMP-2 induction and TGF-β1 modulation of rat periosteal cell chondrogenesis. *J. Cell Biochem.* **81,** 284–294.
55. Lennon, D. P., Haynesworth, S. E., Bruder, S. P., Jaiswal, N., and Caplan, A. I. (1996) Human and animal mesenchymal progenitor cells from bone marrow: identification of serum for optimal selection and proliferation. *In Vitro Cell. Dev. Biol.* **32,** 602–611.
56. Jaiswal, N., Haynesworth, S. E., Caplan, A. I., and Bruder, S. P. (1997) Osteogenic differentiation of purified culture-expanded human mesenchymal stem cells in vitro. *J. Cell. Biochem.* **64,** 295–312.
57. Ballock, R. T. and Reddi, A. H. (1994) Thyroxine is the serum factor that regulates morphogenesis of columnar cartilage from isolated chondrocytes in chemically defined medium. *J. Cell Biol.* **126,** 1311–1318.
58. Pittenger, M. F., Mackay, A. M., Beck, S. C., et al. (1999) Multilineage potential of adult human mesenchymal stem cells. *Science* **284,** 143–147.

6

Semiquantitative Analysis of Gene Expression in Cultured Chondrocytes by RT-PCR

Gaëlle Rolland-Valognes

Summary

Reverse transcriptase-polymerase chain reaction (RT-PCR) is a powerful, sensitive, and rapid method to monitor small amounts of nucleic acids. This is of particular interest for small amounts of cells, as in cartilage. We present here two protocols to isolate total RNA and a protocol to study matrix metalloproteinase and type II collagen gene expression from chondrocytes of human origin. Specific gene expression is revealed on an ethidium bromide-containing agarose gel on an ultraviolet plate and normalized to that of a housekeeping gene.

Key Words: RT-PCR; gene; chondrocytes; cartilage; MMP.

1. Introduction

Cartilage is composed of specific cells (chondrocytes) embedded in an extra-cellular matrix primarily composed of collagen (mainly type II), proteoglycans, and water. In osteoarthritis, this matrix is degraded mainly by enzymes that are secreted by the chondrocytes themselves, such as the matrix metalloproteinases (MMPs), regulated at both protein and gene levels.

Because of the relatively small number of cells in cartilage, it is useful to employ powerful methods to study chondrocyte gene expression. Reverse transcriptase-polymerase chain reaction (RT-PCR) is a powerful, sensitive, and rapid method to monitor the expression of specific mRNAs.

We first discuss total RNA extraction from human chondrocytes. The expression of stromelysin-1 (MMP-3), collagenase-3 (MMP-13), and type II collagen is then used to illustrate the study of gene expression by RT-PCR in human chondrocytes. Total RNA extracted from tissues or cultured cells is first transcribed in DNA that is called complementary (cDNA). Amplification of cDNA

From: *Methods in Molecular Medicine, Vol. 100: Cartilage and Osteoarthritis, Vol. 1: Cellular and Molecular Tools*
Edited by: M. Sabatini, P. Pastoureau, and F. De Ceuninck © Humana Press Inc., Totowa, NJ

copies of the target mRNA is carried out in a controlled manner, so that the products of the PCR reaction remain proportional to the amount of mRNA target in the cell (before the product reaches the plateau). Once deposited on an agarose gel, relative amounts of mRNAs can be studied by densitometric analysis.

2. Materials

2.1. Equipment

1. Centrifuge for 1.5- and 2-mL Eppendorf tubes (Eppendorf 5417R).
2. Mini-Gel Electrophoresis unit (MUPID-2 for DNA, RNA & Proteins, Eurogentec).
3. 0.5-, 1.5- and 2-mL Eppendorf tubes.
4. Filter-tips, presterilized and nucleic acid- and nuclease-free (ART-10, -20, -200 and 1000, Molecular BioProducts).
5. Pipets (Eppendorf P2, P10, P20, P200, and P1000).
6. Spectrophotometer (GeneQuant II, RNA/DNA Calculator, Pharmacia Biotech).
7. Thermocycler GeneAmp PCR System 2400/2700 (Applied Biosystem).

2.2. Cells

1. Human humerus chondrosarcoma cells (SW1353, ATCC HTB-94; Biovalley).
2. Chondrocytes of human origin. For isolation and culture procedures, *see* Chapters 1, 2, and 14.

2.3. Total RNA Isolation

2.3.1. TRIzol® Method

1. Chloroform (Sigma Aldrich).
2. Isopropyl alcohol (Sigma Aldrich).
3. Diethyl pyrocarbonate-treated water (DEPC-water; 0.1% [v/v] DEPC; Sigma Aldrich) (*see* **Note 1**).
4. 75% Ethanol (in DEPC water).
5. TRIzol reagent (Invitrogen).

2.3.2. RNeasy Mini Kit Method

1. QIAshredder™ spin column (Qiagen).
2. RNeasy® Mini Kit, containing RNeasy Mini spin columns; collections tubes (1.5 and 2 mL); buffers RLT, RW1, and RPE; RNase-free water; and handbook (Qiagen).

2.3.3. RNA Gels

1. Agarose (Electrophoresis grade, Invitrogen).
2. 3-(N-morpholino)propanesulfonic acid 10× (MOPS; Sigma Aldrich).
3. Formaldehyde, 37% (Sigma Aldrich).
4. RNA sample loading buffer (Sigma Aldrich).

2.4. Reverse Transcription

1. 25 U Oligo-(dT)$_{12-18}$ (Amersham Biotech).
2. 5000 U RNAGuard (Amersham Biotech).
3. 4×25 μmol dNTPs (Eurogentech).
4. Superscript™ II Rnase H⁻ Reverse Transcriptase Kit (200 U/mL), containing 0.1 M dithiothreitol (DTT) and 5X First Strand Buffer (Invitrogen).

2.5. Polymerase Chain Reaction

1. 4×25 μmol dNTPs (Eurogentech).
2. 20 μM Primer 3' (Eurogentech).
3. 20 μM Primer 5' (Eurogentech).
4. HotStarTaq DNA polymerase Kit (5 U/mL) containing 10X buffer (Qiagen).
5. Distilled ultrapure H_2O.

2.6. Primer Sequences

Gene-specific primers were choosen from corresponding sequences, as shown in **Table 1**. Sequence determinations were performed by dideoxy-chain termination using an automated fluorescent dye ABI 377 DNA sequencer (Applied Biosystems, France).

2.7. DNA Gels

1. 10 mg/mL Ethidium bromide (Sigma Aldrich).
2. 10X Blue Juice Gel Loading Buffer (Invitrogen).
3. Electrophoresis grade agarose (Invitrogen).
4. 10X Tris-borate EDTA (TBE) electrophoresis buffer (Invitrogen).

3. Methods

The method given here describes extraction and quantification of total RNA from cells, reverse transcription (RT), polymerase chain reaction (PCR), and PCR products analysis.

3.1. Extraction and Quantification of Total RNA

When handling RNA, several important precautions must be taken (*see* **Notes 2–5**), as RNA is subject to degradation by intracellular RNases, until it is flash frozen or homogenized in a lysis buffer.

3.1.1. Extraction Using the RNeasy Mini Kit

A new, rapid, and convenient way of isolating total RNA from cells or tissue is to use the Qiagen RNeasy Mini Kit, which permits total RNA isolation by binding to silica gel-based membranes.

Table 1
Sequence, Reference, PCR Product Size, and Cycle Number of Primers Used

Gene	Sequence	Position	Size (bp)	Cycles	Accession No.	Ref.
MMP-3	5'-TCA-CTC-ACT-CAC-AGA-CCT-GAC-TCG-3' 5'-CCT-TAT-CAG-AAA-TGG-CTG-CAT-CG-3'	763–786 1207–1229	467	25–30	X05232	2
MMP-13	5'-GGA-ATT-AAG-GAG-CAT-GGC-GAC-3' 5'-TAT-GCA-GCA-TCA-ATA-CGG-TTG-G-3'	506–526 996–1017	512	30–35	X75308	3
Pro (α1) II Collagen	5'-AGA-TGG-CTG-GAG-GAT-TTG-AT-3' 5'-CTT-GGA-TAA-CCT-CTG-TGA-CCT-3'	702–721 1018–1038	336	35–40	NM_001844	4
β2M	5'-CTC-GCG-CTA-CTC-TCT-CTT-TCT-GG-3' 5'-GCT-TAC-ATG-TCT-CGA-TCC-CAC-TTA-A-3'	1–24 525–550	335	20–25	V00567 J00105	5

β2M, β2-microglobulin; MMP, matrix metalloproteinase.

72

Before starting:
1. Add 10 µL β-mercaptoethanol per mL of buffer RLT.
2. Add 4 volumes of 96–100% ethanol to buffer RPE.

Then
1. Aspirate the culture medium.
2. Lyse cells directly by adding 350 µL (vessel diameter <6 cm) or 600 µL (usual diameter between 6 and 10 cm) to the cell culture vessel.
3. Pipet the lysate directly onto a QIAshredder Spin column placed in a 2-mL collection tube.
4. Centrifuge for 3 min at maximum speed (20,000*g*).
5. Add 600 µL of 70° ethanol to the lysate, and homogenize by pipeting.
6. Apply 700 µL of the sample to an RNeasy column.
7. Centrifuge for 15 s at 8000*g*.
8. Discard the flowthrough material.
9. If the sample exceeds 700 µL, go back to **step 6**, and centrifuge as above. Discard the flowthrough material each time.
10. Add 700 µL of buffer RW1 onto the RNeasy column.
11. Centrifuge for 15 s at 8000*g*.
12. Transfer the column to a new 2-mL collection tube.
13. Add 500 µL of buffer RPE to the column.
14. Centrifuge for 15 s at 8000*g*, to wash the column.
15. Discard the flowthrough material.
16. Add 500 µL of buffer RPE onto the column.
17. Centrifuge for 2 min at maximum speed (20,000*g*), to dry the column.
18. Transfer the RNeasy column into a 1.5 mL sterile Eppendorf tube.
19. Pipet 25 µL of Rnase-free water directly onto the membrane.
20. Centrifuge for 1 min at 8000*g*, to eluate the RNA.

3.1.2. Extraction Using TRIzol®

Alternatively, you can use the protocol derived from Chomczinsky and Sacchi *(1) (see* **Note 6**).
1. Lyse cells directly by adding 1 mL of TRIzol reagent per 10 cm² culture plate.
2. Incubate the homogenate for 5 min at room temperature (to permit the complete dissociation of nucleoprotein complexes).
3. Add 0.2 mL of chloroform per tube.
4. Shake tubes vigorously by hand for 15 min.
5. Incubate them for 2–3 min at room temperature.
6. Centrifuge at 12,000*g* for 15 min at 4°C.
7. RNA is located in the upper-aqueous phase, wich represents about 60% of the volume of the TRIzol reagent used for homogeneization.
8. Transfer the aqueous phase into a new tube, and precipitate the RNA by mixing with 0.5 mL of isopropyl alcohol.
9. Incubate the tubes at room temperature for 10 min.

Table 4
Preparation of PCR Mix

	Concentration		
RT Mix Components	Initial	Final	For 1 tube (µL)
Ultrapure-H$_2$O			39.75
Buffer	10×	1×	5
dNTPs	10 mM	200 µM	1
Primer 3'	20 µM	0.4 µM	1
Primer 5'	20 µM	0.4 µM	1
HotStart Taq			
DNA Polymerase	5 U/µL	1.25 U	0.25
		Total volume	48
cDNA	≤1 µg		2
		Final volume	50

1. Add 2 µL of RT reaction mix in a PCR tube.
2. Prepare PCR mix, as indicated in **Table 4**. (Prepare the mix for an extra; *see* **Note 9**.)
3. Add 48 µL of mix to each tube, and mix smoothly by pipeting. The final volume is 50 µL.
4. Place the tubes into a thermocycler, and start the Hot Start PCR program: 15 min at 94°C and then 30 at 94°C, 30 s at annealing temperature, and 1 min at 72°C. Repeat for 20–35 cycles (*see* **Table 1**). Then perform the final elongation for 10 min at 72°C. To be sure to be in the linear range, it is useful to prepare several identical PCR reactions and remove them from the thermocycler at different numbers of cycles. Alternatively, you can remove an aliquot of the PCR reaction, by stopping the thermocycler and restarting it (*see* **Note 10**).
5. Store PCR products at 4°C or –20°C (for long-term conservation) (*see* **Note 11**).

3.5. PCR Product Analysis

Prepare a 1% agarose gel.

1. Mix 1 g of agarose with 100 mL of 0.5X TBE.
2. Heat in a microwave oven until the agarose is completely dissolved (5–10 min).
3. Let cool down for 2–3 min.
4. Add 1 µL of BET and mix.
5. Pour the liquid in the electrophoresis plate.
6. Allow 30–45 min for the gel to polymerize.
7. Take off the comb.

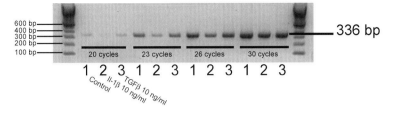

Fig. 2. Amplification of α1 type II collagen. One microgram of total RNA isolated from human chondrocytes has been reverse transcribed and amplified. Lanes 1, non-treated cells (control); lanes 2, cells treated with interleukin-1β (IL-1β) at 10 ng/mL; lanes 3, cells treated with transforming growth factor-β (TGF-β) at 10 ng/mL. Ten microliters of the reaction was taken out of each tube at cycles 20, 23, 26, and 30, and deposited on a 1% gel.

Prepare the samples.

1. Place 10 μL of the PCR reaction in a new tube.
2. Add 3 μL of loading buffer.
3. Mix gently by pipeting.
4. Load 1 μg of molecular weight (mol wt) marker in the first well (1 μL of mol wt marker + 9 μL TE + 3 μL loading buffer).
5. Load 13 μL of each sample in each well.
6. Allow to migrate for 30 min at 100 V.
7. Once migration is over, put the gel on a UV plate.
8. Photograph the gel.

The number of cycles used for amplification must be within the linear range for both the housekeeping gene and the gene of interest (**Fig. 2**). A plot of band intensity vs cycle number should be linear for both. The intensity of the band can then be quantified by Image Analysis Software and normalized to that of the housekeeping gene.

4. Notes

1. DEPC is a strong but not absolute ribonuclease (RNase) inhibitor that inactivates RNases by covalent modification. **Caution:** DEPC should be handled with great care, as it is a suspected carcinogen.
2. RNases are very stable and active enzymes, and they are difficult to inactivate. Always wear latex or vinyl gloves (as hands and dust particles are a source of RNAses), and keep tubes closed whenever possible. Use sterile plasticware (generally RNAse-free) or glassware (which should be cleaned with a detergent, rinsed, and baked at 240°C for several hours). Alternatively, glassware can be treated with DEPC. Fill glassware with 0.1% DEPC in water, allow to stand overnight at room temperature, and then autoclave for 15 min to eliminate residual DEPC.

3. Solutions or water should also be treated with 0.1% DEPC. Add 0.1 mL DEPC to 100 mL solution and water, shake vigorously to bring DEPC into solution, and allow the bottle to stay overnight at room temperature. Then autoclave for 15 min to remove any trace of DEPC.

4. Cell pellets or tissue should be stored at −70°C for several months, for later use.

5. RNA is not protected after harvesting until the cells are lysed in a guanidinium-based buffer (such as buffer RLT or TRIzol).

6. When using the TRIzol protocol for RNA extraction, you can also isolate DNA and proteins from the same sample. Please refer to the TRIzol protocol, **Subheading 3.1.2.**

7. High quality and concentration of the RNA sample will reduce optimization of the PCR reactions.

8. Housekeeping genes, such as β2-microglobulin or GAPDH are expressed at very high levels compared with the genes of interest and will require 20–25 cycles for detection on gels. On the other hand, MMP or collagen mRNAs are expressed at considerably lower levels and thus require more cycles (25–35). Optimal PCR cycle numbers have to be determined empirically (as mentioned in the text).

9. Performing HotStart PCR increases the specificity of primer-mediated amplification and reduces nonspecific amplifications.

10. If you open PCR tubes during the amplification step, in order to take an aliquot of the reaction, be careful of crosscontamination owing to aerosols. It is essential to discard the pipet tips following each operation to prevent carry over contamination.

11. Keep the final PCR products away from the PCR setup area to reduce the possibilities of crosscontamination. Use aerosol-resistant tips (filtered tips), and use dedicated pipets for sample preparation and PCR product analysis.

References

1. Chomczynski, P. and Sacchi, N. (1987) Single-step method of RNA isolation by acid guanidinium thiocyanate phanol chloroform extraction. *Anal. Biochem.* **162**, 156–159.

2. Whitham, S. E., Murphy, G., Angel, P., et al. (1986) Comparison of human stromelysin and collagenase by cloning and sequence analysis. *Biochem. J.* **240(3)**, 913–916.

3. Freije, J. M., Diez-Itza, I., Balbin, M., eta l. (1994) Molecular cloning and expression of collagenase-3, a novel human matrix metalloproteinase produced by breast carcinomas. *J. Biol. Chem.* **269(24)**, 16,766–16,773.

4. Cheah, K. S., Stoker, N. G., Griffin, J. R., Grosveld, F. G., and Solomon, E. (1985) Identification and characterization of the human type II collagen gene (COL2A1). *Proc. Natl. Acad. Sci. USA* **82(9)**, 2555–2559.

5. Suggs, S. V., Wallace, R. B., Hirose, T., Kawashima, E. H., and Itakura, K. (1981) Use of synthetic oligonucleotides as hybridization probes: isolation of cloned cDNA sequences for human β2-microglobulin. *Proc. Natl. Acad. Sci. USA* **78(11)**, 6613–6617.

7

Quantification of mRNA Expression Levels in Articular Chondrocytes With PCR Technologies

Audrey McAlinden, Jochen Haag, Brigitte Bau,
Pia M. Gebhard, and Thomas Aigner

Summary

Unlike any other technology in molecular biology, the polymerase chain reaction (PCR) has changed the technological armamentarium of molecular scientists working on cartilage, in terms of outstanding sensitivity and accuracy. Four approaches to determine mRNA expression levels by PCR amplification of specific cDNA sequences are currently in use and are discussed in this chapter: conventional PCR with end-point determination, conventional PCR in the logarithmic amplification phase, conventional PCR using internal competitive DNA fragments, and real-time PCR as offered by TaqMan™ technology and others. The determination of mRNA expression levels by real-time quantitative PCR appears to be the most reliable method for accurate determination of gene expression levels within cartilage and cultured chondrocytes, as in other tissues and cell types. This technology offers outstanding sensitivity and accuracy in terms of determination of the amount of cDNA molecules. However, this method cannot account for factors such as efficiency of RNA isolation and reverse transcription conditions. Thus, normalization of the acquired data is required, with all its limitations as described.

Key Words: PCR; cartilage; chondrocytes; mRNA quantification; expression analysis; TaqMan.

1. Introduction

Unlike any other technology in molecular biology, the polymerase chain reaction (PCR) has changed the technological armamentarium of molecular scientists working on articular cartilage. In addition to the amplification of DNA fragments for cloning, sequencing, and a large variety of other applications, the determination of mRNA expression levels of genes in cartilage and chondrocytes is a widely used PCR application that provides outstanding sensitivity (up to 5–10 molecules per assay) and accuracy (*see* **Subheading 3.4.**).

From: *Methods in Molecular Medicine, Vol. 100: Cartilage and Osteoarthritis, Vol. 1: Cellular and Molecular Tools*
Edited by: M. Sabatini, P. Pastoureau, and F. De Ceuninck © Humana Press Inc., Totowa, NJ

In general, four approaches to determine mRNA expression levels by PCR amplification of specific cDNA sequences are currently in use and are discussed in this chapter: (1) conventional PCR with end-point determination, (2) conventional PCR in the logarithmic amplification phase, (3) conventional PCR using internal competitive DNA fragments, and (4) real-time PCR as offered by TaqMan™ technology and others.

2. Materials

1. GeneAmp, PCR System 9700 (Applied Biosystems, Foster City, CA).
2. ABI PRISM® 7700 (Applied Biosystems).
3. RNeasy kit (Qiagen, Hilden, FRG).
4. Random hexamer primers (e.g., Promega, Madison, USA).
5. RNasin (Promega).
6. Moloney murine leukemia virus (MMLV) reverse transcriptase, RNase H Minus, 5X reaction buffer (Promega).
7. Nucleotide mix (dTTP, dCTP, dATP, dGTP; Carl Roth, Karlsruhe, FRG).
8. AmpliTaq Gold® DNA Polymerase, 10X PCR Gold buffer (Applied Biosystems).
9. Silver-Star DNA polymerase; 10X polymerase buffer (Eurogentec, Seraing, Belgium).
10. qPCR™Core Kit-No Rox; Rox-buffer (Eurogentec).
11. Sachem® LE agarose (BioWhittaker Molecular Applications, Rockland, ME).
12. QIAquick gel extraction kit (Qiagen).
13. Cloning vectors; e.g., pGEM-T Easy (Promega), pCRII TOPO (Invitrogen, Karlsruhe, FRG).
14. Picogreen® data quantitation kit (Molecular Probes, Eugene, OR).

3. Methods
3.1. Conventional PCR for Detection of mRNA Expression of SOX9 in Normal and Osteoarthritic Cartilage
3.1.1. Principles

The first step to evaluate the expression of a certain gene is to test for its presence in a cDNA preparation by conventional PCR. However, it should be emphasized that conventional PCR is not quantitative, as it mostly determines the presence or absence of the expression of a certain gene. In addition, levels of amplified product do not necessarily reflect the total amount of cDNA/mRNA present in the sample tested owing to the PCR amplification plateau phase. This effect is largely independent of the amount of starting template. For accurate detection, more quantitative methods as outlined below should be used or other mRNA quantification technologies, such as Northern blotting.

The detailed theory of PCR has been described in numerous textbooks *(1,2)* and is not the subject of this chapter. Basically, sequence-specific primers induce the exponential amplification of a region of interest within a template molecule.

3.1.2. Primer Selection

One of the most crucial aspects for designing a PCR is the appropriate selection of the amplification primers. In this respect some general rules have to be envisaged, but by using standard computer programs adequate primers can easily be selected (e.g., Primer Express™, ABI Biosystems):

1. Length of primer: 18–30 bp.
2. The amplification product (as determined by measuring the number of bases amplified by the 5' forward and 3' reverse primers) should be 150–800 bp (Note: products smaller than 150 bp may be difficult to detect by conventional agarose gel electrophoresis, whereas larger products may be more difficult to amplify.)
3. Primers should not display significant complementarity (neither sequence similarity to themselves nor to the other primer).
4. Both forward (5') and reverse (3') primers should have similar melting temperatures (T_m approx 55–70°C; ΔT_m below 1°C).
5. A homology search using public databases and programs (e.g., BLAST, NCBI: Website: www.ncbi.nlm.nih.gov/blast) allows one to check for potential crossreaction of the primers to other genes. This problem is usually minimal, as both primers would need to possess high homology, at least at the 3'-end, to result in a coamplification product. Crossreactivity may occur, however, if the annealing and amplification temperature of both primers is not well defined.

3.1.3. Experimental Protocol for Detection of SOX9 mRNA Expression

A typical protocol for an amplification procedure is given below using primers against human SOX9 (SOX9-fw 5'-primer: 5'-ACCGGCCTCTACTCC ACCTT-3'; SOX9-dw 3'-primer: 5'-TGGGTACGAGTTGCCTTTAGCT-3'). These primers amplify a product of 331 bp. Conventional PCR showed abundant expression of SOX9 in all cartilage samples investigated, with a lower signal detected in the osteoarthritic samples (**Fig. 1**). In fact, quantitative real-time PCR confirmed this pattern and provided exact values *(3)*.

3.1.3.1. REVERSE TRANSCRIPTION: SYNTHESIS OF cDNA

For all work with RNA, RNAse-free apparatus and material should be used and gloves should be worn throughout the procedure. The method is described for components supplied by Promega, but it can be easily adapted for components from other suppliers. For RNA preparation from cultured chondrocytes, *see* Chapter 6 and for RNA preparation from cartilage, *see* Chapters 8 and 10.

1. Add 1 μg total RNA into a microtube and 2 μL random hexamers (100 ng/μL; for poly[dT] primers, *see* **Note 1**). Add diethyl pyrocarbonate (DEPC)-treated (RNAse-free) water to a total volume of 17.25 μL.
2. Incubate for 10 min at 70°C (for denaturation of RNA secondary structures) and cool immediately on ice for 5 min. Centrifuge briefly.

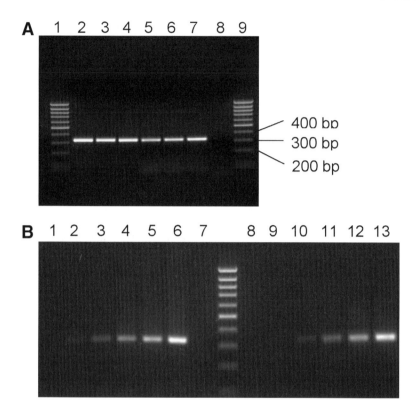

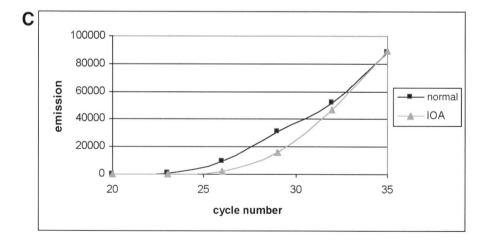

3. Add 5 µL MMLV reverse transcriptase (RT) 5X reaction buffer, 1.25 µL dNTP mix (10 m*M* each), 0.5 µL RNasin (40 U/µL), 1 µL MMLV RT (H–) (200 U/µL; *see* **Note 2**).
4. Mix gently and incubate at room temperature for 10 min and then at 37°C for 1 h.
5. Incubate for 15 min at 70°C (to inactivate the enzyme).

3.1.3.2. PCR

1. Prepare a master mix and adjust to a final PCR volume of 20–24 µL with H_2O (depending on the volume of cDNA added): 2.5 µL 10X DNA-polymerase buffer, 2 µL 5'-primer (10 µ*M*), 2 µL 3'-primer (10 µ*M*), 0.25 µL dNTP mix (10 m*M* each), 0.75 µL $MgCl_2$ (50 m*M*), 0.1 µL Taq DNA-polymerase (5 U/µL). Adjust volume with H_2O.
2. Add 1–5 µL of the cDNA reaction (depending on the assay sensitivity).
3. PCR cycle program:
   a. Initial denaturation step: 94°C, 4 min (using hot-start polymerase: 10 min).
   b. Then 35–40 cycles of: (i) denaturation step: 94°C, 30 s; (ii) annealing step: approx 60°C (needs to be tested for the respective primers), 30 s; and (iii) extension step: 72°C, 1 min (followed by a final extension step: 8 min at 72°C).

3.1.3.3. AMPLIFICATION PRODUCT BY AGAROSE GEL ELECTROPHORESIS EVALUATION

Electrophorese an aliquot of the amplification product through a conventional 1–1.5% agarose gel (the optimal agarose concentration depends on the expected size of the amplification product) and compare the resulting cDNA band size with appropriate DNA standards. Evaluate the results by ultraviolet (UV) detection (**Fig. 1A**). In particular, the size of the cDNA band, the presence of additional amplification products and the overall intensity of the band should be noted. The intensity of the band gives some indication of the gene expression level within the specimen investigated.

Fig. 1. *(opposite page)* (**A**) Conventional PCR analysis showing the presence of SOX9 in normal (lanes 2–4) and osteoarthritic (lanes 5–7) articular cartilage. Amplification product is 331 bp. The SOX9 signals are somewhat less intense in the osteoarthritic specimens. Lanes 1 and 9, 100 bp DNA ladder standards (MBI Fermentas, FRG). Lane 8, negative control (no cDNA added). (**B,C**) Comparative analysis of cDNA from normal (lanes 1–6) and osteoarthritic (lanes 8–13) cartilage during the logarithmic phase of the PCR amplification (lanes 1 and 8, 20 cycles; lanes 2 and 9, 23 cycles; lanes 3 and 10, 26 cycles; lanes 4 and 11, 29 cycles; lanes 5 and 12, 32 cycles; lanes 6 and 13, 35 cycles). Lane 7, negative control. (**C**) Intensities of the amplification bands determined by gel densitometry. Note that at low cycle numbers (20 and 23×), no amplification product is visible, whereas after a high cycle number (35×) both PCRs have reached the plateau phase, revealing a similar amount of amplified product, despite differences in starting concentrations of both samples. Quantification analysis is only possible during the logarithmic amplification phase. OA, osteoarthritic.

3.2. Semiquantitative PCR in the Logarithmic Amplification Phase to Measure SOX9 Expression in Articular Chondrocytes

A more quantitative method to evaluate the amount of cDNA present in a sample is to titrate the number of amplification cycles in order to detect the product during the exponential amplification phase of the PCR. This is demonstrated in **Fig. 1B** and **C**: SOX9 was amplified using the same primers and experimental procedures as described in **Subheading 3.1.3.** Only the amplification cycle numbers differed between experiments. In normal cartilage, more amplified product is shown at lower cycle numbers compared with that amplified from osteoarthritic cartilage (compare cycle number 26 and 29 between normal and osteoarthritic samples). This method should be considered semiquantitative, as it only allows an approximate estimation of gross differences in expression levels. Note that the intensities of the product bands at the plateau phase are identical.

3.3. Semiquantitative PCR Measurement of Anabolic Chondrocyte Activity Using Competitor Fragments

A more exact, but time-consuming technology for quantifying mRNA expression levels in chondrocytes is the use of DNA competitor fragments. Basically, these competitors are similar to the cDNA to be amplified (i.e., they contain identical primer recognition sites and related internal sequences), thus ensuring identical amplification efficiency *(4)*. In order to distinguish the amplified competitor bands from the cDNA amplification products, the internal competitor sequence should contain either a short deletion or insertion of additional sequences or a restriction site sequence. This enables one to distinguish both products by gel electrophoresis directly, or after digestion with the specific restriction enzyme.

The experimental concept is based on the addition of a known number of DNA competitor fragments to the amplification reaction in order to coamplify them in a competitive manner with the cDNA of interest. The ratio of cDNA/ competitor of the PCR products allows us to calculate the amount of cDNA originally present in the sample. The basic protocol is very similar to the standard PCR approach described in **Subheading 3.1.** After reverse transcription of RNA, one adds to a series of aliquots of the obtained cDNA a defined number of competitor fragment molecules and subsequently compares both amplification products (fragment of interest and competitor fragments) by conventional gel electrophoresis and densitometry. The number of competitor fragments that results in a similar amount of amplification product represents a good estimate for the amount of cDNA molecules present in the starting material.

3.3.1. Experimental Protocol

The selection of primers should be followed as outlined above in **Subheading 3.1.2** (*see* also **Table 1**). Care should be taken to optimize the reaction conditions, such as the annealing temperature, primer concentration, nucleotide concentration, and optimal number of cycles to be used in order to maximize visualization and quantitation of the cDNA bands. Different amounts of the competitor fragments should be added at twofold dilution steps over two orders of magnitude depending on the abundance of cDNA fragments present within the sample to be measured. These conditions have to be established empirically.

Generation of internal competitor fragments can be performed according to a protocol originally published by Celi et al. *(5)*, and this is shown in **Fig. 2**. In brief, the competitor fragments are shortened versions of the original sequence of interest (i.e., collagen type II or aggrecan), which are synthesized using specifically designed internal primers. The competitor fragment generated for collagen type II is 587 bp (instead of 670 bp) and 377 bp for aggrecan (instead of 533 bp). This size difference allows clear distinction by conventional gel electrophoresis. A typical experimental result using these competitors is shown in **Fig 2C**.

3.4. Determination of Collagenase mRNA Expression in Articular Chondrocytes by Real-Time Quantitative PCR

The determination of mRNA expression levels by real-time quantitative PCR appears to be the most reliable method for accurate determination of gene expression levels within tissues and cells. This technology offers outstanding sensitivity and accuracy in terms of determination of the amount of cDNA molecules. However, this method cannot account for factors such as efficiency of RNA isolation and reverse transcription conditions. Thus, normalization of the acquired data is required with all its limitations, as described below (*see* **Note 3** and **Subheading 3.5.**). Also, as with all mRNA detection methods, the ability to deduce protein levels from mRNA data is very limited (*see* **Note 4**).

The following section highlights the principles of the TaqMan technology. (For more detailed information, the reader is referred to the manufacturer's manual.) For other real-time PCR technologies, *see* **Note 5**.

3.4.1. Principles

The TaqMan assay is a conventional PCR that uses the 5'-exonuclease activity of Taq DNA polymerase to digest a gene-specific probe (**Fig. 3**). The degradation of this probe is measured online (i.e., in "real-time") after each PCR amplification cycle (**Fig. 4A**). The probe represents a third oligonucleotide that contains at its 5'-end a *reporter* and at its 3'-end a *quencher* fluorochrome, as well as a phosphate group to inhibit further elongation during the PCR.

Table 1
Sequence of Primers Used for Competitive Polymerase Chain Reaction (PCR) Experiments in Order to Evaluate Chondrocyte Anabolic Activity [a]

Target-cDNA	Primer	Sequence	T_m (°C)	T_a (°C)	Amplificate (bp)
COL2A1	col2a1-up	5'-CTC-GTC-GCC-GCT-GTC-CTT-CG-3'	67.1	63.0	670
	col2a1-low	5'-TCA-CAC-CAG-GAG-CAC-CCG-CC-3'	67.5		
	col2a1-int	5'-CGC-CGC-TGT-CCT-TCG-**AAG-GAC-CTC-CTG-GGC-C**-3'	48.8		582
aggrecan	agg-up	5'-TCC-CTC-ACC-ATC-CCC-TGC-TA-3'	60.5	62.0	533
	agg-low	5'-TCT-CCA-TAG-CAG-CCT-TCC-CG-3'	60.6		
	agg-int	5'-TCC-CTC-ACC-ATC-CCC-TGC-TAC-**CTG-CCC-AAC-TAC-CCG-G**-3'	56.7		377

[a] T_m, theoretical melting temperature (in case of the internal primers, the melting temperature of the sequence specific inner portion); T_a, optimized annealing temperature. Bold sequence of the internal primers ("...-int") represents the portions hybridizing to the internal sequence of the cDNA, whereas the remaining sequence represents the binding sites of the external primers (or part of it).

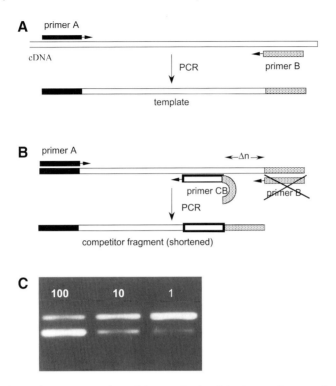

Fig. 2. Schematic representation of the synthesis of the internal competitor fragments for quantitative polymerase chain reaction (PCR) analysis. After normal amplification of the target fragment from the cDNA template **(A)**, the target fragment is then reamplified with an internal primer (primer CB), which replaces one of the external primers **(B)**. This internal primer contains part of the target sequence and usually the sequence of the replaced external primer. The amplification product represents the shortened competitor fragment, which is finally added to the PCR. **(C)** A typical result of a competitive PCR. Gel electrophoretic analysis shows two amplification products (lower bands represent the shortened competitor fragment; upper bands represent the original amplified templates). Three different concentrations of the added competitor fragments were assayed in 10× dilution steps (artificial numbers: 100, 10, and 1). The concentration of cDNA is shown to correspond approximately to the intermediate concentration (i.e., 10).

As long as the reporter and the quencher are closely linked by the oligonucleotide backbone, no fluorescence signal is detected. However, after degradation of the oligonucleotide, the reporter is separated from the quencher and can then be detected by the integrated fluorescence detection system. Importantly, only probes that are fully hybridized to the template are digested by the Taq DNA polymerase, whereas free, unhybridized probe is not digested and therefore does not impede measurement.

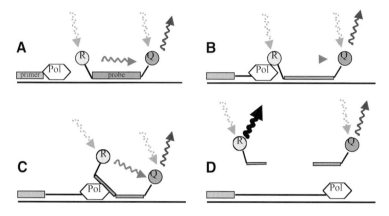

Fig. 3. The physical principle of probe detection in the TaqMan technology. This is based on the FET (fluorescence energy transfer) phenomenon (**A**). If a fluorochrome Q (i.e., the quencher) is very close to another fluorochrome R (i.e., the reporter) and if the absorption spectrum of the former is similar to the emission spectrum of the latter, then after excitation of R, the emitted electron is adsorbed by Q and an electron corresponding to the emission spectrum of Q is emitted. Despite exciting R, no emitted electrons of R are detectable and, thus, R is quenched by Q. Because this effect relies very much on the close proximity of R to Q, it is directly linked to the integrity of the oligonucleotide backbone of the TaqMan probe. (**B–D**) During the amplification procedure the polymerase cleaves the backbone (**B,C**) and R and Q are released and diffuse off. (**D**) Thereafter, emission photons of R are detectable.

The quantification is usually done in comparison with intra-assay standard curves (**Fig. 4B**) and normalized to a housekeeping gene such as GAPDH (glyceraldehyde phosphate dehydrogenase; *see* also **Note 6** and **Subheading 3.5.**). The point of measurement is the C_T-value of the probe, i. e. the first amplification cycle at which the measured signal, representing hydrolyzed probe, exceeds a certain threshold level (**Fig. 4A**). Usually, quantification is done using a calibration curve of standard fragments (*see* **Subheading 3.4.2.4.**). Assays are best performed in triplicate in order to account for pipeting errors (*see* **Note 7**). Another quantification method is the $\Delta\Delta C_T$ method (*see* **Note 8**), which is not described in this chapter as it is not commonly used.

3.4.2. Primer and Probe Selection and Synthesis

Primers and probes as well as assay conditions need to be carefully selected, empirically optimized, and tested for the TaqMan assay in order to obtain optimal results.

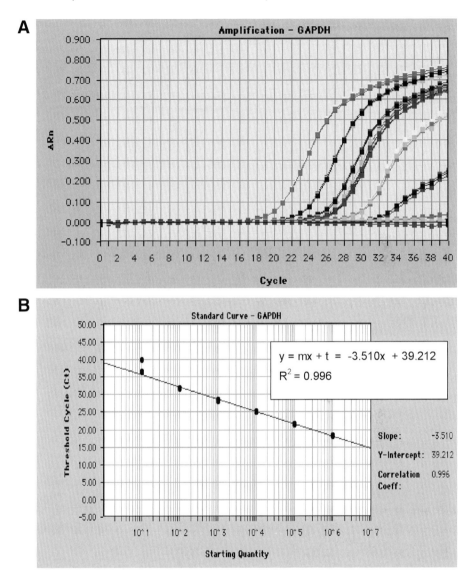

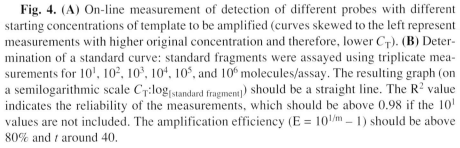

Fig. 4. (A) On-line measurement of detection of different probes with different starting concentrations of template to be amplified (curves skewed to the left represent measurements with higher original concentration and therefore, lower C_T). **(B)** Determination of a standard curve: standard fragments were assayed using triplicate measurements for 10^1, 10^2, 10^3, 10^4, 10^5, and 10^6 molecules/assay. The resulting graph (on a semilogarithmic scale C_T:$\log_{[standard\ fragment]}$) should be a straight line. The R^2 value indicates the reliability of the measurements, which should be above 0.98 if the 10^1 values are not included. The amplification efficiency ($E = 10^{1/m} - 1$) should be above 80% and t around 40.

3.4.2.1. PRIMER SELECTION

Primer selection is best performed using the Primer Express® software supplied by ABI Biosystems. In general, primers should fulfill the following criteria:

1. Length: 18–30 bp.
2. Length of amplified product: 75–150 bp.
3. GC content: 20–80%.
4. T_m: approx 60°C.
5. No poly-T regions (to avoid nonspecific binding to the poly[dT]-tails of cDNAs).
6. No palindromic sequences.
7. Wherever possible, the amplified product should span an exon–intron boundary (*see* **Note 9**).

3.4.2.2. PROBE SELECTION

The TaqMan probes need to be specifically designed using the Primer Express software, and they can be ordered from a company offering the required modifications for the assay. They should generally conform to the following criteria:

1. The 5'-end of the probe should be located close to the 3'-end of one of the PCR primers.
2. Length: 20–30 bp.
3. GC content: 40–60%.
4. T_m of the probe should be 5–10°C above the T_m of the primers to ensure efficient and complete probe binding.
5. Position of the quencher should be at the 3'-end.
6. No G nucleotide at the 5'-end.
7. Avoid GGGs or CCCs in the probe sequence.
8. No complementarity in between primers and probe.

3.4.2.3. OPTIMIZATION OF ASSAY CONDITIONS

The optimal annealing temperature is usually kept at 60°C according to the Primer Express program. Generally, two PCR parameters should be tested in order to identify the optimal amplification conditions, i.e., conditions that correspond to the lowest C_T values for the samples tested:

1. Primer concentrations (test 0.05, 0.3, and 0.9 µM for both primers).
2. $MgCl_2$ concentrations (test 3–7 mM in 0.5-mM steps; *see* **Note 10**).

3.4.2.4. GENERATION OF STANDARD PROBES (*SEE* **NOTE 6**)

In order to calculate absolute copy numbers per assay, one can use gene-specific standard curves of cloned cDNAs that contain the identical sequence to be amplified. Alternatively, amplified PCR products can be used: this is less time-consuming to establish but can be more difficult to manage experimentally. These standard fragments are then assayed in separate tubes to give a concentration curve, usually 10^1, 10^2, 10^3, 10^4, 10^5, and 10^6 molecules/reaction.

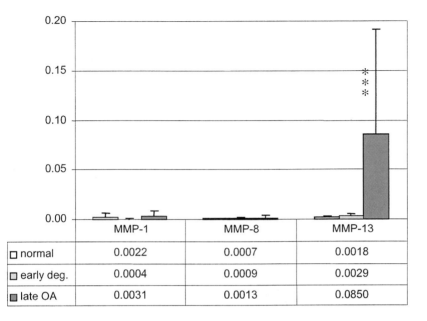

	MMP-1	MMP-8	MMP-13
□ normal	0.0022	0.0007	0.0018
□ early deg.	0.0004	0.0009	0.0029
▨ late OA	0.0031	0.0013	0.0850

Fig. 5. Quantificative TaqMan analysis for mRNA expression levels of MMP-1 (collagenase A), MMP-8 (collagenase B), and MMP-13 (collagenase C) in normal, early degenerative, and late-stage osteoarthritic (OA) cartilage. Ratios of each protease normalized to GAPDH are shown. Stars indicate the significance levels compared to normal articular cartilage (***, $p < 0.001$).

The resulting C_T values should produce a straight line result on a semilogarithmic plot that can subsequently be used to calculate the exact copy number of cDNA present in a sample (**Fig. 4B**). Additionally, the parameters of the standard curve reflect assay reliability (R should be above 0.98), and amplification efficiency (m should optimally be between –3.3 and –3.8) and are also indicative of concentration errors in the standard stocks (t should be about 40) (**Fig. 4B**).

3.4.3. Determination of Collagenase mRNA Expression by Real-Time Quantitative PCR: Experimental Protocol

In order to understand the molecular basis of osteoarthritic cartilage degeneration, knowledge of proteases that are able to cleave the main constituent of adult articular cartilage, collagen type II, are of particular interest. Such candidate molecules are collagenases A, B, and C (MMP-1, MMP-8, and MMP-13, respectively). Expression data obtained by real-time PCR using the protocol outlined in the following steps clearly support the hypothesis that an important player in osteoarthritic cartilage degradation is MMP-13 (**Fig. 5**) *(6,7)*.

The sequences of primers and probes, as well as the optimal assay conditions, for matrix metalloproteinases (MMPs)-1, -8, and –13, as well as a number of other genes relevant to cartilage function, are shown in **Table 2**. For standardization purposes, ratios relative to GAPDH were calculated. The primers (obtained from MWG Biotech, Germany) and TaqMan probes (obtained from Eurogentec, Belgium) were designed using Primer Express software. In order to obtain quantitative results, gene-specific standard PCRs using sequence-specific control probes were performed in parallel (*see* **Subheading 3.4.2.4.**). All experiments were performed in triplicate to minimize inaccurate measurements caused by pipeting errors (*see* **Note 7**). The recommended assay volume is 50 µL, but 25 µL can also be used to save on expensive material. The experimental protocol is described in the following sections.

3.4.3.1. REVERSE TRANSCRIPTION

Reverse transcription is performed as described for conventional PCR (*see* **Subheading 3.1.3.1.**). Again, we prefer the use of random oligo primers to avoid a bias toward 3'-end amplification.

3.4.3.2. TAQMAN ASSAY

1. Preparation of a pre-master mix containing all reagents apart from buffer, Taq DNA polymerase, and cDNA. This can be stored at –20°C for months in, e.g., 500-µL aliquots:

   a. Upstream primer: 0.25–4.5 µM (optimized according to **Subheading 3.4.2.3.**).
   b. Downstream primer: 0.25–4.5 µM (optimized according to **Subheading 3.4.2.3.**).
   c. TaqMan probe: 0.5 µM.
   d. dNTPs: dATP, dTTP, dCTP and dGTP (1 mM of each).
   e. ROX buffer: 3 µM.
   f. MgCl$_2$: 3–7 mM (use the optimized concentration according to **Subheading 3.4.2.3.**).
   g. Adjust the final volume with H$_2$O.

2. Final master mix for a 25-µL reaction. This is prepared immediately prior to the experiment (*see* **Note 11**):

   a. Premaster-mix: 5 µL.
   b. 10X polymerase buffer: 2.5 µL.
   c. Taq polymerase (5 U/µL): 0.1 µL.
   d. Adjust volume to 20 µL with H$_2$O.

3. PCR assay: Usually we use two-step PCR, i.e., the annealing and extension steps are performed at the same (low) temperature to ensure efficient binding of the probe to the template during amplification.

a. Add 5 µL of the diluted cDNA to 20 µL master mix. (Dilution of the cDNA depends on the sensitivity of the assay.)
b. Initial denaturation: 94°C, 4 min (If hot-start enzyme is used, the denaturation step should be carried out for 10 min; *see* **Note 12.**)
c. 40 cycles of: (i.) annealing and extension (**Note 13**): 60°C, 1 min; and (ii.) denaturation step: 94°C, 30 s.

3.4.3.3. EVALUATION OF THE REACTION QUALITY

To analyze the quality of the TaqMan reaction, the following parameters should be considered:

1. Standard deviation of the replicates should be below 0.16. The variations between replicates are mainly owing to pipeting errors, which can be minimized using master mixes.
2. Amplification efficiencies can be calculated: $AE = 10^{-1/m} - 1$ (**Fig. 4B**). The efficiency should be above 70% (optimally above 85%).
3. The mean squared error (MSE) curve displayed in the multicomponent view should be flat and below 200.

3.5. Normalization of Gene Expression Data

Present technology does not permit the measurement of absolute numbers of mRNA species within specimens. Therefore, it is necessary to standardize relative values to internal cellular standards such as the commonly known housekeeping genes. However, this is dependent on the fact that the expression of housekeeping genes, e.g., GAPDH or β-actin, does not change significantly with respect to the biological condition being studied. This assumption, however, may not be correct, at least in some conditions, although regulation of these genes appears to be low compared with other genes (**Fig. 6**); (**8**). Thus, for defined cell types such as articular chondrocytes analyzed in similar conditions it is a suitable method. It was suggested recently that multiple housekeeping genes could be used in order to reduce the risk of regulation of housekeeping genes; however, this is much more time consuming, and significant benefits have not been reported to date.

3.6. Conclusion

Quantitative online PCR is one of the most powerful tools to evaluate gene expression levels. However, care should to be taken with respect to selecting the normalization procedure. Despite being rather expensive, the high sensitivity levels of real-time PCR renders this method appealing if one works with cartilage, from which the isolation of large amounts of RNA is difficult (**9**). This is particularly the case if one is interested in analyzing focal lesions such as those found in osteoarthritic cartilage degeneration (**10**).

Table 2
Nucleotide Sequences of Primers and Probes for Real-Time PCR Quantification Experiments of Genes Relevant to Cartilage and Chondrocyte Function

Gene	Acc. no.	Primers	Probe	$MgCl_2$ conc. (mM)	Ref.
β-actin	M10277	Up: GCCCTGAGGCACTCTTCCA Low: TTGCGGATGTCCACGTCA	AGTTTCGTGGATGCCACAGGACTCCAT	6	
ADAMTS1	NM_006988	Up: GCCAAAGGCATTGGCTACTTC Low: GTGGAATCTGGGCTACATGGA	CGTTTTGCAGCCCAAGGTTGTAGATGGT	7	12
ADAMTS4 (Aggase1)	AF148213	Up: TGCCCGCTTCATCACTGA Low: CAATGGAGCCTCTGGTTTGTC	ACAGTGCCCATAGCCATTGTCCAGGA	4	6
ADAMTS5 (Aggase2)	AF142099	Up: CGCTGCCACCACACTCAA Low: CGTAGTGCTCCTCATGGTCATCT	AAGTGGCAGCACCAACACAACCAGC	4.5	6
Aggrecan	NM_013227	Up: ACTTCCGCTGGTCAGATGGA Low: TCTCGTGCCAGATCATCACC	CCATGCAATTGAGAACTGGCGCC	6	10
Chitinase39	NM_004000	Up: CCTCCTGTCCTTTGACTTCCAT Low: CCTTGCTCAGAGGGCTGTTG	TTGGGAAAAGCCCCTTATCACTG	3.5	13
Chitinase40	NM_001276	Up: CGGAGCCACAGTCCATAGAATC Low: CGTCGTATCCTACCCACTGGTT	CGGCCAGCAGGTCCCCTATGC	4.5	13
Col1A1	NM_000088	Up: AGGGCCAAGACGAAGACATC Low: AGATCACGTCATCGCACAACA	AATCACCTGCGTACAGAACGGCCTCA	6.5	11
Col 2A1	NM_001844	Up: CAACACTGCCAACGTCCAGAT Low: CTGCTTCGTCCAGATAGGCAAT	ACCTTCCTACGCCTGCGTCCACG	5.5	10

94

Gene	Acc. no.	Primers	Probe	MgCl$_2$ conc. (mM)	Ref.
ColIIA Col2-2.exon	L10347	Up: AGAGGTATAATGATAAGGATGTGTGGAAG Low: GTCGTCGCAGAGGACAGTCC	CACAGACACAGATCCGGCAGGGC	6	11
Col 3A1	NM_000090	Up: TGGCTACTTCTCGCTCTGCTT Low: CGGATCCTGAGTCACAGACACA	TTCTGGCTTCCAGACATCTCTATCCGCAT	5	11
Col 10A1	NM_000493	Up: TGCTAGTATCCTTGAACTTGGTTCAT Low: CTGTGTCTTGGTGTTGGGTAGTG	ACGCTGAACGATACCAAACGCCAC	5.5	11
GAPDH	NM_002046	Up: GAAGGTGAAGGTCGGAGTC Low: GAAGATGGTGATGGGATTTC	CAAGCTTCCCGTTCTCAGCC	5.5	9
MMP1	NM_002421	Up: CTGTTCAGGGACAGAATGTGCT Low: TCGATATGCTTCACAGTTCTAGGG	ACGGATACCCCAAGGACATCTACAGCTCC	6.5	6
MMP3	NM_002422	Up: TTTTGGCCATCTCTTCCTTCA Low: TGTGGATGCCTCTTGGGTATC	AACTTCATATGCGGCATCCACGCC	4	6
MMP8	NM_002424	Up: GCTCGCTCACTCCTCTGACC Low: CATCTTGAGGGAGTGAGTAGTTGCT	TGGTGCCTTGATGTATCCCAACTATGCTTTC	6	14
MMP13	NM_002427	Up: TCCTCTTCTTGAGCTGGACTCATT Low: CGCTCTGCAAACTGGAGGTC	TCCTCAGACAAATCATCTTCATCACCACCAC	7	6
MMP14	NM_004995	Up: TGCCTGCGTCCATCAACACT Low: CATCAAACACCCAATGCTTGTC	AAGACGAATTTGCCATCCTTCCTCTCGT	7	6
SOX9	Z46629	Up: ACACACAGCTCACTGACCTTG Low: GGAATTCTGGTTGGTCCTCTCTT	TTAGGATCATCTCGGCCATCGTCGC	7	3

6. Theoretically, RNA standards can also be used and added to the RNA sample before reverse transcription. This allows accurate determination of the number of RNA molecules present within, e.g., RNA isolated from the cells of interest. However, one is still not be able to account for different efficiencies of reverse transcription of different mRNAs. Also, to generate a standard curve one would need to perform multiple reverse transcriptions per assay with different concentrations of standards, which would make the assay time-consuming and expensive under normal conditions. The use of specific polymerases with intrinsic reverse transcriptase activity such as Tth DNA polymerase is advantageous, but they are less optimal in the TaqMan assay. Also, the standards in this case should be different from the probe to be amplified, as they need to be coamplified in one tube (Multiplex TaqMan PCR, a method not further discussed in this chapter).

7. We usually perform assays in triplicate, which allows one to account for pipeting errors. If the standard deviation of the results is below 20%, then an average value can be used for further calculations. Obvious values out of range are excluded from further calculations. If all three results deviate significantly (more than 50%), then the measurement is excluded.

8. The $\Delta\Delta C_T$ technology theoretically avoids the use of standard curves in order to quantify relative template amounts. Therefore, this technique is less time-consuming and less expensive. In practice, however, this approach is based on several assumptions that need to be met rather strictly and that need to be tested carefully: most importantly, the efficiency of the amplification reaction of both templates needs to be nearly the same. This is often hard to achieve and even if this is the case in pilot experiments this is not necessarily true for subsequent assays according to our experience.

9. The selection of intron spanning primers and probes for TaqMan PCR avoids amplification of genomic DNA that may be contaminating the specimen to be measured (either because the primers or the probe are no longer binding, if the exon–exon boundary is within their sequence, or because the intron is too long to be amplified during the PCR reaction; therefore the intron should be longer than 2 kb if possible). However, in most cases, genomic DNA is not a major problem if one is measuring transcripts that are present in reasonable abundance. Also, a DNAse step during/after RNA isolation might be used to avoid this problem.

10. Since binding of the probe to the template is not stabilized during the amplification step (it does not get elongated by the polymerase enzyme), one needs to take precautions in order to ensure optimal binding. Primarily, the T_m of the probe should be approx 5–10°C higher than that of the primers. If possible, the high temperature extension step (i.e., usually carried out at 72°C) should be avoided by, for example, using a two-step PCR assay combining the annealing and the elongation step. Furthermore, a higher $MgCl_2$ concentration can be applied in order to stabilize probe binding.

11. In our experiments we use the ABI PRISM 7700, which provides a 96-well plate format for the assays using either 50 μL or a 25 μL reaction volume. Recently, ABI PRISM 7900H was introduced based on a 384-well plate format allowing

the reaction volume to be scaled down to 5 µL. Although this saves on expensive consumables, it requires a more precise method for pipeting, as offered by specific robotic systems.

12. Different types of DNA polymerases are available for PCR assays: in principle one can distinguish conventional DNA polymerases, such as silver star polymerase (Eurogentec) and the so-called hot-start DNA polymerases. The latter enzymes are more expensive but have the advantage that they are only activated after an extended initial heat treatment (94°C for 10 min). This is of particular advantage if one intends to store pipetted assays at 4°C for some days before commencing the experiment. Overall, polymerases should be tested prior to an experiment in order to select the most sensitive and reliable one. In addition, the same batch of a chosen polymerase enzyme should be used for all the experiments if possible.

13. The extension time is usually not a critical point in TaqMan analysis as the amplified products are short (less than 150 bp) and the extension rates of conventional DNA polymerases exceed 500 bp per min (at 60°C).

Acknowledgments

This work was supported by the BMBF (grant 01GG9824).

References

1. Anonymous (1997) *The PCR Technique: Quantitative PCR*. Eaton Publishing.
2. Köhler, T., Laßner, D., Rost, A.-K., Thamm, B., Pustowoit, B., and Remke,H. (1995) *Quantitation of mRNA by Polymerase Chain Reaction*. Springer-Verlag, Berlin, Germany.
3. Aigner, T., Gebhard, P. M., Schmid, E., Bau, B., Harley, V., and Pöschl, E. (2003) Sox 9 expression does not correlate with type II collagen expression in adult articular chondrocytes. *Matrix Biol.* **22,** 363–372.
4. Gilliland, G., Perrin, S., Blanchard, K., and Bunn, F. H. (1990) Analysis of cytokine mRNA and DNA: Detection and quantitation by competitive polymerase chain reaction. *Proc. Natl. Acad. Sci. USA* **87,** 2725–2729.
5. Celi, F. S., Zenilman, M. E., and Shuldiner, A. R. (1993) A rapid and versatile method to synthesize internal standards for competitive PCR. *Nucleic Acids Res.* **21,** 1047.
6. Bau, B., Gebhard, P. M., Haag, J., Knorr, T., Bartnik, E., and Aigner, T. (2002) Relative messenger RNA expression profiling of collagenases and aggrecanases in human articular chondrocytes in vivo and in vitro. *Arthritis Rheum.* **46,** 2648–2657.
7. Mitchell, P. G., Magna, H. A., Reeves, L. M., et al.. (1996) Cloning, expression, and type II collagenolytic activity of matrix metalloproteinase-13 from human osteoarthritic cartilage. *J. Clin. Invest.* **97,** 761–768.
8. Zien, A., Aigner, T., Zimmer, R., and Lengauer, T. (2001) Centralization: a new paradigm for the normalization of gene expression data. *Bioinformatics* **17,** S323–S331.

9. McKenna, L. A., Gehrsitz, A., Soeder, S., Eger, W., Kirchner, T., and Aigner, T. (2000) Effective isolation of high quality total RNA from human adult articular cartilage. *Anal. Biochem.* **286**, 80–85.

10. Gehrsitz, A., McKenna, L. A., Soeder, S., Kirchner, T., and Aigner, T. (2001) Isolation of RNA from small human articular cartilage specimens allows quantification of mRNA expression levels in local articular cartilage defects. *J. Orthop. Res.* **19**, 478–482.

11. Gebhard, P. M., Gehrsitz, A., Bau, B., Söder, S., Eger, W., and Aigner, T. (2003) Quantification of expression levels of cellular differentiation markers does not support a general shift in the cellular phenotype of osteoarthritic chondrocytes. *J. Orthop. Res.* **21**, 96–101.

12. Wachsmuth, L., Bau, B., Fan, Z., Pecht, A., Gerwin, N., and Aigner, T. (2003) ADAMTS-1 is a gene product of articular chondrocytes in vivo and in vitro and is down-regulated by Il-1β. *J. Rheumatol.* **31**, 315–320.

13. Knorr, T., Obermayr, F., Bartnik, E., Zien, A., and Aigner, T. (2003) YKL-39 (chitinase 3-like protein 2), but not YKL-40 (chitinase 3-like protein 1) is up-regulated in osteoarthritic chondrocytes. *Ann. Rheum. Dis.* **62**, 995–998.

14. Stremme, S., Duerr, S., Bau, B., Schmid, E., and Aigner, T. (2003) MMP-8 is only a minor gene product of human adult articular chondrocytes of the knee. *Clin. Exp. Rheumatol.* **21**, 205–209.

8

RNA Extraction From Cartilage

Frédéric Mallein-Gerin and Jérôme Gouttenoire

Summary

The direct isolation of RNA from cartilage has often proved difficult owing to a number of factors. Cartilage has a low cell content and contains an extracellular matrix rich in proteoglycans, which copurify with the RNA as they are large and negatively charged macromolecules. In our laboratory, we are interested in searching for genes differentially expressed in chondrocytes in diverse in vivo situations, for instance during maturation of chondrocytes in the growth plate or during cartilage degeneration. We found that treatment by proteinase K in 1 M guanidinium isothiocyanate prior to cesium trifluoroacetate ultracentrifugation was crucial to increase the yield and purity of RNA extracted from cartilage matrix. This protocol indeed led to reproducible patterns of differential display reverse transcriptase-polymerase chain reaction (RT-PCR) and should be useful for identifying genes differentially expressed by chondrocytes in situ.

Key Words: RNA; extraction; cartilage; chondrocyte; RT-PCR.

1. Introduction

The use of molecular biology techniques has helped elucidate the metabolism of normal and many pathological processes. Application of these techniques to human adult articular cartilage has been hampered by a number of factors. Cartilage has a low cell content and a highly crosslinked extracellular matrix containing a high concentration of proteoglycans entrapped in a collagenous network. Separation of RNA from the aggregating proteoglycans poses a problem because both classes of molecules are extremely large and highly negatively charged. Therefore, most gene expression studies are based on RNA extracted from cultured chondrocytes. *In situ* hybridization can represent an alternative technique for studying chondrocyte gene expression in cartilage, but this technique is not quantitative. In our laboratory, we are interested in studying gene expression during cartilage development or progression of osteoarthritis in human and different animal models. We describe here a reliable protocol, developed by modi-

From: *Methods in Molecular Medicine, Vol. 100: Cartilage and Osteoarthritis, Vol. 1: Cellular and Molecular Tools*
Edited by: M. Sabatini, P. Pastoureau, and F. De Ceuninck © Humana Press Inc., Totowa, NJ

fying existing procedures, to isolate DNA-free RNA from cartilage. Purified total RNA is suitable for analysis of gene expression by quantitative reverse transcriptase-polymerase chain reaction (RT-PCR) or differential display RT-PCR.

2. Materials

To prevent RNase contamination, gloves are worn when handling tissue and materials. RNase-free glassware and plasticware are used. Solutions are made with diethyl pyrocarbonate (DEPC)-treated water and autoclaved.

2.1. Equipment for RNA Extraction

1. Mortar and pestle.
2. Liquid nitrogen.
3. Ultracentrifuge (e.g., Beckman).
4. Rotor (e.g., SW60Ti).

2.2. Reagents for RNA Extraction

1. Guanidinium isothiocyanate (GIT).
2. Homogeneization buffer: 4 M GIT, 25 mM sodium citrate, pH 7.0, 0.5% N-lauroyl-sarcosine, 0.1% β-mercaptoethanol.
3. Phenol (Rnase-free).
4. Chloroform/Isoamyl alcohol (24:1).
5. Proteinase K.
6. Cesium trifluoroacetate (CsTFA).
7. RNase-free DNase (Promega).
8. Rnase inhibitor RNasin (PE Applied Biosystems).
9. Sodium acetate.
10. DEPC-treated water: dissolve 1 g DEPC in 1 L distilled water, and then autoclave for 40 min at 128°C. (DEPC inactivates Rnases.)

3. Methods

3.1. RNA Extraction

1. Freeze and store cartilage samples (50–150 mg) into liquid nitrogen.
2. Reduce the frozen samples to powder with a mortar and pestle previously cooled in liquid nitrogen.
3. Isolate total RNA by using a combination and modification of GIT procedures *(1,2)*. Homogenize the frozen samples in 5 mL of homogeneization buffer for 3 h at 4°C.
4. Phenol/chloroform extraction: add to the sample 5 mL of phenol and 2.5 mL of chloroform/isoamyl alcohol. Mix by vortex and centrifuge at 10,000g for 1 h at 4°C. Carefully remove the upper phase.
5. Precipitation: add 1/10 vol of 3 M sodium acetate, pH 5.2, and 2 vol of frozen 100% ethanol. Mix and incubate at –20°C overnight. Centrifuge at 10,000g for 30 min at 4°C.

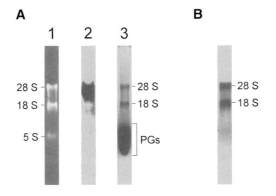

Fig. 1. Agarose-gel resolution patterns of total RNA isolated from bovine cartilage without **(A)** or with **(B)** CsTFA centrifugation. **(A)** Frozen cartilage samples were homogeneized in a solution containing 4 *M* GIT. After phenol-chloroform extraction and precipitation, the pellets were resuspended in 1 *M* GIT with 200 µg/mL proteinase K and incubated at 40°C until complete dissolution. The samples were again phenol-chloroform extracted and precipitated. RNA preparations were electrophoresed in formaldehyde-agarose (1%) minigel and stained with ethidium bromide (lane 1) or transferred to nylon membranes for Northern blot hybridization with a type II collagen probe (lane 2). Note that this RNA is suitable for a good-quality hybridization. After ethidium bromide staining, the sample shown in (lane 1) was further stained with toluidine blue. Toluidine blue reveals contamination of proteoglycans (PGs) in an RNA preparation (lane 3). **(B)** Electrophoresis and toluidine blue staining of RNA isolated as indicated in **Subheading 3.1.** Note that PGs have been eliminated by ultracentrifugation. The positions of the 28S, 18S, and 5S ribosomal RNAs are shown.

6. Resuspend the pellets in 0.8 mL of 1 *M* GIT with 200 µg/mL proteinase K, and incubate at 40°C until complete dissolution (*see* **Note 1**).
7. Adjust GIT concentration to 4 *M* by adding 1.2 mL of 6 *M* GIT, layer the samples on a cushion of CsTFA with a density of 1.6 g/mL, and ultracentrifuge in a Beckman SW60Ti rotor at 88,000*g* for 18 h at 18°C.
8. To eliminate possible traces of genomic DNA, resuspend RNA pellets in a total volume of 200 µL for digestion with 6 U of RNase-free DNase in the presence of 80 U of RNasin, for 30 min at 37°C.
9. Finally recover total RNA after a further phenol-chloroform extraction and sodium acetate precipitation. Resuspend the pellet in 10–15 µL DEPC-treated water and assay 1 µL for concentration and purity of RNA by measuring A_{260}/A_{280}.

4. Notes

1. For our preliminary analyses of gene expression by RT-PCR in human or animal cartilages, we used classical protocols described in the literature for RNA extraction. We obtained extremely low yields of RNA, and our RT-PCR amplification

reactions were poorly reproduced, very likely because of contamination by remaining proteoglycans. We found that a treatment by proteinase K in 1 *M* GIT prior to CsTFA ultracentrifugation was crucial to increase the yield and purity of RNA extracted from human, bovine, mouse, rabbit, or chick cartilage. An example is shown in **Fig. 1**. In particular, this method led to reproducible patterns of conventional PCR after reverse transcription of minute amounts of RNA, which is especially convenient for human samples, which are difficult to obtain in high quantities *(3,4)*. Moreover, this protocol allowed us to obtain reproducible patterns of differential display RT-PCR and should be useful for identifying genes differentially expressed by chondrocytes *in situ (5)*.

References

1. Chomczinski, P. and Sacchi, N. (1987) Single-step method of RNA isolation by acid guanidinium thiocyanate-phenol-chloroform extraction. *Anal. Biochem.* **162,** 156–159.
2. Adams, M. E., Huang, D. Q., Yao, L. Y., and Sandell, L. J. (1992) Extraction and isolation of mRNA from adult cartilage. *Anal. Biochem.* **202,** 89–95.
3. Bluteau, G., Labourdette, L., Ronzière, M. C., et al. (1999) Type X collagen in rabbit and human meniscus. *Osteoarthritis Cartilage* **7,** 498–501.
4. Bluteau, G., Conrozier, T., Mathieu, P., Vignon, E., Herbage, D., and Mallein-Gerin, F. (2001) Matrix metalloproteinase-1, -3, -13 and aggrecanase-1 and -2 are differentially expressed in experimental osteoarthritis. *Biochim. Biophys. Acta* **1526,** 147–158.
5. Bluteau, G., Gouttenoire, J., Conrozier, T., et al. (2002) Differential gene expression analysis in a rabbit model of osteoathritis induced by anterior cruciate ligament (ACL) section. *Biorheology* **39,** 247–258.

9

Gene Expression Analysis in Cartilage by *In Situ* Hybridization

Frédéric Mallein-Gerin and and Jérôme Gouttenoire

Summary

In situ hybridization allows detection and localization of specific nucleic acid sequences directly within a cell or tissue. We present an *in situ* hybridization protocol using double-stranded DNA or single-stranded RNA probes labeled with [^{32}P] to localize and visualize the temporal and spatial distribution of cartilage-characteristic mRNAs. Probes labeled with this high-energy isotope provide good resolution at the tissue level with relatively low background; as a result of the probes that can be obtained that have a higher specificity to emulsion activity, very short exposure times are required.

Key Words: *In situ* hybridization; gene; cartilage; chondrocyte; mRNA.

1. Introduction

Rather than analyze an RNA sample after its extraction from a heterogeneous cell population, detection of RNA by *in situ* hybridization identifies specific cells that contain particular messages and, moreover, makes it possible to determine biochemical and morphological characteristics of the same cells. In vitro, it helped us to determine that aggrecan and type II collagen gene expressions are not necessarily correlated with shape changes during chondrocyte dedifferentiation *(1)*. In vivo, this technology complements and supplements gene expression analysis by Northern blotting or reverse transcriptase-polymerase chain reaction (RT-PCR), in the sense that it can distinguish two types of situation: one in which a gene is expressed in all cells at a low level and one in which a gene is expressed in a few cells at a high level.

From: *Methods in Molecular Medicine, Vol. 100: Cartilage and Osteoarthritis, Vol. 1: Cellular and Molecular Tools*
Edited by: M. Sabatini, P. Pastoureau, and F. De Ceuninck © Humana Press Inc., Totowa, NJ

2. Materials

2.1. Equipment for In Situ Hybridization

1. 60°C oven.
2. Heating block.
3. Embedding molds.
4. Microscope slides.
5. Microtome.
6. Vacuum dessicator.
7. Slide racks.
8. Water bath.
9. Facilities for handling radioactivity.
10. Darkroom.

2.2. Reagents for In Situ Hybridization

1. 4% Paraformaldehyde (PFA) fixative.
2. Paraffin wax (e.g., Paraplast).
3. Ethanol.
4. Xylene.
5. Triethanolamine.
6. Acetic anhydride.
7. Proteinase K solution: proteinase K in 50 mM Tris-HCl, pH 7.6, 5 mM ethylene-diamine tetraacetic acid (EDTA). Concentrations of proteinase K are adjusted from 1 to 10 μg/mL for optimal signal and tissue preservation, depending on the sample (embryonic or adult cartilage).
8. Hybridization solution: 50% formamide, 10 mM Tris-HCl, pH 7.0, 0.15 M NaCl, 1.0 M EDTA, 1X Denhardt's solution, 80 μg/mL denatured salmon sperm DNA, 500 μg/mL yeast tRNA, 10% dextran sulfate.
9. Phosphate-buffered saline (PBS).
10. 1X SSC: 0.15 M NaCl, 0.015 M trisodium citrate.
11. Autoradiographic emulsion (e.g., Kodak NTB-3 nuclear track emulsion).
12. Developer (e.g., Kodak D-19 developer).
13. Fixer (e.g., Kodak rapid fixer).
14. [^{32}P]dCTP (3000 Ci/mmol).

3. Methods

3.1. In Situ Hybridization

1. Place dissected tissues in glass vials. Allow fixation of the samples in freshly prepared PFA. Optimal fixation time is that which gives good morphology as well as good signal-to-noise ratio after *in situ* hybridization and must be determined empirically for each sample.

2. Dehydrate samples in a graded series of ethanol, clear in xylene, embed in 56–57°C Paraplast, section at 7 or 10 μm, and mount the sections on microscope slides.

3. Dry sections overnight on a slide warmer at 37°C, and store at 4°C in the presence of Drierite until hybridization is performed.

4. Deparaffinize the sections, prior to hybridization, in two changes of xylene for 15 min each. Wash twice in ethanol for 5 min, and allow to air-dry.

5. Treat sections with 4% formaldehyde in PBS for 10 min. Wash in three changes of PBS for 5 min each and two changes of 70% ethanol for 5 min each, and let dry.

6. Treat the dried tissue sections with proteinase K solution for 10 min at room temperature, and then rinse in PBS.

7. Treat sections with 4% formaldehyde in PBS for 20 min, wash in two changes of PBS for 5 min each, treat with 0.1 *M* triethanolamine for 5 min, and incubate for 10 min in 0.25% acetic anhydride in 0.1 *M* triethanolamine solution that was prepared immediately before use.

8. Following acetylation, wash sections twice in 2X SSC for 5 min each, twice in 70% ethanol for 5 min each, and once in 95% ethanol for 5 min, and then air dry prior to addition of the hybridization solution.

9. Add to the hybridization solution the appropriate labeled probe (*see* **Note 1**).

10. Perform hybridization by applying 20- to 40-μL aliquots of the hybridization solution containing 250,000 cpm of probe onto the sections and covering them with siliconized cover slips, the edges of which are then sealed with rubber cement. Incubate the slides at 50–52°C for about 20 h.

11. After hybridization, remove the cover slips in 2X SSC, and consecutively wash the sections twice in 2X SSC for 10 min each at room temperature, once in 0.5X SSC for 10 min at 50°C, and three times in 0.1X SSC for 15 min each at 50°C. Then dehydrate the sections in two changes of 70% ethanol for 5 min each and one change of 95% ethanol for 5 min and let dry.

12. For autoradiography, dip the slides in autoradiographic emulsion diluted 1:1 with water at 42°C. After drying vertically at room temperature for at least 1 h, expose the slides in the dark at 4°C in the presence of Drierite for 3–8 d.

13. Develop autoradiographs for 3 min at 18°C, fix, and wash in running tap water. Stain the slides with hematoxylin, dehydrate them with a graded series of alcohols, clear in xylene, and mount with Permount.

4. Notes

1. For our *in situ* hybridization experiments, we obtained very similar results using either the double-stranded DNA probes or single-stranded RNA probes (*2*), each of which offers certain advantages. For instance, benefits of using single-stranded RNA probes are that posthybridization RNase digestion can be used to eliminate mismatched duplexes resulting from the hybridization of the probe to homologous regions of other mRNAs. On the other hand, double-stranded DNA probes are easier to prepare and utilize than RNA probes, and lower hybridization and washing conditions are required to provide sufficiently stringent conditions to limit crosshybridization. An example is shown in **Fig. 1**.

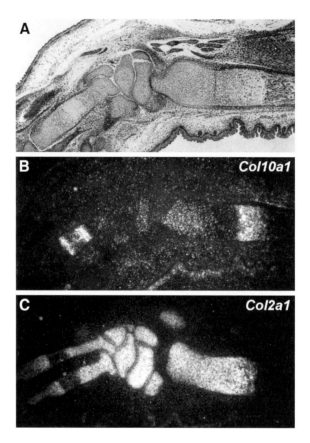

Fig. 1. Autoradiographs of frontal sections through an hindlimb of a 17.5-d-old mouse embryo that were hybridized with ^{32}P-labeled probes. At this stage, cartilage rudiments form prospective long bones. (**A**) Brightfield and corresponding darkfield (**B**) images of a section hybridized with a type X collagen DNA probe. (**C**) Darkfield image of a section adjacent to that in A and B that was hybridized with a type II collagen DNA probe. Note the intense accumulation of silver grains representing hybridizable type II collagen mRNA sequences over the well-differentiated cartilage rudiments and the restricted hybridization of type X collagen mRNA sequences in the regions where chondrocytes undergo hypertrophic maturation.

References

1. Mallein-Gerin, F., Ruggiero, F., and Garrone, R. (1990) Proteoglycan core protein and type II collagen gene expressions are not correlated with cell shape changes during low density chondrocyte cultures. *Differentiation* **43,** 204–211.
2. Mallein-Gerin, F., Kosher, R. A., Upholt, W. B., and Tanzer, M. L. (1988) Temporal and spatial analysis of cartilage proteoglycan core protein gene expression during limb development by in situ hybridization. *Dev. Biol.* **126,** 337–345.

10

Analysis of Differential Gene Expression in Healthy and Osteoarthritic Cartilage and Isolated Chondrocytes by Microarray Analysis

Thomas Aigner, Joachim Saas, Alexander Zien, Ralf Zimmer, Pia M. Gebhard, and Thomas Knorr

Summary

The regulation of chondrocytes in osteoarthritic cartilage and the expression of specific gene products by these cells during early-onset and late-stage osteoarthritis are not well characterized. With the introduction of cDNA array technology, the measurement of thousands of different genes in one small tissue sample can be carried out. Interpretation of gene expression analyses in articular cartilage is aided by the fact that this tissue contains only one cell type in both normal and diseased conditions. However, care has to be taken not to over- and misinterpret results, and some major challenges must be overcome in order to utilize the potential of this technology properly in the field of osteoarthritis.

Key Words: Microarray; differential gene expression; cartilage; chondrocyte; osteoarthritis.

1. Introduction

The regulation of cartilage cells (chondrocytes) in osteoarthritic cartilage and the expression of specific gene products by these cells during early-onset and late-stage osteoarthritis are not well characterized. However, with the introduction of cDNA-array technology *(1)*, the measurement of thousands of different genes in one small tissue sample can be carried out. Interpretation of gene expression analyses in articular cartilage is aided by the fact that this tissue contains only one cell type in normal and diseased conditions. Thus, changes in gene expression in osteoarthritic cartilage will be an effect produced only by the chondrocytes and not by other inflammatory cells, which may be present in the surrounding synovial fluid, for example.

From: *Methods in Molecular Medicine, Vol. 100: Cartilage and Osteoarthritis, Vol. 1: Cellular and Molecular Tools*
Edited by: M. Sabatini, P. Pastoureau, and F. De Ceuninck © Humana Press Inc., Totowa, NJ

2. Materials

1. 12X MES (2-[*N*-Morpholino]ethanesulfonic acid), 1.22 *M*, pH 6.6, 0.89 *M* [Na⁺]
(Sigma, St. Louis, MO).
2. 5X RNA fragmentation buffer: 200 m*M* Tris-acetate, pH 8.1, 500 m*M* KOAc,
150 m*M* MgOAc.
3. Phase lock gel (Brinkman Instruments, Westbury, NY).
4. DNAse (RNAse free; Qiagen, Hilden, Germany).
5. 20X SSPE: 3 *M* NaCl, 0.2 *M* NaH₂PO₄, 0.02 *M* EDTA.
6. Diethyl pyrocarbonate (DEPC; Carl Roth, Karlsruhe, Germany).
7. T7 (dT)₂₄ primer (5'-GGCCAGTGAATTGTAATACGACTCACTATAGGGAG
GCGG(dT)₂₄-3' and SuperScript Choice System for cDNA synthesis (Invitrogen
Life Technologies, Karlsruhe, Germany).
8. Herring sperm DNA (Promega, Madison, WI).
9. RNeasy kit (Qiagen).
10. Human cancer 1.2 cDNA arrays (BD Bioscience Clontech, Heidelberg, Germany).
11. Salmon testes DNA (Sigma-Aldrich Chemie GmbH, München, Germany).
12. Wash solution 1: 2X SSC (15 m*M* NaCl/1.5 m*M* Na₃ citrate) ,1% sodium dodecyl
sulfate (SDS).
13. Wash solution 2: 0.1X SSC (0.75 m*M* NaCl / 0.075 m*M* Na₃ citrate), 0.5% SDS.
14. [α-³²P]dATP: 3000 Ci/mmol, 10 µCi/µL (Amersham, Uppsala, Sweden).
15. Enzo BioArray HighYield RNA transcript labeling kit (Enzo Diagnostics,
Farmingdale, NY).
16. GeneChip® Eukaryotic Hybridization control kit (Affymetrix, Santa Clara, CA).
17. Affymetrix GeneChips® (Affymetrix).
18. Antibody solution mix: 1X MES stain buffer (100 m*M* MES, 1 *M* [Na⁺], 0.05%
Tween-20), 2 mg/mL acetylated bovine serum albumin (BSA; Invitrogen Life
Technologies), 0.1 mg/mL normal goat IgG (Sigma-Aldrich), 3 µg/mL
antistreptavidin antibody (Vector, Burlingame, CA).
19. SAPE (streptavidin/phycoerythrin) solution mix: 1X MES stain buffer (100 m*M*
MES, 1 *M* [Na⁺], 0.05% Tween-20), 2 mg/mL acetylated BSA, 10 µg/mL R-phy-
coerythrin streptavidin; Molecular Probes, Leiden, Netherlands).
20. GeneChip® Fluidics Station 400, GeneChip® Hybridization Oven, GeneChip®
Scanner (Affymetrix).
21. 6800 Freezer/Mill (SPEX CertiPrep, Metuchen, NJ).
22. PhosphorImager (e.g., Molecular Dynamics, Sunnyvale, CA, or Bio-Rad, Her-
cules, CA).

3. Methods

3.1. RNA Isolation

The effective isolation of sufficient amounts of high-quality RNA is of primary importance for gene expression analyses (e.g., Clontech: 2–50 µg total
RNA; Affymetrix: 5–10 µg total RNA). There are preamplification methods

available that reduce the starting amount of RNA required, but these methods can cause some technical problems and thus are not yet well established.

3.1.1. Isolation of RNA From Cultured Chondrocytes

The isolation of RNA from chondrocyte cultures can be done using conventional isolation protocols (e.g., Qiagen RNeasy isolation kits).

3.1.2. Isolation of RNA From Normal and Osteoarthritic Adult Cartilage

The isolation of large quantities of good-quality RNA directly from human adult articular cartilage is difficult owing to two main factors: (1) low cell number (2–3% chondrocytes per total mass of cartilage tissue) and (2) the presence of a proteoglycan-rich, highly crosslinked extracellular matrix. The major proteoglycan in articular cartilage, aggrecan, tends to copurify with the RNA because it is also a large, negatively charged macromolecule. The following protocol describes a reliable method for the isolation of reasonably high amounts of pure RNA from adult articular cartilage *(2)*.

3.1.2.1. TISSUE PREPARATION

Remove cartilage from the joint and freeze immediately in liquid nitrogen (slow freezing leads to degradation of RNA). Store the cartilage at –80°C until further use.

3.1.2.2. TISSUE HOMOGENIZATION

This is done in our laboratory using a SPEX CertiPrep freezer mill 6800 (*see* **Note 1**).

1. Precool a vial and tissue grinder apparatus in liquid nitrogen.
2. Fill SPEX CertiPrep 6751 vial with frozen cartilage tissue (approx 2.5 g maximum).
3. Insert two to four vials into the freezer mill. Following a precooling phase (2 min), grind the sample for five cycles of impact (2 min, at a frequency of 10 Hz) and cooling (2 min).
4. Homogenized tissue can be stored at –80°C prior to RNA isolation.

3.1.2.3. RNA ISOLATION

We use the RNeasy-kit from Qiagen with some modifications to the manufacturer's protocol.

1. Mix 1 g of milled cartilage powder with 5 mL of RLT lysis buffer (containing 10 µL/mL β-mercaptoethanol) at room temperature. Vortex to homogeneity (15 s) and centrifuge at 10,000g for 1 h.
2. To the cleared lysate, add an equal volume of 70% ethanol and vortex for 15 s.
3. Apply aliquots (3 mL) of the cleared lysate/ethanol mix sequentially to Qiagen RNeasy midi-columns. Centrifuge at 3360g for 1 min and repeat until all the lysate has been applied to the column (*see* **Note 2**).

4. DNAse digestion: add 3 mL (instead of the recommended 4 mL) of wash buffer RW1 to the column followed by 80 Kunitz units DNAse I in 210 µL RNAse-free DNAse buffer. Following digestion for 25 min at room temperature, apply another 3 mL of RW1 washing-buffer to the column and centrifuge at 3360g for 5 min.

5. Wash the column with 2.5 mL of RPE wash buffer and centrifuge twice at 3360g for 2 min. Centrifuge for a further 5 min to ensure complete removal of ethanol (present in wash buffer RPE) from the column.

6. Elute the RNA twice in 160 µL aliquots of DEPC-treated water by centrifugation at 3360g for 3 min.

3.1.2.4. RNA ANALYSIS AND QUANTIFICATION

1. Agarose gel electrophoresis: analyze two aliquots of isolated RNA (1 and 5 µL) on either 1.2% formaldehyde-agarose denaturing gels or on 1.2% agarose gels. (Conventional DNA gels are usually sufficient.) Gel electrophoresis will determine whether the RNA is degraded or whether there is contamination of genomic DNA as well as provide a rough estimation of RNA concentration.

2. Spectrophotometry: measure an aliquot of RNA at 260 and 280 nm (or, if needed, perform a full spectrum analysis from 230 to 400 nm). This allows quantification of RNA concentration as well as RNA purity (i.e., a low OD_{260}/OD_{280} ratio suggests protein contamination; *see* also **Note 3**).

3.2. cDNA Array Analysis

A DNA microarray, or gene-chip, is defined as a matrix of hundreds or thousands of DNA fragments (>200 bp) or oligonucleotides (20–80 bp) bound to a solid support (e.g., nylon membranes or glass slides). Labeled cDNA from the tissue or cell type of interest is hybridized to its complementary sequence on the gene-chip and then the relative abundance of mRNA in the sample is estimated. The final readout from this hybridization experiment gives what is referred to as an *expression profile* of genes in a given sample. A flow chart summarizing the gene profiling approach is shown in **Fig. 1**.

3.2.1. Gene Expression Analysis Parameters

Some basic parameters have to be considered when performing gene expression analysis:

1. *Complexity of the array:* the number and selection of genes on the array chip will determine the success in identifiying genes of interest. Gene-chips are available containing less than 100 different genes (often custom-made according to the needs of the user) up to more than 10,000 genes.

2. *Type of cDNA labeling:* radioactive as well as fluorescent (e.g., rhodamine, fluorescein, Cy3, or Cy5) labeling can be used depending on the array type. Utilizing two different-colored fluorochromes allows direct visualization of samples showing different expression profiles. Radioactive labeling of cDNA offers greater

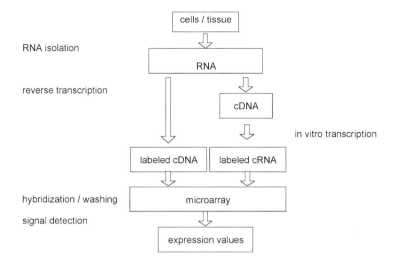

Fig. 1. Basic workflow scheme of a gene profiling approach. After isolation of total RNA from the cells or tissues of interest, cDNA is generated by reverse transcription. Usually, this step is directly combined with labeling of the cDNA. In some protocols (e.g., Affymetrix) an amplification step is introduced using an additional in vitro transcription step of the cDNA for probe labeling. The labeled cDNA/cRNA is hybridized to the immobilized DNA on a microarray. After stringent washing the amount of bound target DNA is determined by counting the radioactivity on the microarray.

sensitivity but lacks the ability to compare two different sets of mRNA pools directly.

3. *RNA quality:* the quality of RNA used to make probes is the most important factor influencing the sensitivity and reproducibility of the hybridization results (for RNA isolation, *see* **Subheading 3.1.**). Contaminated or partially degraded RNA may lead to high background and thus, inaccurate hybridization patterns.

    Both total RNA or poly(A)⁺RNA have been used successfully as a starting material for the generation of probes. In our laboratory, we usually use total RNA.

4. *cDNA synthesis:* the reverse transcription reaction usually starts from the poly(A)-tail of the oligo(dT)-primed mRNA molecule. Since all oligo(dT)-primed-mRNAs are not reverse-transcribed with the same efficiency (a process that begins at the 3'end of the RNA molecule), random primers are sometimes preferred since reverse transcription can be initiated throughout the mRNA molecule. However, use of random primers can also lead to reverse transcription (and hence labeling) of irrelevant mRNA species such as ribosomal RNA and transfer RNA; these are not labeled if oligo(dT)-primers are used. The use of gene-specific primers for reverse transcription (e.g., Clontech Cancer array) ensures only the synthesis of cDNAs corresponding to genes present on the particular array. Therefore, the

hybridization probes created here are significantly less complex than those generated using oligo(dT) or random primers. This results in increased sensitivity with a concomitant reduction of nonspecific background in the array experiment.

It should be noted that, since the reverse transcription reaction is not equally efficient for all genes under analysis, the intensities of hybridized probes ("spots") can only be compared for the same gene between different assays and not between different genes in one assay.

5. *Hybridization and posthybridization conditions:* these important parameters are provided by the manufacturer. Particularly, the sensitivity and specificity of probes are of major concern in all array systems (*see* **Note 4**).

3.2.2. Nylon Membrane-Based cDNA Arrays: Experimental Protocol

Nylon membranes may contain hundreds to more than a thousand different cDNAs. For our studies, we used the Human Cancer 1.2 cDNA AtlasTM arrays (Clontech), which are nylon membranes containing 1185 cDNAs (a typical result is shown in **Fig. 2A**).

3.2.2.1. PROBE SYNTHESIS FROM TOTAL RNA: REVERSE TRANSCRIPTION

The reverse transcription reaction described below converts 2–5 µg of total RNA into radioactive-labeled first-strand cDNA (one can use ^{32}P-, ^{33}P- or ^{35}S-labeled deoxyribonucleotides). All components are contained in the Human Cancer 1.2 cDNA Atlas kit.

Fig. 2. *(opposite page)* **(A)** RNA (5 µg total) was isolated from human articular cartilage and hybridized with the Atlas human cancer 1.2 cDNA array (Clontech). The detected dots correspond to the amount of labeled probes hybridized to cDNAs representing the arrayed genes. **(B–D)** The study of chondrocyte gene expression is always linked to the main function of this cell type, which is the preservation and turnover of the cartilage matrix. Thus, matrix components and matrix-degrading proteases were a focus of interest in this study. In our analysis of the extracellular matrix proteins *(21)*, we could confirm an absence of cartilage collagen expression in normal cartilage. mRNA levels of several collagen genes were identified in advanced osteoarthritis, however **(B)**. With regard to the cartilage matrix-degrading metalloproteinases, MMP-3 (stromelysin) was surprisingly downregulated in the diseased tissue **(C)**. Instead, other degradation pathways appeared to be more important involving proteases such as MMP-2 (gelatinase A) and MMP-13 (collagenase 3) **(D)**. Both MMP-2 and MMP-13 are known to be involved in terminal breakdown of cartilage collagen fibers. Bars, means with indicated standard deviations; significance levels: *, $p < 0.05$; **, $p < 0.01$; ***, $p < 0.001$). OA, osteoarthritis.

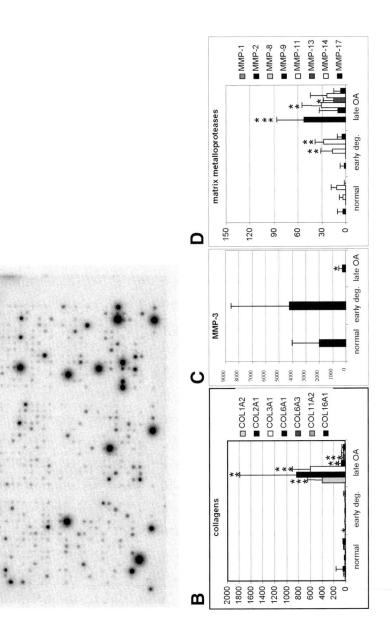

1. Preparation of the "reaction mix" (carried out at room temperature):

5X reaction buffer (for the specific enzyme)	2.0 μL
10X dNTP mix	1.0 μL
(for dATP labeling, the dNTP mix contains *5 mM each of dCTP, dGTP and dTTP)*	
[α-^{32}P]dATP (3000 Ci/mmol, 10 μCi/μL)	3.5 μL
Dithiothreitol (DTT; 100 m*M*)	0.5 μL
Total volume/assay	7.0 μL

2. Preparation of the RNA/primer mix (in a 0.5-mL PCR tube):

5X reaction buffer (for the specific enzyme)	2.0 μL
RNA	2–5 μg (1–2 μL)
Primer mix	1 μL
H$_2$O	X μL
Total volume/assay	3 μL

3. Reverse Transcription.
   a. Mix the RNA/primer mix by pipeting followed by a brief centrifugation step.
   b. Incubate at 70°C for 2 min. (We use a PCR cycler, which allows rapid cooldown to 50°C.)
   c. Incubate at 50°C for 2 min. During this incubation step, add 1 μL murine Moloney leukemia virus (MMLV) reverse transcriptase and mix by pipeting. The reaction mix is at room temperature at this stage.
   d. Immediately add 7 μL of the reaction mix to 3 μL RNA/primer mix.
   e. Incubate at 50°C for 25 min.
   f. Stop the reaction by addition of 1 μL 10X termination mix (provided by the manufacturer).
   g. Labeled probes can be stored on ice at 4°C for a few hours, if necessary.

3.2.2.2. Hybridization Procedure

The hybridization procedure is performed as described in the manufacturer's hybridization protocol (all components are contained in the Human Cancer 1.2 cDNA Atlas kit.):

3.2.2.2.1. Preparation of Hybridization Solution

1. Prewarm 5 mL of BD ExpressHyb solution to 68°C.
2. Heat 0.5 mg of the sheared salmon testes DNA at 95–100°C for 5 min, and then chill quickly on ice.
3. Mix heat-denatured sheared salmon testes DNA with prewarmed BD ExpressHyb solution.
4. Store at 68°C until use.

3.2.2.2.2. Preincubation

1. Place the membrane into a bottle filled with deionized H_2O. After discarding the water, the membrane should adhere around the inside of the bottle without creating air bubbles.
2. Add 5 mL of the hybridization solution prepared as described in **Subheading 3.2.2.2.** (Ensure that the solution is evenly distributed over the membrane.)
3. Prehybridize the nylon membrane for 30 min with continuous agitation at 68°C.

3.2.2.2.3. Probe Preparation

1. Heat the radiolabeled probe (95–100°C) in a water bath for 2 min.
2. Transfer immediately onto ice for 2 min.
3. Add the labeled probe to the prehybridization solution coating the nylon membrane inside the bottle. Ensure that the probe is equally distributed over the membrane.
4. Hybridize the membrane overnight with continuous agitation at 68°C. If necessary, add an extra 2–3 mL of prewarmed BD ExpressHyb solution in order to ensure even coverage of the filter during the incubation period.

3.2.2.2.4. Washing Procedure

1. Prewarm wash solution 1 (2X SSC, 1% SDS) and wash solution 2 (0.1X SSC, 0.5% SDS) at 68°C.
2. Carefully remove the hybridization solution.
3. Wash the membrane four times in 200 mL of prewarmed wash solution 1 for 30 min at 68°C with continuous agitation.
4. Wash twice in 200 mL of prewarmed wash solution 2 for 30 min at 68°C with continuous agitation.
5. Finally, wash twice with 200 mL SSC for 5 min at room temperature.

3.2.2.2.5. Signal Detection

1. Remove the membrane from the bottle and wrap in plastic cling-film to keep it moist.
2. Expose the membrane array to a storage phosphor screen.

3.2.2.3. IDENTIFICATION OF LABELED, HYBRIDIZED "SPOTS"

Different software tools can be used for the detection and quantification of hybridized cDNA spots, depending on the array systems. For the Atlas Nylon cDNA Expression Arrays, we use the Clontech Atlas Image 1.01 software. Updated versions of this software are now available. It is also useful to analyze the spots by eye, if possible, in order to confirm the accuracy of the detection methodology. A spot is considered positive if it is easily located, "roundish," and has an intensity more than twofold above the background level.

Other parameters of data acquisition such as technical reproducibility, assay sensitivity, and signal quantification are not discussed in this chapter. The reader should see recently published reviews describing these issues in more

3. Wash the GeneChip with nonstringent wash buffer at 25°C (10 cycles of 2 mixes/ cycle).
4. Wash with stringent wash buffer (100 mM MES, 0.1 M [Na$^+$], 0.01% Tween-20) at 50°C (four cycles of 15 mixes/cycle).
5. Stain with SAPE solution for 30 min at 25°C .
6. Wash with nonstringent wash buffer at 25°C (10 cycles of 4 mixes/cycle).
7. Incubate with antibody solution for 10 min at 25°C .
8. Stain with SAPE solution for 10 min at 25°C.
9. Wash the GeneChip with nonstringent wash buffer at 30°C (15 cycles of 4 mixes/ cycle).
10. The gene-chip arrays are then analyzed twice with a confocal scanner (Hewlett-Packard Gene Array scanner) using an argon laser ($\lambda_{excitation}$ = 488 nm, $\lambda_{emission}$ = 570 nm).

3.2.3.4. PRIMARY DATA ANALYSIS

1. The array images are acquired and quantitated with Affymetrix Microarray Suite 4.0.1.
2. The images (saved as .dat files) are initially controlled visually, and subsequently the files for cell intensity (.cel) and chip intensity (.chp) are generated.
3. Next, the scans to be compared are normalized ("globalized": *see* **Subheading 3.3.**). For each gene, the average difference intensity (ADI) is calculated, which reflects the transcript level of a gene. Essentially, for each probe pair, the mismatch (MM) intensity is subtracted from the perfect match (PM) intensity, and the average for all the probe pairs for a specific gene is calculated excluding outliers (**Fig. 3**).
4. In addition, a decision matrix is employed to render a gene either absent (A), present (P), or marginal (M). Data files containing intensity values as well as A and P information can be exported and processed further using available software packages (*see* also **Note 5**).
5. In a recent experiment, we analyzed the effect of interleukin-1β (Il-1β) on cultured human articular chondrocytes (**Fig. 4B**) and found a significant alteration in gene expression. In comparison, **Fig. 4A** shows the technical scatter of genes using identical control RNAs in two independent analyses.

3.3. Normalization

A prerequisite for biologically meaningful comparisons between microarrays is that the data have to be adjusted to the same scale (i.e., "normalized"). In large-scale gene expression biotechnology, "globalization" is the most commonly used normalization method: for each array, all measured values are divided by their sum (or average). This method is based on the assumption that the amount of mRNA per cell is constant. However, the sum of all expression signals is often dominated by the strongest signals *(10,11)*. Such highly expressed genes are most likely to be regulated as they represent the major expression products of specialized cells (e.g., immunoglobulin chains for plasma cells, hemoglobin for erythro-

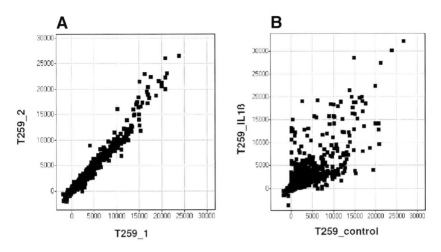

Fig. 4. (A) The same target material (prepared from T259 RNA of in vitro cultured primary chondrocytes) was hybridized consecutively onto two HG-U95Av2 GeneChips. The intensities (ADI; *see* **Subheading 3.2.3.**, Primary data analysis) for each gene (represented as squares) are plotted for the two scanned GeneChips. High technical reproducibility is recognizeable since most genes reside on a diagonale. **(B)** Diagram showing the effect of IL-1β treatment on primary human chondrocytes in vitro. RNA from nontreated primary chondrocytes (T259_control) and cells treated with IL-1β for 24 h (T259_IL1) was labeled and hybridized onto HG-U95Av2 GeneChips.

blasts). For this reason, we recently proposed a method ("centralization": http://www.scai.fhg.de/bio/centralization.html) that rests on the weaker assumption that the regulation of gene expression is well behaved, i.e., that most genes are either not regulated or only moderately regulated. The choice of normalization method is important in order to avoid false findings *(11)*.

3.4. Evaluation of Gene Expression Data: How to Proceed From Data to Understanding

Given reliable data on gene expression levels, the real challenge of functional genomics then has to be addressed, i.e., how to interpret results from a mass of data and relate them to an understanding of the processes in a biological system or disease. Fundamentals of such efforts, as outlined below, include:

1. Pre-existing knowledge of relevant biological systems (*genes of known relevance*; an example for cartilage research is outlined in **Fig. 2B–D**).
2. Ranking genes according to biostatistical significance (p-*value-approach*).
3. The comparison of gene expression patterns with those found in vivo (*evo-devo-approach*) or in vitro models.

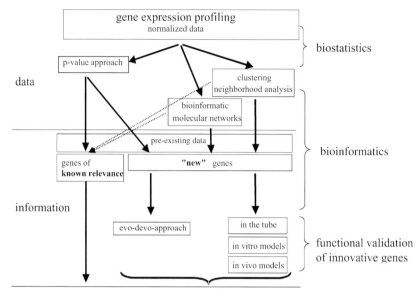

knowledge   integrated concepts of physiology and pathology

Fig. 5. "Functional genomics" in many cases starts from gene expression analysis, which yields a huge amount of unstructured primary data. Biostatistical evaluation then allows one to highlight directly the significance levels of differentially expressed genes of defined interest. Genes also become a focus of interest if they show significant differential regulation or show close clustering to other well-defined genes. Improved computational tools will further allow us to search specifically for biologically relevant molecular networks, or parts of them. These "new" genes will have to be validated for their relevance in the respective disease process, e.g., osteoarthritis. Analyzing both gene expression and function during evolution and development (evo-devo-approach) as well as pursuing functional assays of the genes in a test tube (molecular approaches), in vitro (cell culture) or in vivo (animal models, transgenic approaches) will establish the roles of these molecules in physiology and pathology.

4. Bioinformatical tools (*clustering and neighborhood-analyses*).
5. A combination of preexisting knowledge and computational processing of obtained data (i.e., bioinformatical pathway modeling. A possible workflow diagram is shown in **Fig. 5**).
6. Final confirmation of a revealed pattern then requires functional validation so that the molecular networks can be identified.

3.4.1. Search for Novel Genes of Interest

1. *The p-value approach.* A basic but useful method of analysis is the search for differentially expressed genes between groups of samples (e.g., normal vs dis-

eased tissue). Parametric tests are most commonly used but are based on the assumption that the data follow a specific distribution, e.g., the *t*-test assumes a normal distribution. Although gene expression levels seem to follow other distributions, transformations have been proposed in order to achieve normal distributions. Another solution is offered by distribution-free tests, e.g., the rank sum test and new tests developed specifically for expression data *(12,13)*. Either way, one should be aware that, owing to the high numbers of genes assayed, low *p* values may still lead to many false positives. Therefore derived measures, such as the false discovery rate *(14)*, may be more helpful in practice.

2. *Clustering and neighborhood analyses.* In addition to analyses at the single-gene level, many algorithms are available to cluster genes or tissue samples, or to perform neighborhood analyses with the whole dataset in an attempt to identify coregulated genes. In fact, depending on the stringency of the clustering criteria applied, one can find various numbers of gene clusters such as those containing most of the ribosomal genes and others containing regulated collagen genes, etc. *(15)*. However, clustering and neighborhood analyses as such are only of limited value as long as they lack integration with overall knowledge on the genes involved.

3. *Validation of novel genes.* Regardless of what successful bioinformatical analysis is performed, validation of the cellular role and molecular function of a detected gene is of primary importance. This area of "functional genomics" represents the most challenging task in terms of study design and manpower required. Even when the functions of well-characterized gene products are known in other contexts, it is not guaranteed that they will fulfill similar functions in the system under study.

   a. *The evo-devo-approach.* One way to attempt to understand regulatory patterns of mature cells and tissues in the adult is to exploit the fact that in many conditions, processes that occurred during evolution and individual development are recapitulated. Although an evolutionary model for cartilage has not really been established, the fetal growth plate of cartilage has served as a long-standing model in the study of chondrocyte behavior during development. In addition, the established chondrocyte phenotypes are mainly based on observations of events that occur in the growth plate. Furthermore, processes known to be central in osteoarthritic cartilage degeneration, such as matrix anabolism and catabolism and, in particular, cellular differentiation, are observed within the fetal growth plate. It remains a challenging task to delineate which patterns are found in which spatiotemporal sequence in the diseased tissue as well.

   b. *In vivo and in vitro models.* Clearly, in vivo (animal) models are of paramount importance for any disease area in order to understand the disease processes clearly and what happens if these processes are modified. Unfortunately, no generally accepted animal model for osteoarthritis is available at the moment. Isolated articular chondrocytes (in vitro models) have been known for a long time to be susceptible to drastic alterations of their gene expression pattern. This is in response to modulating factors such as cytokines and growth factors

2. McKenna, L. A., Gehrsitz, A., Soeder, S., Eger, W., Kirchner, T., and Aigner, T. (2000) Effective isolation of high quality total RNA from human adult articular cartilage. *Anal. Biochem.* **286,** 80–85.

3. Grant, E. P., Pickard, M. D., Briskin, M. J., and Gutierrez-Ramos, J. C. (2002) Gene expression profiles: creating new perspectives in arthritis research. *Arthritis Rheum.* **46,** 874–884.

4. Lockhart, D. J. and Winzeler, E. A. (2000) Genomics, gene expression and DNA array. *Nature* **405,** 827–836.

5. Quackenbush, J. (2001) Computational analysis of microarray data. *Nat. Rev. Genet.* **2,** 418–427.

6. Schulze, A. and Downward, J. (2001) Navigating gene expression using microarrays—a technology review. *Nat. Cell Biol.* **3,** E190–E195.

7. Lipshutz, R. J., Fodor, S. P., Gingeras, T. R., and Lockhart, D. J. (1999) High density synthetic oligonucleotide arrays. *Nat. Genet.* **21,** 20–24.

8. Lockhart, D. J., Dong, H., Byrne, M. C., et al. (1996) Expression monitoring by hybridization to high-density oligonucleotide arrays. *Nat. Biotechnol.* **14,** 1675–1680.

9. Eberwine, J., Yeh, H., Miyashiro, K., et al. (1992) Analysis of gene expression in single live neurons. *Proc. Natl. Acad. Sci. USA* **89,** 3010–3014.

10. Velculescu, V. E., Madden, S. L., Zhang, L., et al. (1999) Analysis of human transcriptomes. *Nat. Genet.* **23,** 387–388.

11. Zien, A., Aigner, T., Zimmer, R., and Lengauer, T. (2001) Centralization: a new paradigm for the normalization of gene expression data. *Bioinformatics* **17,** S323–S331.

12. Ben Dor, A., Bruhn, L., Friedman, N., Nachman, I., Schummer, M., and Yakhini, Z. (2000) Tissue classification with gene expression profiles. *J. Comput. Biol.* **7,** 559–583.

13. Manduchi, E., Grant, G. R., McKenzie, S. E., Overton, G. C., Surrey, S., and Stoeckert, C. J., Jr. (2000) Generation of patterns from gene expression data by assigning confidence to differentially expressed genes. *Bioinformatics* **16,** 685–698.

14. Benjamini, Y., Drai, D., Elmer, G., Kafkafi, N., and Golani, I. (2001) Controlling the false discovery rate in behavior genetics research. *Behav. Brain Res.* **125,** 279–284.

15. Erickson, G. R., Gimble, J. M., Franklin, D. M., Rice, H. E., Awad, H., and Guilak, F. (2002) Chondrogenic potential of adipose tissue-derived stromal cells in vitro and in vivo. *Biochem. Biophys. Res. Commun.* **290,** 763–769.

16. Goldring, M. B., Birkhead, J. R., Sandell, L. J., Kimura, T., and Krane, S. M. (1988) Interleukin 1 suppresses expression of cartilage-specific types II and IX collagens and increases types I and III collagens in human chondrocytes. *J. Clin. Invest.* **82,** 2026–2037.

17. Benya, P. D. and Shaffer, J. D. (1982) Dedifferentiated chondrocytes reexpress the differentiated collagen phenotype when cultured in agarose gels. *Cell* **30,** 215–224.

18. von der Mark, K., Gauss, V., von der Mark, H., and Müller, P. K. (1977) Relationship between cell shape and type of collagen synthesized as chondrocytes lose their cartilage phenotype in culture. *Nature* **267,** 531–532.

19. Kolettas, E., Buluwela, L., Bayliss, M. T., and Muir, H. I. (1995) Expression of cartilage-specific molecules is retained on long- term culture of human articular chondrocytes. *J. Cell Sci.* **108,** 1991–1999.
20. Attur, M. G., Dave, M. N., Tsunoyama, K., et al. (2002) "A system biology" approach to bioinformatics and functional genomics in complex human diseases: arthritis. *Curr. Issues Mol. Biol.* **4,** 129–146.
21. Aigner, T., Zien, A., Gehrsitz, A., Gebhard, P. M., and McKenna, L. A. (2001) Anabolic and catabolic gene expression pattern analysis in normal versus osteoarthritic cartilage using complementary DNA-array technology. *Arthritis Rheum.* **44,** 2777–2789.

11

High-Efficiency Nonviral
Transfection of Primary Chondrocytes

Jean F. Welter, Luis A. Solchaga, and Matthew C. Stewart

Summary

The introduction of foreign DNA into mammalian cells is an essential investigative tool in molecular biology. Nonviral approaches to transfection offer the advantage of relatively simple vector design, production, and purification and, for tissue engineering applications, avoid many of the potential risks associated with virus-mediated transfection methods. Unfortunately, primary cells, and in particular chondrocytes, are notoriously refractory to conventional transfection approaches, and optimized transfection efficiencies in these cells are extremely low (1–1.5%). In this chapter, we present three protocols that have proved useful in transfecting primary chondrocytes at high efficiency (~70%). The first uses radiofrequency electroporation, a transfection method that frequently works extremely well in cell types that are difficult to transfect. It should be noted that electroporation is not limited to DNA but that essentially any molecule can be introduced into the cell using this approach. In addition to the primary protocol, we present two additional reliable, albeit less efficient backup protocols, the first using exponential decay electroporation and the second FuGENE™ 6 transfection.

Key Words: Chondrocytes; transfection; nonviral transfection; electroporation; radio frequency electroporation; exponential decay electroporation; FuGENE™ 6 transfection.

1. Introduction

The introduction of foreign DNA into mammalian cells is an essential investigative tool in molecular biology. It is used analytically for the study of gene promoter function and functional testing of proteins, and has the potential to be used therapeutically to augment tissue engineering endeavors. Nonviral approaches to transfection offer the advantage of relatively simple vector design, production, and purification, and, for tissue engineering appli-

From: *Methods in Molecular Medicine, Vol. 100: Cartilage and Osteoarthritis, Vol. 1: Cellular and Molecular Tools*
Edited by: M. Sabatini, P. Pastoureau, and F. De Ceuninck © Humana Press Inc., Totowa, NJ

cations, avoidance of many of the potential risks associated with virus-mediated transfection methods *(1)*.

Highly efficient methods for transfecting established cell lines are used routinely in the laboratory; commercially available, off-the-shelf systems easily achieve transfection efficiencies on the order of 70% for many established cell lines. Unfortunately, some cell types, in particular primary cells, respond poorly to these approaches. Chondrocytes are notoriously recalcitrant, and optimized transfection efficiencies in these cells are on the order of only 1–5% using conventional approaches *(2)*. Higher efficiencies have been reported using more complex delivery methods *(3,4)*.

Electroporation is a transfection approach that frequently works well for cell types that are refractory to other methods of transfection. In this approach, cells are subjected to a brief electric field pulse of appropriate waveform, amplitude, and duration *(5–8)*. This exposure results in the transient permeabilization of the cytoplasmic membrane, which allows extracellular molecules to enter the cell. However, a subset of the cells does not recover from the membrane breakdown, and a high rate of cell death may occur *(9)*. Depending on the subsequent disposition of the cells, the survival rate may become important. For example, to initiate pellet *(10)* or micromass *(11)* chondrogenesis, a minimum concentration of viable cells is required. Usually, cells are electroporated in suspension in a specialized cuvet that incorporates a pair of planar electrodes. However, it can be applied to adherent cells or even used in vivo *(12–18)*. Furthermore, it should be noted that electroporation is not limited to DNA, but that essentially any molecule can be introduced into the cell using this approach *(8)*.

An electroporation variant, known as radiofrequency (RF) electroporation, which combines squarewave and radiofrequency (5–50 kHz) AC pulses to transfect the cells, was introduced by Donald Chang in the late 1980s *(19,20)*. The primary advantages of this method over conventional (exponential decay) electroporation are equal or better transfection efficiencies, lower cell death, and lower DNA requirements *(21,22)*. Transfection efficiencies of better than 30% can be achieved routinely, and with cell type-specific optimization and careful handling of the cells, the efficiency can exceed 70% of the surviving cells. This system has proved extremely valuable for transfecting otherwise difficult cell types.

Our primary approach to high-efficiency transfection of primary chondrocytes utilizes RF electroporation and is discussed in this chapter. We use a commercial system, the Bio-Rad Gene Pulser II with the RF module. In addition to the primary protocol, we present two additional reliable, albeit less efficient backup protocols, the first using exponential decay electroporation, and the second, FuGENE™ 6 transfection.

2. Materials

2.1. Primary Protocol: RF Electroporation

1. A Bio-Rad Gene Pulser II with RF module or equivalent device (Bio-Rad cat. no. 165-2105 and 165-2112; *see* **Note 1**).
2. Sterile electroporation cuvets: 2-mm electrode gap electroporation cuvets (Bio-Rad cat. no. 165-2086, or similar).
3. Electroporation buffer: 272 m*M* sucrose, 7 m*M* sodium phosphate, pH 7.4, 1 m*M* MgCl$_2$. Prepare the solution, and then filter sterilize using a 0.2-µm filter. Store frozen aliquots at –20°C.
4. Chondrocytes.
5. Plasmid DNA.
6. Complete growth medium without antibiotics (*see* **Note 2**): 0.25% trypsin (Invitrogen Life Technologies, Carlsbad, CA, cat. no. 15050057), calcium- and magnesium-free Hanks' balanced salt solution (HBSS; Invitrogen Life Technologies, CA, cat. no. 14170112), sterile T$_{10}$E$_1$ (10 m*M* Tris HCl, 1 m*M* EDTA in sterile water, pH 8.0) or water.
7. Standard tissue culture equipment and supplies: incubator, cell culture hood, inverted microscope, hemacytometer, tissue culture plasticware, sterile Pasteur pipets (any supplier).

2.2. Backup Protocol 1: Exponential Decay Electroporation

1. A Bio-Rad Gene Pulser II with the Capacitance Extender II and (optionally) Pulse Controller Plus modules (Bio-Rad cat. no. 165-2105, 165-2107, and 165-2110)
2. Sterile 4-mm electrode gap electroporation cuvets (Bio-Rad cat. no. 165-2088, or similar).
3. Electroporation buffer: Ca^{2+} and Mg^{2+}-free Tyrode's solution supplemented with 5% calf serum.
4. Chondrocytes, plasmid DNA, growth medium, trypsin, HBSS, sterile T$_{10}$E$_1$ or water, standard equipment and supplies: *see* **Subheading 2.1.**, items **4–7**.

2.3. Backup Protocol 2: FuGENE 6 Transfection

1. FuGENE 6 Transfection Reagent (Roche Diagnostics, Indianapolis, IN, cat. no. P/N 1 814 443).
2. Chondrocytes, plasmid DNA, standard equipment and supplies: *see* **Subheading 2.1.**, items **4**, **5**, and **7**.
3. Opti-MEM I® reduced serum medium (Invitrogen Life Technologies, cat. no. 31985070).
4. Sterile 1.5-mL Eppendorf tubes.
5. Ultra Low Attachment plates (Corning Costar, Acton, MA, cat. no. 3473)

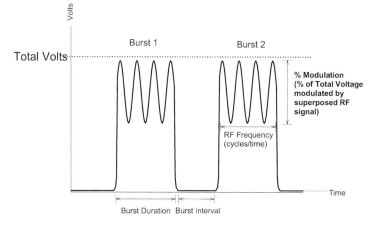

Fig. 1. Schematic of principal components of an radio frequency (RF) electroporation burst train. Two representative bursts are shown.

3. Methods

3.1. Primary Protocol: RF Electroporation

In this approach, the cells are exposed to an electrical field that varies over time in a complex, preprogrammed waveform, or burst, resulting from the superposition of a RF and a DC pulse of the same width. Trains of identical bursts can be delivered. The critical parameters are illustrated in **Fig. 1**, and include total voltage, RF frequency,% modulation, and burst duration, number, and interval. This approach works best in low conductivity buffers.

3.1.1. Planning

Determine the total number of transfections required for the experiment. Usually, we use 3×10^5 to 1×10^6 cells per transfection, with 6×10^5 working best for human chondrocytes.

3.1.2. Setting up
3.1.2.1. GENERAL

Wipe down the work area in the cell culture hood with 70% ethanol. Prepare and label a sterile conical tube for each cell-plasmid combination to be tested, and the required number of cell culture plates to receive the transfected cells. Time requirements will, of course, vary with the scale of the experiment, but they are minimal. In general, the apparatus can be set up in 5 min. Trypsinizing, washing, and counting the cells can be accomplished in 45 min, and the actual electroporation step takes about 1 min for each cuvet.

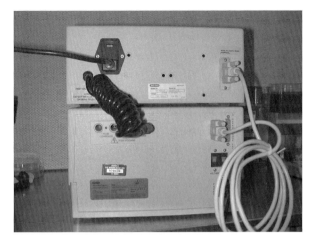

Fig. 2. Rear panel electrical connections for RF electroporation using the Bio-Rad Gene Pulser II and RF modules.

3.1.2.2. SETTING UP THE ELECTROPORATOR

(These instructions refer to the Bio-Rad Gene Pulser II equipment. Refer to the appropriate user's manual if you are using a different unit.)

1. Place the electroporation apparatus in a corner of the cell culture hood.
2. At the back of the machine, connect the 9-pin D connector from the RF module port labeled *Gene Pulser II Rear* to the base unit port labeled *Accessory*. This should be the only D connector cord connected to the base unit.
3. Connect the high voltage leads (thick black coiled cord) from the RF module to the socket labeled *Capacitance Extender* on the base module. This should be the only coiled cord connected to the base unit.
4. Plug both power cords into grounded outlets. When done, the setup should look like **Fig. 2**.
5. Connect cuvet holder to the RF module, not to the base module. Set the rotary switch on the base unit to *High Cap*. Now, turn on the electroporator base unit and RF modules.

3.1.2.3. PROGRAMMING THE ELECTROPORATOR

(These instructions refer to the Bio-Rad Gene Pulser II equipment. Refer to the appropriate user's manual if you are using a different unit.)

1. On the RF unit, make sure the black knob is pointing to any position other than OFF, and then press both red buttons on the base unit simultaneously. The base unit is now in RF mode, and the display should read -*rf*- (**Fig. 3**).
2. Program the electroporator to run the desired parameters using the front panel controls on the RF module (**Fig. 3**). We have optimized the following parameters for human chondrocytes:

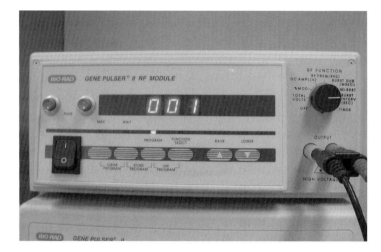

Fig. 3. Front panel of the RF module. Rotary function selector at right, and touch keys at left. Note high-voltage connection to the electroporation cuvet at the lower right. This connection should not be made to the similar set of output jacks on the base unit.

Total Volts	25 V (125 V/cm)
% Modulation	100
RF frequency	30 kHz
Burst duration	2 ms
No. of bursts	10
Burst interval	0.1 s

3. Program each parameter in turn by selecting it with the *Function Select* knob and using the *Raise* and *Lower* buttons to adjust the setting to the desired value (**Fig. 3**). When done, save the program, using the *Save Program* buttons on the front panel (*see* also **Note 3**).

3.1.3. DNA

The DNA should be highly purified. We have found Qiagen column purification to be adequate. The DNA should be washed thoroughly with 70% ethanol to remove residual salts.

1. Resuspend the DNA in a sterile, low ionic strength vehicle ($T_{10}E_1$ or water), at high concentration (1 µg/µL or greater) to minimize the volume contribution of the plasmid to the overall transfection mix. Ten micrograms per transfection works well, but considerably less will also yield positive transfections. The amount of DNA will impact on the transfection efficiency, so it is important to maintain a consistent concentration between experiments.
2. Heat the plasmid DNA solution to 70°C for 5–10 min, vortex briefly, and then, using sterile technique, deposit the plasmid volume required at the bottom of a sterile conical tube prepared as in **Subheading 3.1.2.1.**

3.1.4. Cells

For human chondrocytes, 6×10^5 cells per electroporation work best. One can expect approx 70% survival at the recommended parameters. Cells that are subconfluent just before the electroporation seem to survive the process better. The cells should be treated gently: prolonged trypsinization, vigorous pipeting, high g-forces during centrifugation, and prolonged dwell time in the electroporation buffer all have a negative impact on transfection efficiency and viability.

1. Trypsinize the cells after rinsing with HBSS. Check the plates every few min, and stop the trypsinization using complete medium once the cells are free floating.
2. Centrifuge the cell suspension in 50-mL conical tubes ($250g$, 6 min) and remove the supernatant. Resuspend the cells in the electroporation buffer.
3. Centrifuge ($250g$, 6 min) and remove the supernatant. Repeat this washing step once, and then resuspend the cells in electroporation buffer.
4. Count the cells using a hemacytometer and adjust the volume with electroporation buffer so that there are 1.5×10^6 cells/mL (6×10^5 cells per 400 µL—the volume between the cuvet electrodes in a 2-mm cuvet).

3.1.5. Electroporation

Select the desired electroporation program (*see* **Subheading 3.1.2.3.**). To switch between stored programs, adjust the program number using up and down arrows, and then press the two buttons labeled *USE PROGRAM* simultaneously. U*nn* will be displayed, with *nn* being the number of the program now in use. The following steps should be completed quickly, so the cells do not have time to sediment.

1. Gently mix the required volume of cells with the DNA in the labeled conical tubes.
2. Transfer 400 µL of the cell/DNA mixture to an electroporation cuvet, and place the cuvet in the slider of the electroporation cuvet holder. The cuvet is keyed and will fit easily in one orientation only. Push the slider into the holder until it engages with a click.
3. Press and hold both red buttons on the RF unit simultaneously until a beep sounds. Release the buttons.

3.1.6. Post Electroporation

Best results are achieved if the time between trypsinization of the cells and their return to normal medium after the electroporation is kept at a minimum (*see* **Note 4**).

1. Immediately remove the cuvet from the holder and add 1 mL of antibiotic-free medium to the cuvet.
2. Gently aspirate the cell suspension from the cuvet using a sterile pipette and plate it in the desired final volume of antibiotic-free medium.
3. Return the plated cells to the cell culture incubator. If stable tranfectants are desired, selection can begin after 24–48 h (*see* **Note 5**).

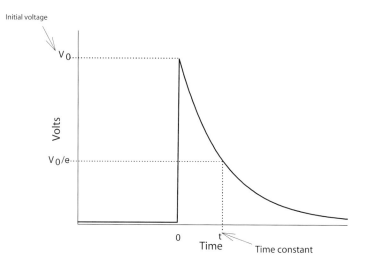

Fig. 4. Schematic of principal components of an exponential decay electroporation pulse. V_0 = initial voltage, τ = time constant = time for voltage to decay from V_0 to V_0/e.

3.2. Backup Protocol 1: Exponential Decay Electroporation

In this approach, the cells are exposed to a single pulse which decays exponentially through time. The pulse is defined by two pulse parameters, the initial field strength (kV/cm) and the time constant (τ) (**Fig. 4**). Both of these must be optimized for each cell type. The field strength is the initial voltage V_0 input into electroporator divided by the distance between the cuvet electrodes. The time constant τ is equivalent to the amount of time it takes for V_0 to drop to V_0/e (i.e., about 37% of V_0). τ is also the product of the total resistance and capacitance of the pulse circuit ($\tau = R \times C$) in ms, Ω, μF, respectively. It is thus dependent on the conductivity and the amount of buffer between the electrodes.

3.2.1. Planning (see **Subheading 3.1.1.**)

3.2.2. Setting Up

3.2.2.1. SETTING UP THE ELECTROPORATOR

(These instructions refer to the Bio-Rad Gene Pulser II equipment. Refer to the appropriate user's manual if you are using a different unit.)

1. Place the electroporation apparatus in a corner of the cell culture hood.
2. At the back of the unit, optionally connect the high-voltage leads (thick black coiled cord) from the Pulse Controller module to the socket labeled *Pulse Controller* on the base module.
3. Connect the high-voltage leads (thick black coiled cord) from the Capacitance Extender II module to the socket labeled *Capacitance Extender* on the base mod-

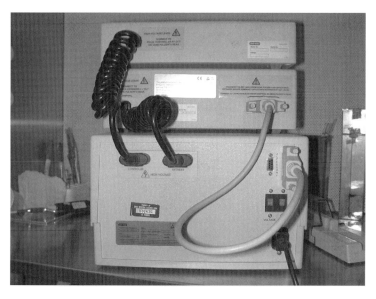

Fig. 5. Rear panel electrical connections for exponential decay electroporation using the Bio-Rad Gene Pulser II and Capacitance Extender and Pulse Controller modules.

ule. Connect the 25-pin D connector on the Capacitance Extender module to the 25-pin D connector on the base unit.

4. Plug the power cord into a grounded outlet. When done the setup should look like **Fig. 5**.

5. Connect the cuvet holder to the base module. Now, turn on the electroporator base unit.

3.2.2.2. Programming the Electroporator

(These instructions refer to the Bio-Rad Gene Pulser II equipment. Refer to the appropriate user's manual if you are using a different unit.)

The electroporator must be programmed to run the desired parameters using the front panel controls. Set the rotary control to *High Cap* to connect the capacitance extender module (**Fig. 6**). If connected, set the knobs on the pulse Controller Plus to *High Range* and ∞. For human chondrocytes, the following parameters work well: 0.400 kV, 250 µF (base unit), and ∞Ω (Pulse Controller Plus in open circuit mode; *see* **Note 6**). The parameters are entered using the front panel buttons.

3.2.3. DNA

The DNA should be prepared as described in **Subheading 3.1.3.** Exponential decay electroporation requires large amounts of DNA for maximum efficiency;

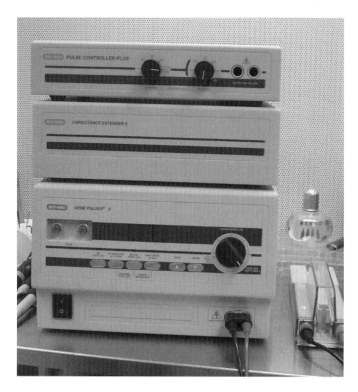

Fig. 6. Front Panel view of the exponential decay electroporation setup using the Bio-Rad Gene Pulser II and Capacitance Extender and Pulse Controller modules. The latter is in open circuit ($\infty\Omega$), and the high-voltage connection to the electroporation cuvet is made to the base unit.

40 μg per transfection works well, but considerably less will also yield positive transfections. Heat the plasmid DNA solution to 70°C for 5–10 min, and then, using sterile technique, deposit the total volume of plasmid required at the bottom of a sterile conical tube prepared as in **Subheading 3.2.2.1.**

3.2.4. Cells

Some 3×10^5 to 1×10^6 cells can be transfected at a time, with 6×10^5 working best for human chondrocytes. Exponential decay electroporation kills many more cells than RF electroporation. Expect only about 30% survival at the recommended parameters. Cells that were subconfluent seem to survive the electroporation process better. As described in **Subheading 3.1.4.**, the cells should be treated gently to enhance viability. Additionally, keeping the cells on ice before and immediately after electroporation improves viability.

The cells should be prepared as described in **Subheading 3.1.4.** with the final resuspension being in *cold electroporation buffer*. Count the cells using a hemacytometer and adjust the volume with cold electroporation buffer so that there are 0.75×10^6 cells/mL.

3.2.5. Electroporation

1. Gently mix the required volume of cells with the DNA in the labeled conical tubes.
2. Transfer 800 µL of the cell/DNA mix to a sterile cuvet and place the cuvet in the slider of the electroporation cuvet holder. The cuvet is keyed and will fit easily in one orientation only. Push the slider into the holder until it engages with a click.
3. Press and hold both red pulse buttons simultaneously until the beep sounds (*CHg* will flash and then *PLS* will be displayed during this process).
4. Release both pulse buttons after the beep. The time constant is automatically displayed after every pulse. Record it, as well as the actual volts and sample resistance (*see* **Note 7**). This information can be useful for troubleshooting and for verifying interexperimental consistency.

3.2.6. Post Electroporation

Results improve if the time between trypsinization of the cells and their return to normal medium after the electroporation is kept at a minimum (*see* **Note 4**). However, the cells are fragile immediately after electroporation.

1. Remove the cuvet from the holder and add 1 mL of cold, antibiotic-free medium to the cuvet.
2. Place the cuvet on ice and wait for 10–15 min *(7)*, before gently aspirating the cell suspension from the cuvet using a sterile pipette. It has been reported that reheating the cells to 37°C instead of keeping them on ice at this stage improves transfection efficiency *(23)*, but we have not verified this in our system.
3. Plate the cells in the desired final volume of antibiotic-free medium, and return the plates to the incubator.

3.3. Backup Protocol 2: FuGENE 6 Transfection

This protocol was developed for the transfection of chondrocytes maintained under nonadherent culture conditions; however the procedure is also applicable to monolayer cultures. FuGENE 6 is a proprietary, lipid-based transfection reagent that has been shown to provide significantly higher transfection efficiencies in chondrocytes than similar cationic liposome-based alternatives in two comparative analyses *(3,24)*. The transfection efficiency using this protocol is generally 10–40%. This is not sufficient to assess the effects of specific gene expression on the entire target cell populations without selection, owing to the high negative-cell background. It is adequate for promoter/reporter-based experiments, establishing stable transfectants and creating positive control lysates and media.

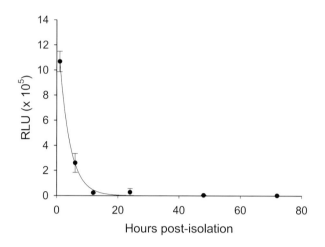

Fig. 7. Effect of time after isolation on chondrocyte transfection efficiency. Primary chondrocytes were transfected with a cytomegalovirus (CMV) promoter-driven luciferase reporter at varying times after isolation from cartilage. Luciferase activities, indicated in relative light units (RLU), were measured 48 h after transfection ($n = 3$).

3.3.1. Setting Up

Wipe down the work area in the cell culture hood with 70% ethanol. Prepare and label sterile tubes for each plasmid combination and the required number of cell culture plates to receive the transfected cells. The chondrocytes should be transfected immediately after collagenase isolation to maximize efficiency (**Fig. 7**). Therefore, the FuGENE 6/DNA complex should be set up concurrently with the final stages of the cell isolation procedure.

3.3.2. DNA

The DNA should be highly purified. We have found Qiagen column purification to be adequate. The DNA should be washed thoroughly with 70% ethanol to remove residual salts. Resuspend the DNA at high concentration (1 µg/µL or greater) to minimize volume contribution, in a sterile vehicle ($T_{10}E_1$ or water).

3.3.3. Cells

The transfection efficiency of primary chondrocytes falls substantially with time after isolation (**Fig. 7**). Therefore, optimal results will be obtained using chondrocytes immediately after being released from cartilage by collagenase digestion (*see* **Note 8**). For reporter-based experiments, we generally aliquot chondrocytes into groups of $2\text{--}3 \times 10^5$ cells, with each group maintained in a 2.0-cm² nonadherent well.

The following protocol details the steps required to transfect a single well of 3×10^5 cells. The quantities and volumes can be scaled up as necessary, to accommodate larger populations of target cells or to prepare sufficient reagents for replicates. It is advisable to prepare sufficient complex solution for an extra well, to ensure adequate quantities for the entire experimental group.

1. Place 97 µL of Opti-MEM in a 1.5-mL Eppendorf tube.
2. Add 3 µL of FuGENE 6 reagent directly into the medium, so as to prevent the FuGENE 6 from directly contacting the plastic surface of the tube.
3. Mix gently, and then add 1 µg of DNA (usually in 1–2 µL) to the Opti-MEM containing the FuGENE 6.
4. Mix by gently tapping the tube, and incubate at room temperature for 15–30 min.
5. Chondrocyte isolation from the digestion buffer can be completed during this interval. After isolation, washing, and counting, place 3×10^5 cells in 500 µL of Opti-MEM I into a 2-cm-diameter, ultra-low attachment well. Do not supplement the medium with ascorbic acid until the transfection has been carried out.
6. Add the FuGENE 6/DNA complex to the well and swirl the dish to disperse the complex and cells evenly.
7. Return the cells to an incubator and maintain in the FuGENE 6/DNA medium for at least 3 h.

3.3.4. Post Transfection

The cultures can be supplemented with appropriate medium after 3 h. It is not necessary to remove the medium containing the FuGENE 6/DNA complex. We routinely maintain chondrocyte cultures in serum-free Opti-MEM, so this only entails adding a further 500 µL of medium, with the required ascorbic acid supplementation. Using this protocol, we have found that constitutive luciferase expression is maximal 48–72 h after transfection and persists at detectable (24-h equivalent) levels for at least 9 d (**Fig. 8**). These data were obtained from chondrocytes maintained in serum-free Opti-MEM. Maintenance in serum-supplemented medium may alter these parameters.

4. Notes

1. Unfortunately, although (or perhaps because) the Gene Pulser II RF is an extremely versatile, configurable, and thus complex system, this particular model was discontinued by Bio-Rad in 2002. Many of them are still in operation, however, and they can occasionally be found on the used equipment market. It has been replaced by a less versatile square-wave capable electroporation system (Gene Pulser Xcell); this and other devices, e.g., from BTX, or Amaxa *(2)*, may be able to produce similar transfection efficiencies *(25)*. Alternately, a competent electronics shop may be able to produce a device with capabilities similar to those of the commercial RF system *(19)*.
2. Deleting antibiotics from the post transfection medium improves cell survival.

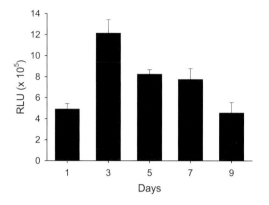

Fig. 8. Persistence of luciferase activity in chondrocyte aggregates. Luciferase activity, indicated in relative light units (RLU), was assessed at varying time points after transfection of a cytomegalovirus (CMV) promoter-driven reporter in chondrocytes maintained in serum-free medium ($n = 3$).

3. Optimizing RF electroporation: the parameters presented work well for cultured primary human chondrocytes (and, incidentally, for human bone marrow-derived mesenchymal stem cells). Other parameters may work better for passaged chondrocytes or for chondrocytes from different species. The following guidelines may be useful in optimizing RF electroporations.

   a. We have found that 30 kHz 100% modulation appears to work well for most cell types.
   b. Also, in general, both transfection efficiency and cell death rise with the number of bursts, so an optimal tradeoff will have to be found empirically.
   c. Focusing on optimizing the Total Voltage and Burst Durations seems to be the most expedient approach. Assuming a 2 mm cuvet, a good starting point would be setting up an experimental grid of nine conditions, e.g.,

Burst duration	Total volts		
(ms)	25	50	100
0.5	1	2	3
1	4	5	6
2	7	8	9

while maintaining the RF frequency at 30 kHz, percent modulation at 100%, burst number at 5 and burst interval at 1 s. Pick the condition that results in the highest transfection efficiency, and then increase the burst number.

Preliminary optimization is most conveniently done by transfecting with a luciferase reporter vector. Assessing transfection efficiency can be conveniently done using a green fluorescent protein (GFP) reporter vector, e.g., pEGFP-N1

(Clontech, BD Biosciences, Franklin Lakes, NJ, http://www.clontech.com/techinfo/vectors/vectorsE/pEGFP-N1.shtml). The transfected cells are plated onto chamber slides, e.g., Nunc™ Lab-Tek™ (Nalge Nunc International, Rochester, NY, cat. no. 155380,). Percent efficiency is determined by dividing the number of GFP-positive cells by the total number of cells counted on several random 10× fields, × 100. Peak expression of GFP usually occurs on the third day after transfection. A bacterial β-galactosidase reporter system followed by X-gal detection can also be used; however, the sensitivity of this assay is several orders of magnitude lower than that of either luciferase- or GFP-based systems.

4. Leaving the cells in the electroporation buffer for an extended period decreases both transfection efficiency and viability. Therefore, complete all the electroporator setup and programming steps, quantify the DNA, label the culture dishes, and so on, before harvesting the cells. If a large number of transfections are planned, consider breaking up the experiment into smaller groups. It may be helpful to have an assistant handle the postelectroporation plating in another cell culture hood.

5. Stable transfections: both electroporation protocols yield higher numbers of stable transformants than one would expect using conventional transfection techniques. Selection of stable transformants can begin the day after electroporation. From the literature, selection levels for human chondrocytes transfected with the neomycin resistance marker are in the range of 350–400 μg/mL of G418 *(26)*.

6. The parameters given in **Subheading 3.2.2.3.** work well for human chondrocytes. Other species will probable require further optimization. Cell-specific optimization is important if for no other reason than that the required field strength depends on the diameter of the cell *(27)*. Setting up an optimization grid varying V_0 up and down around 400 V, while maintaining the capacitance, should prove to be a good starting point. Careful washing of the cells in electroporation buffer, and use of the Pulse-Track system (*see* **Note 7**) will help ensure reproducible results.

7. The Gene Pulser II unit incorporates a system called Pulse-Track that monitors the resistance of the sample and delivers the desired voltage regardless of sample volume or conductivity. Using this system according to the manufacturer's instructions can improve the reproducibility of exponential decay electroporations.

8. When transfection with FuGENE 6 cannot be carried out immediately after chondrocyte isolation, the effects of newly synthesized pericellular matrix can be mitigated by pretreating the chondrocytes with 4 U/mL hyaluronidase for 6 h prior to and during the transfection *(3)*.

References

1. Reid, T., Warren, R., and Kirn, D. (2002) Intravascular adenoviral agents in cancer patients: Lessons from clinical trials. *Cancer Gene Ther.* **9,** 979–986.

2. Hamm, A., Krott, N., Breibach, I., Blindt, R., and Bosserhoff, A. K. (2002) Efficient transfection method for primary cells. *Tissue Eng.* **8**, 235–245.

3. Stove, J., Fiedler, J., Huch, K., Gunther, K. P., Puhl, W., and Brenner, R. (2002) Lipofection of rabbit chondrocytes and long lasting expression of a lacZ reporter system in alginate beads. *Osteoarthritis Cartilage* **10**, 212–217.

4. Goomer, R. S., Deftos, L. J., Terkeltaub, R., et al. (2001) High-efficiency non-viral transfection of primary chondrocytes and perichondrial cells for ex-vivo gene therapy to repair articular cartilage defects. *Osteoarthritis Cartilage* **9**, 248–256.

5. Neumann, E., Schaefer-Ridder, M., Wang, Y., and Hofschneider, P. H. (1982) Gene transfer into mouse lyoma cells by electroporation in high electric fields. *EMBO J.* **1**, 841–845.

6. Wong, T. K. and Neumann, E. (1982) Electric field mediated gene transfer. *Biochem. Biophys. Res. Commun.* **107**, 584–587.

7. Potter, H., Weir, L., and Leder, P. (1984) Enhancer-dependent expression of human kappa immunoglobulin genes introduced into mouse pre-B lymphocytes by electroporation. *Proc. Natl. Acad. Sci. USA* **81**, 7161–7165.

8. Gehl, J. (2003) Electroporation: theory and methods, perspectives for drug delivery, gene therapy and research. *Acta Physiol. Scand.* **177**, 437–447.

9. Kekez, M. M., Savic, P., and Johnson, B. F. (1996) Contribution to the biophysics of the lethal effects of electric field on microorganisms. *Biochim Biophys. Acta* **1278**, 79–88.

10. Lennon, D. P., Haynesworth, S. E., Arm, D. M., Baber, M. A., and Caplan, A. I. (2000) Dilution of human mesenchymal stem cells with dermal fibroblasts and the effects on in vitro and in vivo osteochondrogenesis. *Dev. Dyn.* **219**, 50–62.

11. Ahrens, P. B., Solursh, M., and Reiter, R. S. (1977) Stage-related capacity for limb chondrogenesis in cell culture. *Dev. Biol.* **60**, 69–82.

12. Raptis, L. and Firth, K. L. (1990) Electroporation of adherent cells in situ. DNA *Cell Biol.* **9**, 615–621.

13. Zheng, Q. A. and Chang, D. C. (1991) High-efficiency gene transfection by in situ electroporation of cultured cells. *Biochim. Biophys. Acta* **1088**, 104–110.

14. Wegener, J., Keese, C. R., and Giaever, I. (2002) Recovery of adherent cells after in situ electroporation monitored electrically. *Biotechniques* **33**, 348–357.

15. Saito, T. and Nakatsuji, N. (2001) Efficient gene transfer into the embryonic mouse brain using in vivo electroporation. *Dev. Biol.* **240**, 237–246.

16. Ohashi, S., Kubo, T., Kishida, T., et al. (2002) Successful genetic transduction in vivo into synovium by means of electroporation. *Biochem. Biophys. Res. Commun.* **293**, 1530–1535.

17. Kishimoto, K. N., Watanabe, Y., Nakamura, H., and Kokubun, S. (2002) Ectopic bone formation by electroporatic transfer of bone morphogenetic protein-4 gene. *Bone* **31**, 340–347.

18. Muramatsu, T., Nakamura, A., and Park, H. M. (1998) In vivo electroporation: a powerful and convenient means of nonviral gene transfer to tissues of living animals (Review). *Int. J. Mol. Med.* **1**, 55–62.

19. Chang, D. C. (1989) Cell poration and cell fusion using an oscillating electric field. *Biophys. J.* **56,** 641–652.
20. Chang, D. C., Gao, P. Q., and Maxwell, B. L. (1991) High efficiency gene transfection by electroporation using a radio-frequency electric field. *Biochim. Biophys. Acta* **1092,** 153–160.
21. Zald, P. B., Cotter, M. A., and Robertson, E. S. (2001) Strategy for increased efficiency of transfection in human cell lines using radio frequency electroporation. *Prep. Biochem. Biotechnol.* **31,** 1–11.
22. Zald, P. B., Cotter, M. A., 2nd, and Robertson, E. S. (2000) Improved transfection efficiency of 293 cells by radio frequency electroporation. *Biotechniques* **28,** 418–420.
23. Rols, M. P., Delteil, C., Serin, G., and Teissie, J. (1994) Temperature effects on electrotransfection of mammalian cells. *Nucleic Acids Res.* **22,** 540.
24. Madry, H., and Trippel, S. B. (2000) Efficient lipid-mediated gene transfer to articular chondrocytes. *Gene Ther.* **7,** 286–291.
25. Gehl, J., Skovsgaard, T., and Mir, L. M. (1998) Enhancement of cytotoxicity by electropermeabilization: an improved method for screening drugs. *Anticancer Drugs* **9,** 319–325.
26. Piera-Velazquez, S., Jimenez, S. A., and Stokes, D. (2002) Increased life span of human osteoarthritic chondrocytes by exogenous expression of telomerase. *Arthritis Rheum.* **46,** 683–693.
27. Kotnik, T., Bobanovic, F., and Miklavcic, D. (1997) Sensitivity of transmembrane voltage induced by applied electric fields—a theroetical analysis. *Bioelectrochem. Bioenergetics* **43,** 285–291.

12

In Vitro Gene Transfer to Chondrocytes and Synovial Fibroblasts by Adenoviral Vectors

Jean-Noel Gouze, Martin J. Stoddart, Elvire Gouze, Glyn D. Palmer, Steven C. Ghivizzani, Alan J. Grodzinsky, and Christopher H. Evans

Summary

The major requirement of a successful gene transfer is the efficient delivery of an exogenous therapeutic gene to the appropriate cell type with subsequent high or regulated levels of expression. In this context, viral systems are more efficient than nonviral systems, giving higher levels of gene expression for longer periods. For the application of osteoarthritis (OA), gene products triggering anti-inflammatory or chondroprotective effects are of obvious therapeutic utility. Thus, their cognate genes are candidates for use in the gene therapy of OA. In this chapter, we describe the preparation, the use, and the effect of the transduction of chondrocytes or synovial fibroblasts with an adenoviral vector encoding the cDNA for glutamine: fructose-6-phosphate amidotransferase (GFAT). This is intended to serve as an example of a technology that can be used to evaluate the biological effects of overexpression of other cDNAs.

Key Words: Gene transfer; adenovirus; GFAT; chondrocyte; synoviocyte; gene therapy; osteoarthritis; interleukin-1; glucosamine.

1. Introduction

Osteoarthritis (OA) is the most common joint disorder and is associated with a dramatically impaired quality of life *(1)*. It is increasingly viewed as a disease of the entire joint, involving cartilage, the underlying bone, and the synovial lining of the joint capsule *(2)*. Present treatments for OA remain unsatisfactory. Although many pharmacologies diminish pain and inflammation, none is capable of blocking the progression of the disease *(3,4)*.

Advances in molecular biology combined with a better understanding of the basic biology of OA have opened new therapeutic opportunities for the treatment of this disorder. Many of these potential new drugs with which to treat OA are proteins; although they have potent activities, they are difficult to deliver to OA joints in a manner that achieves sustained therapeutic intra-articular concentration.

From: *Methods in Molecular Medicine, Vol. 100: Cartilage and Osteoarthritis, Vol. 1: Cellular and Molecular Tools*
Edited by: M. Sabatini, P. Pastoureau, and F. De Ceuninck © Humana Press Inc., Totowa, NJ

Because genes are able to produce proteins locally for extended periods, their transfer to specific cells within the joint, such as chondrocytes or synoviocytes, are attractive alternatives to protein delivery in the context of treating OA.

To illustrate this point, the present chapter describes the construction and utilization of an adenoviral vector containing the cDNA for glutamine:fructose-6-phosphate amidotransferase (GFAT). Indeed, based on the recent attention afforded by studies supporting the notion that glucosamine may have beneficial effects in OA *(5–11)*, we have developed an approach using GFAT as a transgene. GFAT is the rate-limiting step of glucosamine synthesis within cells *(12)*; thus, by overexpressing the cDNA for GFAT in certain cells in the joint, it may be possible to elevate the intra-articular levels of glucosamine and its derivatives. Adenoviral vectors have been used to deliver the GFAT cDNA successfully to synoviocytes cocultured with chondrocytes. In the presence of interleukin-1 (IL-1), GFAT gene transfer was found to maintain matrix synthesis by chondrocytes and also significantly reduced production of various inflammatory mediators such as nitric oxide and prostaglandin E_2 *(13)*.

Because of their ease of use, efficiency of gene delivery, and high levels of resulting transgene expression, adenoviral vectors have proved to be valuable tools for evaluating the in vivo or in vitro activities of various transgene products *(14–16)*. These vectors can be readily propagated to high titer and can efficiently infect and transduce many cell types, including those of articular tissues, such as synovial lining cells and chondrocytes. This chapter details the infection of primary articular chondrocytes and synoviocytes with a recombinant adenoviral vector encoding GFAT (Ad.GFAT). The process entails the cloning of human GFAT cDNA, the generation and propagation of a novel recombinant adenovirus, and the large-scale preparation of chondrocytes and/or synoviocytes from joint tissues. Following infection of cell cultures, the effect of GFAT overexpression can be demonstrated by protection against IL-1 challenge assessed by the changes in nitrate oxide (NO) levels.

This chapter describes methods by which the effects of GFAT overexpression following gene transfer may be assessed and is intended to serve as an example; the same technology can be used to evaluate the biological effect of other cDNA overexpression.

2. Materials

1. TRIzol® reagent (Life Technologies).
2. Chloroform.
3. Isopropanol.
4. 70% Ethanol.
5. 95% Ethanol.
6. Dithiothreitol.
7. TE buffer: 10 m*M* Tris-HCl, pH 7.4, 1 m*M* ethylenediaminetetraacetic (EDTA).

8. RQ1 DNase (Promega).
9. Phenol/chloroform/isoamyl alcohol (25:24:1 v/v/v).
10. Reverse transcriptase-polymerase chain reaction (RT-PCR) reagents (Life Technologies, unless otherwise noted).

    a. Random primers.
    b. Murine Moloney leukemia virus (MMLV) RNase H⁻ reverse transcriptase.
    c. RNase OUT, ribonuclease inhibitor.
    d. Deoxynucleotides (100 mM).
    e. Forward and reverse oligodeoxynucleotides.
    f. Vent DNA polymerase (New England Biolabs).

11. Reverse transcription buffer: 50 mM Tris-HCl, pH 8.4, 75 mM KCl, 3 mM MgCl$_2$.
12. PCR buffer: 10 mM Tris-HCl, pH 9.0, 50 mM KCl, 1.5 mM MgCl$_2$.
13. pAdlox adenoviral shuttle plasmid (Genebank accession number U62024; generous gift of Dr. Stephen Hardy; *see* ref. *17*).
14. DH5α™ Competent Cells (Invitrogen).
15. Bacterial culture reagents (e.g., Sigma).

    a. LB media: 1% tryptone, 0.5% yeast extract, 1% NaCl (w/v), pH 7.0.
    b. LB agar: LB media + 15 g/L Bacto-agar.
    c. Ampicillin (50 mg/mL).

16. QIAquick gel extraction kit (Qiagen).
17. Qiagen Tip 2500 plasmid kit (Qiagen).
18. T4 DNA ligase (Life Technologies).
19. *Eco*RI restriction endonuclease (Life Technologies).
20. *Bsa*BI restriction endonuclease (New England Biolabs).
21. *Bam*HI restriction endonuclease (Life Technologies).
22. Tissue culture reagents (e.g., Life Technologies, Sigma-Aldrich).

    a. Ham's F-12/Dulbecco's modified eagle's medium (DMEM).
    b. DMEM.
    c. Trypsin-EDTA: 0.05% trypsin, 0.53 mM EDTA.
    d. Gey's balanced salt solution (GBSS).
    e. Phosphate-buffered saline (PBS).
    f. Fetal bovine serum (FBS).
    g. 10 mg/mL Penicillin /10,000 U/mL streptomycin in 0.85% saline.
    h. Protease type XIV, from *Streptomyces griseus*.
    i. Collagenase type II, from *Clostridium histolyticum*.
    j. Dispase, from *Bacillus polymyxa*.

23. Tissue culture vessels (e.g., Becton Dickinson, NalgeNunc).

    a. 225-cm^2 tissue culture flasks.
    b. 75-cm^2 tissue culture flasks.
    c. 25-cm^2 tissue culture flasks.
    d. 96-well tissue culture plates.
    e. 40-μm sterile cell strainer.

24. 293 Cells (American Type Culture Collection [ATCC] cat. no. CRL 1573).

25. 293 Cre8 cells (generous gift of Dr. Stephen Hardy; *see* ref. *17*).
26. Ψ5 Adenovirus (generous gift of Dr. Stephen Hardy; *see* ref. *17*).
27. DOC lysis buffer: 100 m*M* Tris-HCl, pH 9.0, 20% (v/v) ethanol, 0.4% (w/v) sodium deoxycholate.
28. 0.5 *M*, Spermine-HCl.
29. RNase A (10 mg/mL ; Sigma-Aldrich).
30. Sodium dodecyl sulfate (SDS), 10% (w/v).
31. 0.5 *M* EDTA, pH 8.0.
32. 2 *M* $CaCl_2$.
33. Cesium chloride solutions:
   a. 1.4 g/mL CsCl in 10 m*M* Tris-HCl, pH 7.9.
   b. 1.2 g/mL CsCl in 10 m*M* Tris-HCl, pH 7.9.
34. Thin-walled ultraspeed centrifuge tubes (e.g., 10-mL polyallomer tubes; Sorvall).
35. Dialysis buffer: 10 m*M* Tris-HCl, pH 7.5, 200 m*M* NaCl, 1 m*M* EDTA, 4% (w/v) sucrose.
36. Dialysis tubing, molecular-weight cutoff (MWCO) 50,000 (e.g., Spectra/Por, Spectrum Laboratories).
37. Griess reaction.
   a. Solution I: 1% (w/v) sulfanilamide, 2.5% (v/v) H_3PO_4.
   b. Solution II: 0.1% (w/v) dihydrochloride *N*-ethylendiamine.
   c. $NaNO_2$, for standard curve.
   d. Microplate reader, set at 550-nm wavelength.

3. Methods

The methods described below outline (1) the isolation of a specific cDNA and its insertion into an adenoviral shuttle plasmid, (2) the generation and amplification of recombinant adenovirus, (3) the isolation and culture of articular chondrocytes and synoviocytes, (4) the adenoviral transduction of these cells, and (5) measurement of cellular response to the transgene product.

The adenoviral vector system discussed in the following sections was developed by Hardy et al. *(17)* and makes use of Cre-mediated recombination among an adenoviral shuttle vector, pAdlox, and an adenoviral backbone, Ψ5. The resulting vector is a replication-deficient, type 5 adenovirus lacking the E1 and E3 loci. The gene of interest is contained within a cytomegalovirus (CMV)-driven expression cassette located in the site of the E1 domain.

To illustrate the practical application of these methods, the cDNA for human GFAT will be used as a specific example.

3.1. Insertion of a Novel cDNA Into the Adenoviral Shuttle Plasmid

The shuttle plasmid described here, pAdlox *(17)*, can serve two purposes. The first is as a eukaryotic expression plasmid for verification of expression of the gene product of the cDNA of interest. The second is as a shuttle plasmid for

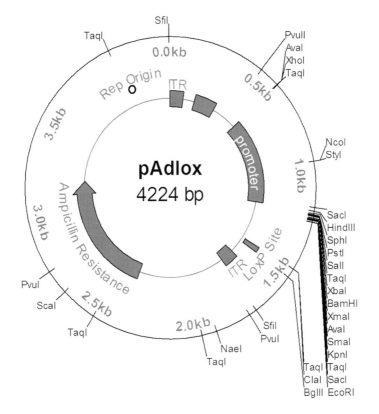

Fig. 1. Schematic of pAdlox expression plasmid (generous gift of Dr. Stephen Hardy; *see* ref. *19*).

the generation of recombinant adenovirus *(17)*. pAdlox contains the left-hand inverted terminal repeat of the adenovirus, viral packaging signal (Ψ), a cDNA expression cassette driven by the CMV promoter/enhancer, and finally, a *loxP* recognition site for the Cre-recombinase (**Fig. 1**). Described below is (1) the isolation of the cDNA for the human form of GFAT, (2) its insertion into pAdlox, and (3) its propagation in a competent strain of *E. coli*, DH5α.

3.1.1. cDNA Cloning

1. Plate one 25-cm² flask with cells that provide robust expression of the gene of interest. For isolation of human GFAT, approx 10⁵–293 cells were cultured in DMEM/10% FBS/1% penicillin–streptomycin.
2. At confluence, remove the media and add 1 mL TRIzol reagent to cells; harvest the lysate using a cell scraper (*see* **Note 1**).
3. Mix with 200 μL chloroform and centrifuge for 10 min at 13,000*g*, 4°C.

4. Remove the aqueous phase (top layer), and precipitate the RNA by addition of 2 vol of isopropanol.
5. Centrifuge for 10 min at 13,000g, 4°C, remove the supernatant, and resuspend the RNA in 20 µL TE buffer.
6. Quantitate RNA by spectrophotometry, and freeze at –80°C.
7. For cDNA synthesis, heat 3 µg of total RNA to 65°C for 5 min and then place it on ice. Reverse transcribe the RNA for 2 h at 37°C in a final volume of 20 µL of reverse transcription buffer, plus 500 µM each of dATP, dCTP, dGTP, and dTTP, 10 mM dithiothreitol, 100 pmol random primer, 40 U Rnase OUT, and 200 U MMLV RNase H$^-$ reverse transcriptase.
8. Amplify the cDNA of interest by incubating 2 µL of the cDNA from **step 7** in a PCR reaction of 50 µL consisting of PCR buffer plus 0.2 mM of each dNTP, 20 pmol of the forward and reverse oligodeoxynucleotide primers, and 2 U of Vent DNA polymerase. Incubate the reaction for 5 min at 95°C and then 35 cycles of 1 min at 95°C, 1 min at 60°C, and 2 min at 72°C. For human GFAT, the forward primer spanned nucleotides 32–54; the reverse primer was complementary to nucleotides 2197–2227 relative to the published human GFAT sequence (Genebank accession no. M90516) (*see* **Note 2**).
9. Following resolution of the reaction products on a 0.8% agarose gel, purify the DNA fragment corresponding to the proper size using a QIAquick gel extraction kit following the manufacturer's instructions.
10. Dilute an aliquot of the purified DNA fragment 100–500 times in TE buffer.
11. Using the same conditions as in **step 8**, amplify by PCR 1 µL of the purified DNA using sequence-specific forward and reverse oligodeoxynucleotide primers engineered to contain endonuclease restriction sites for convenient insertion into the multiple cloning site of pAdlox (20 cycles) (*see* **Fig. 2** and **Note 3**).
12. Digest pAdlox and the amplified DNA with the appropriate endonuclease restriction enzymes (2 h, enzyme-specific temperature) (*see* **Note 4**). Gel-purify the fragments as described in **step 9**.
13. Directionally ligate the DNA fragment and pAdlox (T4 ligase, 14°C overnight) by standard methods *(18)*.
14. Freeze sample at –20°C (optional).

3.1.2. Bacterial Transformation and Plasmid Selection

1. Transform DH5α cells with plasmid Adlox.GFAT using standard methods *(18)*.
2. Plate bacterial cells on an LB agar dish containing ampicillin (50 µg/mL) and incubate overnight at 37°C.
3. Carefully select single colonies and inoculate individual cultures of 10 mL LB media with ampicillin (50 µg/mL). Incubate overnight at 37°C.
4. Following standard miniprep isolation of the plasmid DNA *(18)*, screen each isolate for the presence and orientation of the cDNA insert by strategic restriction digestion.
5. Following identification of a suitable construct, prepare a large-scale culture (500 mL) of the bacteria and incubate overnight at 37°C with vigorous shaking.

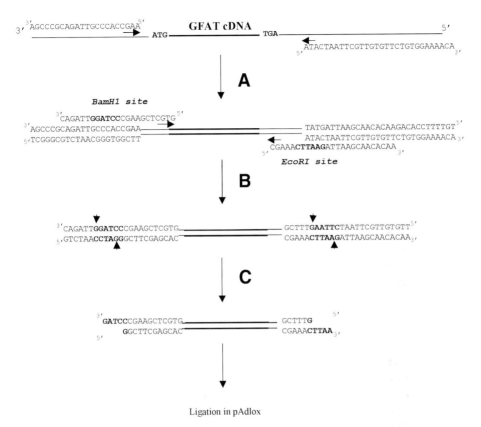

Fig. 2. Schematic of mutagenesis by PCR reaction. (**A**) cDNA cloning using 100% homologous oligonucleotide. (**B**) Amplification using new oligonucleotides with a *Bam*HI or *Eco*RI site in their sequence. (**C**) Digestion with *Eco*RI and *Bam*HI.

6. Purify the plasmid DNA from the bacteria using a Qiagen Tip 2500 Plasmid Kit following the manufacturer's instructions.
7. Freeze at −20°C (optional).

3.2. Recombinant Adenovirus

To generate recombinant virus for large-scale infections, replication-deficient adenovirus is typically amplified in 293 cells, which supply in trans the E1 gene products necessary for viral replication. **Caution:** stringent safety procedures should be followed while working with recombinant adenovirus (*see* **Note 5**) *(19)*. It is also strongly advised that the investigator be familiar with the appropriate federal, state, and institutional regulations concerning microbiological safety.

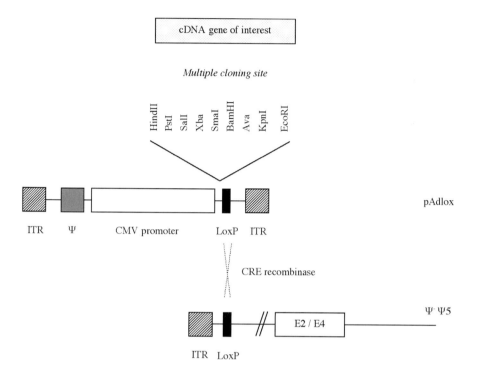

Fig. 3. Construction of an E1-substituted adenovirus by using Ψ5 and a shuttle vector *(19)*. The gene of interest is directionally inserted into the pAdlox plasmid. Cre-mediated recombination between the *loxP* site in the shuttle vector and the *loxP* site in the Ψ5 adenoviral backbone not only allows generation of adenovirus carrying the gene of interest but also avoids the propagation of non-recombinant viruses. The packaging site is labeled Ψ. CMV, cytomegalovirus; ITR, internal tandem repeat.

The procedures described below outline (1) the preparation and amplification of Ψ5 adenoviral DNA, (2) the generation of an adenoviral vector using a system of Cre-lox recombination *(17)* (*see* **Note 6**), and (3) the large-scale preparation of recombinant adenovirus. For this, the pAdlox shuttle plasmid is cotransfected with genomic DNA from the Ψ5 adenoviral backbone into 293 Cre8 cells. This cell line constitutively expresses Cre recombinase, which mediates recombination between *loxP* sites in the shuttle plasmid and the Ψ5 adenoviral backbone, generating a novel recombinant virus. Negative pressure on Ψ5 propagation in these cells is achieved by Cre-mediated intramolecular recombination, which removes the Ψ packaging site from the Ψ5 backbone, preventing its insertion into the viral capsid. Thus, viral particles arising from the transfection typically contain a very high percentage of recombinants (**Fig. 3**).

3.2.1. Preparation and Amplification of Ψ5 Adenoviral DNA

The 293 cell line, which does not express the Cre recombinase, is permissive for replication of the Ψ5 adenovirus. Infection of these cells will allow amplification of the virus for isolation of the genomic DNA and for the generation of Ψ5 viral stocks. Both procedures are described below.

1. Plate approx 5×10^5 293 cells in a 75-cm^2 flask containing 15 mL DMEM/10% FBS/1% penicillin–streptomycin.
2. At confluence, remove media and replace with a minimal volume (4 mL) of fresh DMEM without serum, followed by 50 µL of Ψ5 viral lysate (*see* **step 5**). Incubate for 2–4 h at 37°C, and then supplement with 10 mL of medium.
3. Monitor cells daily for signs of infection (*see* **Note 7**).
4. When the cells are rounded and begin to detach, harvest the cells and media using a cell scraper.
5. Pellet the cells by centrifugation for 10 min at 2000*g*, 4°C and resuspend in 400 µL of TE buffer. (Alternatively, the cell pellet can be resuspended in 5 mL of fresh media and placed through three cycles of freeze-thaw [*see* **Subheading 3.2.3.**]). This lysate is then frozen and stored at –80°C and serves as a stock for future amplification of Ψ5 virus.)
6. For DNA purification, add 400 µL of DOC lysis buffer to the cell pellet. Mix by pipeting 10–15 times through a 1-mL pipet and transfer the lysate to a microcentrifuge tube and add 8 µL of 0.5 *M* spermine-HCl. Incubate on ice for 10 min.
7. Centrifuge for 5 min at 13,000*g* to pellet cellular debris and genomic DNA.
8. Transfer the supernatant to a new microcentrifuge tube. Add 4 µL of 10 mg/mL RNase A and incubate at 37°C for 10 min.
9. To release the viral DNA from the particles, add 60 µL of 10% SDS, 20 µL of 0.5 *M* EDTA, and 40 µL of 50 mg/mL pronase. Incubate for 60 min at 40°C.
10. Extract viral DNA with phenol/chloroform/isoamyl alcohol and then precipitate using standard methods *(18,19)*.
11. Wash the DNA pellet with 70% ethanol. Resuspend the DNA pellet in 25 µL TE buffer. The viral DNA is now suitable for restriction digestion analysis or transfection as needed. For example, digestion of 4–6 µL of the Ψ5 DNA with *Bsa*BI and resolution of the fragments in an 0.8% agarose gel generates a discreet restriction pattern with a limited number of bands (*see* **Note 8** and **Fig. 4**).

3.2.2. Generation of Recombinant Adenovirus

This procedure describes the cotransfection of the pAdlox shuttle plasmid and the Ψ5 adenoviral backbone into 293 Cre8 cells, which results in the generation of a novel recombinant vector.

1. Plate approx 10^6 Cre8 cells in a 75-cm^2 flask to 60% confluence in DMEM/10% FBS/1% penicillin–streptomycin.
2. Cotransfect the Cre8 cells with 3 µg of pAdlox and 3 µg of purified Ψ5 adenoviral DNA using standard methods *(18,19)* (*see* **Note 9**).

4. Resuspend the cartilage fragments in 30 mL Ham's F-12 medium/10% FBS/1% penicillin–streptomycin supplemented with collagenase (2% w/v) and incubate at 37°C overnight with gentle agitation.
5. Filter the digestion mixture using a sterile 40-μm cell strainer (Falcon) to remove the debris from the cell suspension. Collect the liquid suspension and pellet the chondrocytes by centrifugation for 15 min at 2000*g*.
6. Plate the cells in a 25-cm² flask in 3 mL Ham's F-12/10% FBS/1% penicillin–streptomycin. Wash the adherent cells 24 h later to remove debris, and return to culture with fresh media.

3.3.1.2. SYNOVIOCYTES

1. Carefully harvest synovial membrane from the joint capsule under aseptic conditions.
2. Using a razor blade, finely mince the recovered synovial tissue.
3. Transfer the minced tissue into 25 mL of Ham's F12 containing 1.5 mg/mL of collagenase and dispase and incubate for 1 h, at 37°C under gentle agitation.
4. Filter the digestion mixture through a 40-μm sterile cell strainer.
5. Collect the liquid suspension and centrifuge for 15 min at 2000*g* to pellet the synovial cells.
6. Wash the cells twice in PBS and plate them in a 25-cm² flask in 3 mL Ham's F-12 medium/10% FBS/1% penicillin–streptomycin (*see* **Note 13**).

3.3.2. Adenoviral Transduction

Depending on the number of cells used in each experiment, achieving a high percentage (>85%) of transduced synovial fibroblasts or chondrocytes may require the use of large volumes of recombinant adenovirus. Mixing the adenoviral suspension with $CaCl_2$ prior to infection has been shown to increase the transduction efficiency of various cell types *(20)* (*see* **Note 14**). We have recently confirmed that this is also effective for chondrocytes and synovial fibroblasts. Described below are the procedures for $CaCl_2$-enhanced transduction of these cells.

1. Seed two 25-cm² flasks with 4×10^6 bovine articular chondrocytes or synovial fibroblasts in Ham's F-12/10% FBS/1% penicillin–streptomycin. This should result in a near-confluent monolayer.
2. On the day of infection, wash the cells and add 3 mL of fresh medium.
3. Add the appropriate amount of adenoviral stock solution to achieve the desired MOI (the multiplicity of infection is defined as the number of infectious viral particles per cell) to 990 μL of serum-free Ham's F-12 and mix thoroughly.
4. Slowly add 10 μL of a 2 *M* solution of $CaCl_2$ with constant agitation (final concentration 20 m*M*), and then briefly vortex.
5. Leave to stand for 30 min at room temperature with occasional vortexing.
6. Add the 1 mL of viral/calcium mix to the 25-cm² plate and leave infection to proceed overnight.

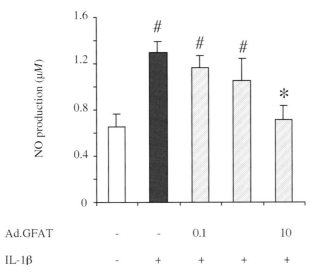

Fig. 5. Nitric oxide(NO) production after interleukin-1 (IL-1) stimulation of glutamine:fructose-6-phosphhate amidotransferase (GFAT)[+] chondrocytes. Chondrocyte cultures were infected with Ad.GFAT at the indicated multiplicity of infection (MOI). After 24 h, cells were treated with 5 ng/mL of human IL-1β. NO production assessed by measurement of nitrite in the medium was measured 24 h later. Results are expressed in mM nitrite (mean ± SD of three different assays). #, $p < 0.05$ vs untransduced control; *, $p < 0.05$ vs untransduced cells treated by IL-1β. Infection with Ad.GFAT decreased NO production after IL-1 stimulation in a dose-dependent manner.

7. Aspirate the viral solution and feed the cells with 5 mL of fresh Ham's F-12 medium/10% FBS/1% penicillin–streptomycin.
8. Verify GFAT mRNA expression in one flask using RT-PCR procedure (*see* **Note 15**), and proceed to experiment further on the second flask.

3.4. NO Measurement

To assess the chondroprotective effect of the Ad.GFAT transduction, the nitrate concentration in the culture medium can be measured 24 h after IL-1α challenge (5 ng/mL) (*see* **Fig. 5**).

1. Produce a standard curve using sodium nitrite (concentration ranging from 0 to 200 μM).
2. Add 100 μL of standard or sample medium to a 96-well plate.
3. To each standard and sample add 50 μL of solution I (sulfanilamide 1% [w/v]; H$_3$PO$_4$ 2.5%), followed by 50 μL of solution II (dihydrochloride N-ethylendiamine 0.1% [w/v]).
4. Read the absorbance within 15 min at 550 nm on an MR5000 microplate reader.

4. Notes

1. Precautions should be taken while working with RNA to avoid RNase contamination. It is strongly recommended to wear disposable gloves and work only with DNase/RNase-free material and supplies.
2. When the coding sequence is not entirely available in the database, 3' and 5' RACE-PCR methods can be used to complete the missing part of the sequence *(21)* (Life Technologies).
3. To achieve RT-PCR amplification of the coding sequence of any gene, two oligonucleotides have to be designed, allowing amplification of all sequences that extend from the translation start site through the stop codon. A second PCR amplification using a new set of oligonucleotide primers containing convenient endonuclease restriction sites allows a directional insertion within the polylinker or multiple cloning sites of the plasmid. Alternatively, a blunt-ended ligation can be performed. However, it will be necessary to confirm the orientation of insertion by specific digestion of the plasmid. Following insertion into the plasmid, the cDNA should be sequenced to verify its accuracy.
4. The choice of the endonuclease restriction enzymes depends on (1) their presence in the polylinker site of pAdlox plasmid and (2) their absence in the cDNA sequence of the gene of interest. Concerning GFAT cDNA, we choose *Eco*RI and *Bam*HI.
5. Wild-type adenovirus has been associated with upper respiratory disease in humans, and recombinant virus is highly infectious for numerous human tissues. First-generation adenoviral vectors are replication-defective and are only able to replicate in permissive cells. The 293 cell lines used here contain the left-hand 11% of the wild-type adenoviral genome, which contains the E1 locus. Because these proteins are provided in *trans*, they can complement the E1 deletion in the adenoviral vector. Recombinant adenovirus is a biosafety level 2 hazardous agent. Whenever possible, work should be performed in a class II biological safety cabinet. In addition, proper protective clothing and eyewear should be worn at all times. Solid waste should be rinsed with 10% bleach solution and placed in biohazard containers. Liquid waste should be decanted or aspirated into a large container of bleach. Likewise, surfaces on which all virus work was performed should be decontaminated with 10% bleach. Extra caution should be used during the handling of sharp objects.
6. Multiple methods can be utilized in the generation of recombinant adenovirus. Several companies have now developed techniques to generate such recombinant vectors (i.e., AdEasy System, Stratagene). The procedure described in this chapter represents only one method among others.
7. Cytopathic effects appear as an increase of granularity, a rounding aspect, and a tendency of the cells to detach from the plates. Monitoring the lytic infection closely is key to obtaining a high yield of adenovirus.
8. Any appropriate restriction enzyme can be used. In the case of *Bsa*BI, the 2249 band is from the left-hand end of the Ψ5 DNA and contains the expression cassette. Thus, its size will be altered by the insertion of a specific cDNA in a recombinant virus. Usually by the second or third passage in CRE8 cells, the Ψ5 helper virus is no longer detectable by restriction analysis of the DNA.

9. Primary digestion of pAdlox with *Sfi*I is recommended. This will release the adenoviral component of the plasmid, and in this linear form, recombination with the Ψ5 backbone is enhanced several fold. This will generate two bands, a 2500-bp fragment and a fragment of 1600 bp plus the cDNA insert *(19)*. However, if the cDNA of interest contains internal *Sfi*I recognition sites, such as the GFAT cDNA, this step can be omitted.

10. When generating new recombinant adenovirus, it is essential to determine that it expresses a functional gene product. This can be done by enzyme-linked immunosorbent assay, Western blot, or bioassay when available. If there is no existing quantitative assay for the protein of interest, transgenic expression can be measured at the RNA level by RT-PCR (*see* also **Note 15**).

11. To measure virus particle concentration, mix a 50-µL aliquot with 950 µL of GBSS and determine A_{260} by spectrophotometry. (One A_{260} is approximately equal to 10^{12} viral particles/mL.) The percentage of infectious virions typically ranges between 1 and 10% of the total number of viral particles. The infectious titer may be determined by performing a plaque assay on confluent cultures of 293 cells.

12. Typically two bands will be seen near the interface of the 1.2- and 1.4-g/mL CsCl layers. The lower band containing the infectious particles is the band that is collected.

13. To isolate the fibroblastic synoviocyte population preferentially, cells can be passaged three times to eliminate nonadherent, type A, macrophage-like cells. The type B synovial fibroblast can then be split into 75-cm^2 flasks and grown until 80% confluence.

14. Compared with adenovirus alone, adenovirus-$CaCl_2$ coprecipitates increase binding of virus to cells. Although the mechanism involved is not yet understood, increased binding is probably responsible for the significant increase in transgene expression *(20)*.

15. Transcriptional expression of the human cDNA delivered by the adenovirus can be distinguished from that of the endogenous homolog of the xenogenic host cell using RT-PCR and a modification of the method of Khiri et al. *(22)*. When available, a restriction site polymorphism between the coding sequences of the two species can allow strategic digestion such that the DNA amplification products of only one of the two species is digested into two fragments, whereas the other species remains uncut.

References

1. Pincus, T. and Callahan, L. F. (1992) Early mortality in RA predicted by poor clinical status. *Bull. Rheum. Dis.* **41,** 1–4.
2. Felson, D. T., Lawrence, R. C., Hochberg, M. C., et al. (2000) Osteoarthritis: new insights. Part 2: treatment approaches. *Ann. Intern. Med.* **133,** 726–737.
3. Smalley, W. E., Ray, W. A., Daugherty, J. R., and Griffin, M. R. (1995) Nonsteroidal anti-inflammatory drugs and the incidence of hospitalizations for peptic ulcer disease in elderly persons. *Am. J. Epidemiol.* **141,** 539–545.

4. Tamblyn, R., Berkson, L., Dauphinee, W. D., et al. (1997) Unnecessary prescribing of NSAIDs and the management of NSAID-related gastropathy in medical practice. *Ann. Intern. Med.* **127,** 429–438.

5. Reginster, J. Y., Deroisy, R., Rovati, L. C., et al. (2001) Long-term effects of glucosamine sulphate on osteoarthritis progression: a randomised, placebo-controlled clinical trial. Lancet **357,** 251–256.

6. Muller-Fassbender, H., Bach, G. L., Haase, W., Rovati, L. C., and Setnikar, I. (1994) Glucosamine sulfate compared to ibuprofen in osteoarthritis of the knee. *Osteoarthritis Cartilage* **2,** 61–69.

7. Bassleer, C., Rovati, L., and Franchimont, P. (1998) Stimulation of proteoglycan production by glucosamine sulfate in chondrocytes isolated from human osteoarthritic articular cartilage in vitro. *Osteoarthritis Cartilage* **6,** 427–434.

8. Gouze, J. N., Bordji, K., Gulberti, S., et al. (2001) Interleukin-1β down-regulates the expression of glucuronosyltransferase I, a key enzyme priming glycosaminoglycan biosynthesis: influence of glucosamine on interleukin-1β-mediated effects in rat chondrocytes. *Arthritis Rheum.* **44,** 351–360.

9. Gouze, J. N., Bianchi, A., Becuwe, P., et al. (2002) Glucosamine modulates IL-1-induced activation of rat chondrocytes at a receptor level, and by inhibiting the NF-κ B pathway. *FEBS Lett.* **510,** 166–170.

10. Sandy, J. D., Gamett, D., Thompson, V., and Verscharen, C. (1998) Chondrocyte-mediated catabolism of aggrecan: aggrecanase-dependent cleavage induced by interleukin-1 or retinoic acid can be inhibited by glucosamine. *Biochem. J.* **335,** 59–66.

11. Shikhman, A. R., Kuhn, K., Alaaeddine, N., and Lotz, M. (2001) N-acetylglucosamine prevents IL-1 β-mediated activation of human chondrocytes. *J. Immunol.* **166,** 5155–5160.

12. Chang, Q., Su, K., Baker, J. R., Yang, X., Paterson, A. J., and Kudlow, J. E. (2000) Phosphorylation of human glutamine:fructose-6-phosphate amidotransferase by cAMP-dependent protein kinase at serine 205 blocks the enzyme activity. *J. Biol. Chem.* **275,** 21,981–21,987.

13. Gouze, J., Ghivizzani, S., Gouze, E., et al. (2004) Adenovirus-mediated gene transfer of glutamine/fructose-6-phosphate amidotransferase antagonizes the effects of interleukin 1 beta in rat chondrocytes. *Osteoarthritic Cartilage* **12,** 217–224.

14. Ghivizzani, S. C., Lechman, E. R., Kang, R., et al. (1998) Direct adenovirus-mediated gene transfer of interleukin 1 and tumor necrosis factor alpha soluble receptors to rabbit knees with experimental arthritis has local and distal anti-arthritic effects. *Proc. Natl. Acad. Sci. USA* **95,** 4613–4618.

15. Ghivizzani, S. C., Oligino, T. J., Glorioso, J. C., Robbins, P. D., and Evans, C. H. (2001) Direct gene delivery strategies for the treatment of rheumatoid arthritis. *Drug. Discov. Today* **6,** 259–267.

16. Yao, Q., Glorioso, J. C., Evans, C. H., et al. (2000) Adenoviral mediated delivery of FAS ligand to arthritic joints causes extensive apoptosis in the synovial lining. *J. Gene Med.* **2,** 210–219.

17. Hardy, S., Kitamura, M., Harris-Stansil, T., Dai, Y., and Phipps, M. L. (1997) Construction of adenovirus vectors through Cre-lox recombination. *J. Virol.* **71,** 1842–1849.

18. Sambrook, J., Fritsch, E. and Maniatis, T. (eds.) (1989) *Molecular Cloning: A Laboratory Manual*, Cold Spring Harbor Laboratory Press, Cold Spring Harbor, NY.
19. Palmer, G. D., Gouze, E., Gouze, J. N., Betz, O. B., Evans, C. H., and Ghivizzani, S. C. (2003) Gene transfer to articular chondrocytes with recombinant adenovirus. *Methods Mol. Biol.* **215,** 235–246.
20. Fasbender, A., Lee, J. H., Walters, R. W., Moninger, T. O., Zabner, J., and Welsh, M. J. (1998) Incorporation of adenovirus in calcium phosphate precipitates enhances gene transfer to airway epithelia in vitro and in vivo. *J. Clin. Invest.* **102,** 184–193.
21. Frohman, M. A., Dush, M. K., and Martin, G. R. (1988) Rapid production of full-length cDNAs from rare transcripts: amplification using a single gene-specific oligonucleotide primer. *Proc. Natl. Acad. Sci. USA* **85,** 8998–9002.
22. Khiri, H., Reynier, P., Peyrol, N., Lerique, B., Torresani, J., and Planells, R. (1996) Quantitative multistandard RT-PCR assay using interspecies polymorphism. *Mol. Cell Probes* **10,** 201–211.

13

Changes of Chondrocyte Metabolism In Vitro
An Approach by Proteomic Analysis

Anne-Marie Freyria and Michel Becchi

Summary

Changes in chondrocyte metabolism in vitro using different support systems and under different culture conditions were studied with a proteomic approach. Qualitative and quantitative modifications in the synthesis of chondrocyte proteins were investigated using two-dimensional (2D) gel electrophoresis. This technique provided a simple way to visualize the most abundant chondrocyte proteins. Proteins were identified after in-gel proteolysis with trypsin and matrix-assisted laser desorption ionization-time of flight mass spectrometry, using peptide mass fingerprinting. Tryptic peptide masses were measured and matched against a computer-generated list from the simulated trypsin proteolysis of a protein database (SwissProt).

Key Words: Proteomics; cartilage; chondrocyte culture; 2D electrophoresis; in-gel protein digestion; MALDI-TOF; peptide-mass fingerprinting.

1. Introduction

Articular cartilage is a tissue that has a limited capacity for repair after trauma or diseases such as osteoarthritis (OA) *(1)*. Among the numerous changes that occur during the course of OA, a modulation of the chondrocyte phenotype that can be reproduced in vitro is observed *(2)*. Most in vitro studies have analyzed chondrocyte growth and the synthesis of cartilage-specific matrix components by chondrocytes of different origins grown under different culture conditions: in monolayer, in a 3D environment and in explants *(3,4)*. More recently, qualitative and quantitative modifications in the synthesis of chondrocyte proteins have been investigated using 2D electrophoresis and microsequencing, to get insights into the mechanisms involved in chondrocyte differentiation and cartilage regeneration *(5–7)*. The applications of proteome analysis in a clinical context were also reported in the secretion medium of OA cartilage explants *(8)* and in the synovial fluids and plasma from OA patients *(9)*.

From: *Methods in Molecular Medicine, Vol. 100: Cartilage and Osteoarthritis, Vol. 1: Cellular and Molecular Tools*
Edited by: M. Sabatini, P. Pastoureau, and F. De Ceuninck © Humana Press Inc., Totowa, NJ

Two-dimensional electrophoresis is a powerful technique for separating proteins from a mixture according to two physical parameters: charge and molecular weight. The identification of proteins may be carried out using immunolabeling when antibodies are available, Edman microsequencing to obtain amino acid sequences that will match known sequences in databases, or mass spectrometry. Matrix-assisted laser desorption (MALDI) *(10)* and electrospray ionization (ESI) *(11)* are two ionization methods frequently used in protein mass spectrometry analyses *(12,13)*. Total protein mass is insufficiently discriminating to identify proteins with confidence; rather, proteins should first be converted into shorter peptides by proteolysis. The usual method involves excision of gel spots of interest, in-gel digestion using trypsin (the enzyme that cleaves the C-terminal to the lysyl and arginyl residues), and finally, mass spectrometric analysis of the peptides produced *(14–16)*. There is a direct relationship between mass spectrometric data and peptide amino acid sequences, and at this stage, two methods are available for protein identification:

1. Peptide mass fingerprinting (PMF), which compares an experimental peptide mass profile with a theoretical profile calculated from the known sequences in a protein database *(17,18)*.
2. Peptide fragmentation information generated by tandem mass spectrometry (MS/MS). Mass spectra produced by collision-induced decomposition of selected peptide ions are compared with theoretical tandem mass spectra in a database *(19)*.

We have used PMF with a MALDI-TOF (time-of-flight) instrument. The efficiency of a PMF search strongly depends on the accuracy of peptide mass measurements. This technique may be sufficient to characterize proteins from completely sequenced genomes, as the masses of all theoretical peptides can be calculated precisely. The PMF strategy is generally completed by combining it with MS/MS to generate additional sequence information. MALDI-TOF mass spectrometry can offer limited information via postsource decay (PSD) mass spectra *(20,21)*, but, for small proteins and for proteins that generate a limited number of peptides in the classical working mass range (600–4000) from trypsin proteolysis, PSD can help confirm their identification.

2. Materials

2.1. Chondrocyte Culture Equipment

1. Hemacytometer (Malassez).
2. Centrifuge (up to 3800*g*).
3. Inverted-phase contrast microscope.
4. 12.5-cm^2 Sterile culture flasks.
5. Orbital shaker (Heidolph, Schwabach, Germany).

2.2. Chondrocyte Culture

When not indicated, prepare the solutions from analytical grade reagents and dissolve in deionized water.

1. Phosphate-buffered saline (PBS; Sigma, Saint Quentin Fallavier, France): one pouch dissolved in 1 L of distilled water yields 0.01 M sodium phosphate, 0.138 M NaCl, 0.0027 M KCl, pH 7.4.
2. 0.4% Trypan Blue solution (Sigma).
3. Cartilage: metacarpophalangeal joints of calves less than 6 mo old, obtained from a local slaughterhouse less than 3 h after death.
4. Chondrocyte isolation solution: 0.2% (w/v) hyaluronidase type I-S (Sigma) dissolved in PBS.
5. 0.1% (w/v) Collagenase type IA (Sigma) + 0.1% (w/v) dispase II (Roche Applied Bioscience, Meylan, France) dissolved in PBS (*see* **Note 1**).
6. Cell culture medium: NCTC 109 medium + RPMI-1640 medium (Sigma; 50/50, v/v) containing 0.25% glutamine (Sigma), 10% fetal calf serum (Seromed, Strasbourg, France), 1% penicillin–streptomycin (PS), and 0.4% amphotericin B (stock solutions; Gibco BRL Life Technologies).
7. Biomaterials: bovine type I collagen sponges (Coletica, Lyon, France) cross-linked using *n*-hydroxysuccinimide/1-ethyl-3(-3-dimethylaminopropyl)carbodiimide hydrochloride (NHS/EDC) methods.

2.3. Protein Preparation and Separation Equipment

1. Sterile 15-mL tubes, Eppendorf tubes, and Petri dishes (35 × 10 mm).
2. Reswelling tray (Amersham Biosciences) for the rehydration of the immobiline drystrips (*see* **Subheading 2.4.**)
3. First-dimension separation: Multiphor™ II system and EPS 3500 XL power supply (Amersham Biosciences). Temperature control provided by a Haake F3 thermostatic circulator (Haake, Bioblock Scientific).
4. Second-dimension separation: power supply (1000/500) and a Criterion cell (Bio-Rad, Life Science).

2.4. Protein Preparation and Separation Reagents

1. Immobiline drystrip, pH 4.0–7.0, 11 cm (Bio-Rad), immobilized pH gradient (IPG) buffer pH 4.0–7.0 (Amersham Biosciences).
2. Criterion precast gel 10% acrylamide (Bio-Rad).
3. Collagenase in PBS (1.5 mg/mL).
4. Trypsin/EDTA (Gibco-BRL Life Technologies) diluted with PBS to obtain final concentrations of 0.1%/0.04%.
5. Dithiothreitol (DTT) and iodoacetamide (Sigma).
6. Molecular mass marker proteins: sodium dodecyl sulfate-polyacrylamide gel electrophoresis (SDS-PAGE) standard (Bio-Rad).
7. Protein lysis buffer: 8 M urea (Bio-Rad), 1 M thiourea (Sigma), 4% CHAPS (3-[(3-cholamidopropyl)dimethylammonio]-1-propane sulfonate; Sigma), 40 mM

Tris base. This buffer can be stored in 250-µL aliquots at –20°C for up to 4 mo. **Do not heat above 30°C to dissolve the different components.**

8. Drystrip rehydration buffer: 8 M urea, 2% CHAPS, 0.2% IPG buffer (same pH range as the drystrip), 50 mM DTT (Sigma), and a trace of bromophenol blue (Bio-Rad). This buffer can be stored in 250-µL aliquots at –20°C for up to 4 mo.

9. SDS equilibration buffer: 0.375 M Tris-HCl, pH 8.8, 6 M urea, 20% glycerol, 2% SDS (Sigma), and a trace of bromophenol blue. The buffer can be stored in 12-mL aliquots at –20°C for up to 4 mo.

10. SDS equilibration buffer containing a reducing agent (equilibration buffer 1): dissolve 130 mM DTT in 6 mL equilibration buffer. Prepare the solution just prior to use.

11. SDS equilibration buffer containing an alkylating agent (equilibration buffer 2): dissolve 135 mM iodoacetamide in 6 mL equilibration buffer. Prepare the solution just prior to use.

12. Running buffer for the second dimension gel: 0.025 M Tris, 0.192 M glycine, 1% SDS, pH 8.3. This buffer can be stored at 4°C for up to 6 mo.

13. Coomassie blue solution: 0.25 g of Coomassie R250 (Roth, Lauterbourg, France) dissolved in 400 mL methanol, 100 mL acetic acid, and 500 mL deionized water.

14. Destaining solution: 30% methanol, 10% acetic acid in deionized water.

2.5. In-Gel Enzymatic Digestion Equipment

1. Heating block for microcentrifuge tubes with shaker (type: Thermomixer comfort, Eppendorf, Fisher Scientific).
2. Water bath at 37°C.
3. Vacuum concentrator (e.g., Speed-Vac Savant, Avantec).
4. Centrifuge (5000–7000g; e.g., Micro 7, Fisher Scientific).
5. Laboratory rotating mixer (Vortex, Fisher Scientific).
6. Scalpel.
7. Tweezers.
8. Glass sheet, 15 × 15 cm.
9. Polypropylene microcentrifuge tubes (0.5 and 1.5 mL).
10. Ultrafine tips (gel loader type pipet tips, VWR International, Strasbourg, France).

2.6. In-Gel Enzymatic Digestion Reagents

When not indicated prepare the solutions from analytical grade reagents.

1. Milli-Q grade water (Millipore).
2. Ethanol/water (20/80, v/v).
3. 100 mM Ammonium bicarbonate (NH_4HCO_3), pH 8.0, stock solution, aliquoted in 1.5-mL Eppendorf tubes and kept at –20°C. Working solutions: 20 and 50 mM NH_4HCO_3 in water.
4. Sequencing-grade modified trypsin (20 µg/vial; Promega).
5. Acetonitrile.
6. Formic acid/water (5/95, v/v).
7. Acetonitrile/water (50/50, v/v).

2.7. MALDI–MS Equipment

1. MALDI-TOF mass spectrometer equipped with delayed source extraction, operating in linear and/or reflector mode. For PSD capability for MS/MS experiments, we use a Voyager-DE™ PRO MALDI-TOF from Applied Biosystems.
2. ZipTip$_{SCX}$ (Millipore) pipet tips containing strong cation exchange resin.

2.8. MALDI–MS Reagents

1. Trifluoroacetic acid (TFA; Sigma); stock solution: 1% TFA in water (v/v). Working solution: 0.1% in water (v/v).
2. Matrix: α-cyano-4-hydroxycinnamic acid (HCCA, purified; Laser Bio Labs, Sophia-Antipolis, France): a saturated solution at 5 mg/0.5 mL of acetonitrile/water (50/50 v/v) containing 0.1% TFA is prepared every d.
3. Methanol.
4. Ammonium hydroxide, 25% stock solution in water.
5. Elution solution for ZipTip$_{SCX}$: 5% ammonium hydroxide/30% methanol in Milli-Q-grade water (in a 1.5-mL centrifuge tube: 500 μL H$_2$O, 300 μL CH$_3$OH, and 200 μL 25% NH$_4$OH).

3. Methods

3.1. Protein Sample Preparation From Cell Cultures

3.1.1. Cell Collection and Solubilization From Monolayer Culture

1. Isolate chondrocytes from minced cartilage by enzymatic digestion with a mixture of 0.2% hyaluronidase and 0.2% collagenase/dispase in PBS at 37°C for 4 h with gentle magnetic stirring.
2. Wash isolated cells three times in culture medium and count them with an hemacytometer. Check viability using the trypan blue solution (1 vol cell suspension + 0.1 vol trypan blue solution).
3. Seed the cells at high-density culture (0.6×10^6 cells/cm^2) and grow them in an incubator at 37°C in a closed flask with 5 mL of culture medium for up to 1 mo, changing the medium every 3 d.
4. Harvest cells (at the chosen time of analysis):
   a. Wash twice in PBS and incubate for 2 min at 37°C in 0.1% trypsin/EDTA (100 μL/flask).
   b. Detach cells with a cell scraper, add 2 mL of culture medium, and suspend the cells by repeated pipeting in a 15 mL tube, so as to obtain a single-cell suspension.
   c. Add 10 mL of culture medium to the suspension and count the cells.
   d. Centrifuge for 6 min at 1400g, discard the supernatant, resuspend the pellet in 1 mL PBS and place it in an Eppendorf tube. Centrifuge and re-suspend the pellet in lysis buffer at 50 μL per 4 million cells (*see* **Subheading 2.4.7.**).

3.1.2. Cell Collection and Solubilization From a 3D Culture

1. Seed collagen sponges with 1×10^6 or 10×10^6 cells per sponge (2.3×10^6 or 23×10^6 cells per cm^3). Culture them in a 37°C incubator in 5 mL of culture medium per sponge, in a closed flask, changing the medium every 3 d.
2. Harvest the cells:
   a. Cut each sponge into four pieces with a scalpel blade in a Petri dish.
   b. Place the pieces in a tube with 1 mL 0.2% hyaluronidase in PBS. Shake for 15 min on the orbital shaker (30 rpm) in the incubator at 37°C.
3. Collect the liquid phase in a 15-mL tube and centrifuge for 4 min at 1400*g*. Discard the supernatant, add 1 mL of PBS to the pellet, and resuspend the cells. Keep this tube (T1) for the cell count.
4. Treat the sponge phase with 1 mL of collagenase at 1.5 mg/mL in PBS for 15 min at 37°C with gentle shaking. Collect the fluid phase, centrifuge, and resuspend the pellet in 2 mL PBS. Keep the tube (T2) for the cell count. Treat the remaining sponge phase in the same way (T3). Wash the sponge phase with 5 mL of culture medium for 15 min at 37°C and collect the liquid phase (T4). Pool all four tubes into a 15-mL tube, and count the cells with a hemacytometer. Centrifuge the tube for 4 min at 1400*g*, and discard the supernatant. Resuspend the pellet in 1 mL PBS, and then transfer it to an Eppendorf tube and centrifuge. Resuspend the pellet in cell lysis buffer (50 µL per 4 million cells) and store at –20°C for the assay.

3.2. 2D Electrophoresis (see Note 2)

3.2.1. First Dimension: Isoelectric Focusing (IEF)

1. Rehydrate the drystrip gel, pH 4.0–7.0, with a mixture of the sample in lysis buffer (50 µL) and rehydration buffer (230 µL), place in one groove of the reswelling tray, and protect by a layer of paraffin oil (3 mL per drystrip) for 12 h at room temperature. (The number of gel strips required corresponds to the samples to be compared in one experiment.)
2. Set the temperature of the Haake F3 thermostatic circulator to 19°C prior to the start of IEF.
3. Place the rehydrated drystrips into the tray of the Multiphor II system and verify that the anodic terminus of the drystrip faces the anode side of the Multiphor II system. Place the electrodes at both ends of the strips. Pour about 80 mL of paraffin oil into the tray. Start the IEF according to the parameters given in **Table 1**, using the gradient mode of the EPS 3500 XL power supply.
4. When IEF is complete, discard the paraffin oil and remove the electrodes and the focused gel strips from the tray using clean forceps.
5. Store the focused gel strips in clean individual tubes (15 mL) at –20°C until the second dimension run.

3.2.2. Drystrip Gel Equilibration

1. Take the tube containing the focused gel out of the freezer.
2. Add equilibration buffer 1 and place the tube on a shaker for 15 min at room temperature. Remove equilibration buffer 1 from the tube.

Table 1
Running Conditions for Drystrips, pH 4.0–7.0, 11 cm

Time	Voltage	Current (mA)	Power (W)
30 min	0–300	1	5
30 min	300	1	5
90 min	300–3500	1	5
5 h[a]	3500	1	5

[a]Adjust the time of the last step of the program to obtain 20.6 kVh at the end.

3. Add equilibration buffer 2 and place the tube on the shaker for another 15 min at room temperature.
4. Rinse the gel briefly with distilled water to remove excess equilibration buffer and place it on a piece of filter paper on the edge of one long side for 2–3 min. (Bending the gel helps to keep it on the long side.)

3.2.3. Second Dimension

1. Prepare the Criterion precast gel for the second dimension according to the manufacturer's instructions while the focused gel strip is equilibrating.
2. Rinse the top of the gel with running buffer and leave buffer in the two wells (one small one for the molecular weight marker and one long one for the focused gel).
3. Load the focused gel strip on top of the Criterion gel, with the plastic sheet facing the top glass plate. Push down on the gel with a spatula, taking care to avoid creating or trapping air bubbles where the two gels meet. Add 10 µL of molecular mass marker protein to the small well.
4. Insert the gel cassette into the electrophoresis chamber of the Criterion cell containing 800 mL of fresh running buffer. Fill the upper chamber with 60 mL of running buffer.
5. Run the machine for 10 min at 100 V and for 45–60 min at 200 V (ensure that the bromophenol blue migrates to the end of the SDS-PAGE gel; *see* **Note 3**).

3.2.4. Staining of the Gel

1. Immediately after electrophoresis, rinse the gel with distilled water for 1–2 min with gentle shaking to remove SDS.
2. Soak the gel in 200 mL of a fresh solution of Coomassie blue for 20–30 min. Rinse briefly with water, and then soak in 200 mL destaining solution until the desired contrast is achieved. Keep gel at 4°C in water for a few d until in-gel protein digestion (*see* **Fig. 1** and **Note 4**).

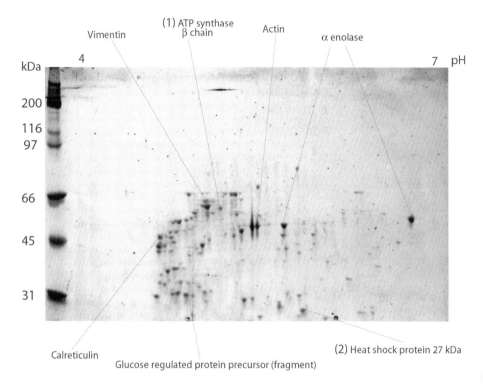

Fig. 1. Two-dimensional electrophoretic separation of intracellular proteins extracted from bovine chondrocytes grown in 3D culture for 3 wk (initial seeding 10×10^6 cells). The protein sample was treated following the procedures given in **Subheadings 3.1.2.** for protein extraction and **3.2.** for protein separation. This figure gives an example of the effectiveness of direct extraction from collagen sponges. The pattern compares with a published pattern obtained after protein extraction from a monolayer culture *(6)*. For spots (1) and (2) see the MALDI-TOF mass fingerprinting results in **Figs. 2** and **3**, respectively.

3.3. In-Gel Protein Digestion (see Note 5)

3.3.1. Excision of Protein Spots

1. Clean work areas and all utensils (scalpel, tweezers, glass sheets, and so on) with methanol.
2. Identify the spot of interest on the gel and excise it with a scalpel. Cut it as close as possible to the protein spot (*see* **Note 6**).
3. Cut the excised spot into roughly 1-mm³ pieces and transfer them to a clean, labeled 0.5-mL microcentrifuge tube.

3.3.2. Destaining of Coomassie Blue-Stained Gel Pieces

1. Add 400 µL 20 mM NH$_4$HCO$_3$ to gel pieces. Let the tubes stand for 15 min at 30°C (in Thermomixer without shaking or water bath). Remove liquid using gel loading pipet tips.
2. Add 400 µL of CH$_3$CN/H$_2$O (50/50, v/v) and incubate for 15 min at 30°C. Remove solvent using gel loading pipet tips. Repeat this step until the blue coloration disappears.
3. Add 400 µL H$_2$O and incubate for 15 min at 30°C. Remove water using gel loading pipet tips and dry the gel pieces in a vacuum centrifuge. If a large volume of gel is used, shrink it by adding CH$_3$CN before drying.
4. Keep dried gel pieces at –20°C until the next step (*see* **Note 7**).

3.3.3. In-Gel Digestion

1. Stock solution of trypsin: dissolve 20 µg of trypsin (*see* **Subheading 2.6.**) in 200 µL 50 mM NH$_4$HCO$_3$ at 25–30°C for 10 min (*see* **Note 8**).
2. Distribute stock solution into 0.5 mL polypropylene centrifuge tubes in 10–20 µL aliquots and keep at –20°C. Thaw the required trypsin solution at room temperature before use. The final concentration of trypsin should be 0.1 µg/µL.
3. Apply trypsin solution directly onto gel pieces. The trypsin/protein ratio in the gel should be about 1:10. Use 0.5–4 µL of trypsin solution, depending on the intensity of the protein spot (i.e., protein concentration): from 0.5 µL for small and lightly colored spots and up to 4 µL for large and intense spots.
4. Centrifuge for 2 min at 5000–7000g to allow trypsin to penetrate inside the gel pieces.
5. Complete rehydration with enough 50 mM NH$_4$HCO$_3$ buffer to just cover the gel pieces. At this stage avoid the absence or excess of NH$_4$HCO$_3$ buffer (*see* **Note 9**).
6. Digest for 6 h at 37°C. Check buffer volume during digestion (especially after about 1 h of digestion) and add fresh buffer, if necessary, to keep the gel pieces completely covered and wet.

3.3.4. Extraction of Tryptic Peptides

1. Spin and shake the microcentrifuge tubes in the Thermomixer Comfort (Eppendorf) at 30°C for 8 min. Centrifuge for 2 min at 4600–5000g (8–9000 rpm).
2. Remove supernatant (digest buffer) with a gel loader pipet tip and keep it in a new labeled 0.5-mL microcentrifuge tube.
3. Extract successively with CH$_3$CN, HCOOH/H$_2$O (5/95, v/v) and CH$_3$CN/H$_2$O (50/50, v/v). For each extraction step, add approximately the same volume of solvent as the volume of trypsin solution plus buffer used for digestion. After adding solvent, shake for 10 min at 30°C in the Thermomixer Comfort (Eppendorf) at 1300 rpm, centrifuge, and remove solvent extract with a gel loader pipet tip. Pool all corresponding extracts in the same labeled microcentrifuge tube.
4. Keep the extract solutions at –20°C until mass spectrometry analysis.

3.4. MALDI-TOF Sample Preparation

3.4.1. Loading of the MALDI-TOF Target

1. Matrix preparation: *see* **Subheading 2.8.2.**
2. Dry down extract solutions of peptides in a vacuum concentrator.
3. Redissolve peptides in 12–15 µL 0.1% TFA, vortex, and then centrifuge.
4. Add 1 µL of sample solution and 1 µL matrix solution to the target and leave to dry in a gentle stream of air. (We use the fans of the MALDI-TOF instrument.)

3.4.2. Sample Clean-Up on ZipTip$_{SCX}$

1. Equilibrate the ZipTip$_{SCX}$ pipet tip by drawing up 10 µL 0.1% TFA (use a 10-µL pipet; *see* **Note 10**). Expel the TFA solution. Repeat this process three times.
2. Bind the peptides from the remaining sample solution used in **Subheading 3.4.1.** by carrying out 12–15 aspirate-dispense cycles of the entire sample (*see* **Note 11**).
3. Wash the ZipTip$_{SCX}$ by drawing up 10 µL 0.1% TFA into the tip and expelling it. Repeat this process five times.
4. Desorb bound peptides by aspirating 2.5 µL elution solution (*see* **Subheading 2.8.**). Deposit eluates directly onto the MALDI-TOF target and pipet up and down three times.
5. Dry spots in a gentle air stream.
6. Overlay each peptide spot with 1 µL matrix solution (*see* **Subheading 2.8.**).

3.5. MALDI-TOF–MS Analysis

MALDI-TOF mass spectra are acquired in the 700-5000-Dalton mass range using a minimum of 200 shots of laser per spectrum.

3.5.1. Internal Calibration

Delayed ion extraction and reflectron MALDI-TOF mass spectrometer equipment allow sufficient resolution to consider monoisotopic masses of singly charged ions [M+H]$^+$. The accuracy of mass measurements depends on the calibration procedures. External calibration is performed with a mixture of known peptides covering the mass range applied (as close as possible to but well separated from the sample deposit). We use internal calibration with autolysis ion fragments of trypsin at m/z 842.5100, 1045.5642, 2211.1046, and 2283.1807, which allow a peptide mass tolerance of ± 30 ppm for peptide mass measurements.

3.5.2. Peptide Mass Fingerprinting

1. Follow the manufacturer's instructions for mass spectra acquisitions (*see* **Subheading 2.7.**, **Note 12**, and **Fig. 2**). MALDI produces only singly charged [M+H]$^+$ peptide ions and is tolerant toward complex mixtures, permitting the mass of many different peptides to be recorded.
2. Carry out a first assay on the sample extract solution (*see* **Subheading 3.4.1.**).

A

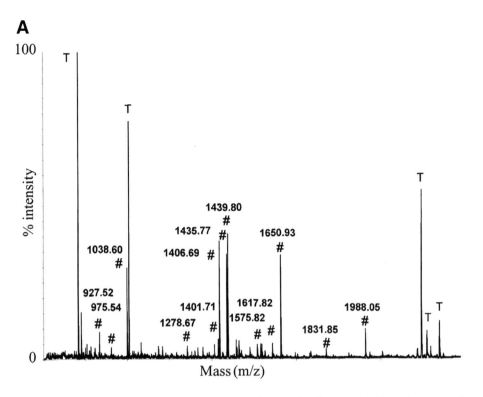

Fig. 2. **(A)** MALDI-TOF mass spectrum of a tryptic digest of a 2D gel separated protein. #, matched peptide ions [M + H]⁺ for the ATP synthase β-chain (SwissProt accession number P00829). T, trypsin autolysis peptide fragments. *(See following page for* **Fig. 2B.**)

3. If the mass spectrum shows a very low ion count then carry out a second assay after ZipTip$_{SCX}$ treatment (*see* **Subheading 3.4.2.**).
4. Obtain a list of monoisotopic [M+H]⁺ masses of tryptic peptides for each protein spot. Remove trypsin autolysis peptides from this list (i.e., peptides used for internal calibration; *see* **Subheading 3.5.1.**) and contaminants from the gel (*see* **Note 13**).

3.5.3. Peptide-Mass Searches

1. Several search engines available on the internet, and these can all be found on the proteomic server of the Swiss Institute of Bioinformatics at http://www.expasy. org/: MS-Fit (ProteinProspector), Mascot, PeptideSearch, Pepident, and so on.

B   **MS-Fit Search Results**

Parameters

Database searched : **SwissProt. 10.25.2002**
Digest Used : **Trypsin**
Max. # Missed Cleavages : **1**
Peptide N terminus : **Hydrogen**
Peptide C terminus : **Free Acid**
Cysteine Modification : **carbamidomethylation**
Instrument Name : **MALDI-TOF**
Sample ID (comment) : **T462 digest**
Minimum Matches : **4**
Sort Type : **Score Sort**
Considered modifications : **Oxidation of M**
Min Parent Ion Matches : **1**
MOWSE On : **1**
MOWSE P Factor : **0.4**

Pre Search Results

Number of entries in the database : **116819**
Molecular weight search (**10000-100000 Da**) selects **99526** entries.
Full pI range : **116819** entries.
Species search (**MAMMALS**) selects **21366** entries
Combined molecular weight, pI and species searches select **18117** entries.
Pre searches select **18117** entries.

Data Set 1 Results

MS-Fit search selects **24** entries (results displayed for top **5** matches).

Results Summary

	MOWSE Score	#/27(%) Masses Matched	% Cov	Mean Err ppm	Data Tol ppm	MS-Digest Index #	Protein MW (Da)/pI	Accession #	Species	Protein Name
1	6.227e+004	12 (44)	30.0	1.57	18.9	86706	56284/5.1	P00829	BOVIN	ATP synthase beta chain, mitochondrial precursor
2	2.237e+004	10 (37)	26.0	2.85	19.7	80369	56301/5.2	P56480	MOUSE	ATP synthase beta chain, mitochondrial precursor
3	2.335e+004	11 (40)	29.0	1.97	19.6	106175	56354/5.2	P10719	RAT	ATP synthase beta chain, mitochondrial precursor
4	2.326e+004	11 (40)	29.0	1.97	19.6	107105	56560/5.3	P06576	HUMAN	ATP synthase beta chain, mitochondrial precursor
5	262	4 (14)	12.0	11.2	24.8	25150	47221/4.9	Q63081	RAT	Protein disulfide isomerase A6 precursor (Protein di sulfide Isomerase P5) (Calcium-binding protein 1) (CaBP1)

Detailed Results

1.   12/27 matches (44 %).
Acc. # : P00829 **Species** : BOVIN **Name** : ATP synthase beta chain, mitochondrial precursor
Index : 86706 **MW**: 56284 Da **pI** : 5.1

m/z Submitted	MH⁺ Matched	Delta ppm	Modifications	Start	End	Missed Cleavages	Database Sequence
927.5238	927.5264	-2.8		125	133	0	(K)VLDSGAPIR (I)
975.5387	975.5627	-25		202	212	0	(K)IGLFGGAGVGK (T)
1038.6002	1038.5948	5.2		134	143	0	(R)IPVGPETLGR (I)
1401.7082	1401.7048	2.4	1Met-ox	144	155	0	(R)IMNVIGEPIDER(G)
1406.6934	1406.6817	8.3		226	239	0	(K)AHGGYSVFAGVGER (T)
1435.7669	1435.7545	8.6		311	324	0	(R)FTQAGSEVSALLGR (I)
1439.7978	1439.7898	5.5		282	294	0	(R)VALTGLTVAEYFR (D)
1575.8223	1575.8165	3.7		110	124	1	(R)TIAMDGTEGLVRGQK (V)
1617.8160	1617.8059	6.2	1Met-ox	265	279	0	(K)VALVYGQMNEPPGAR(A)
1650.9290	1650.9179	6.7		95	109	0	(R)LVLEVAQHLGESTVR (T)
1831.8523	1831.8649	-6.9	1 Met-ox	407	422	0	(R)IMDPNIVGSEHYDVAR(G)
1988.0466	1988.0340	6.3		388	406	0	(R)AIAELGIYPAVDPLDSTSR (I)

The matched peptides cover **30%** (163/528AA's) of the protein.
Coverage Map for This Hit (MS-Digest index #) : 86706

Fig. 2. *(Continued from previous page)* **(B)** MS-Fit search results for peptide mass fingerprinting for the first proposition.

We have MS-Fit in-house and we also use Mascot on the web to confirm results. Whichever one you use, there are several parameters to specify:

a. *Database*: we use the SwissProt database for a PMF search. The NCBInr database may be used to find other sequence homologies or relevant propositions.
b. *Species*: select Mammals from the suggested species.

    c. *MW of protein*: input a ±30 kDa range from the estimated MW from the 2D gel (*see* **Note 14**).

    d. *Protein pI*: select all because proteins may be post-translationally modified (phosphorylation, glycosylation, and so on).

    e. *Digest*: trypsin, with 1 as the maximum number of missed cleavages.

    f. *Cysteine modification*: input carbamidomethylation, as the protein is reduced and alkylated by iodoacetamide (*see* **Subheading 3.2.2.**).

    g. *Possible modifications*: we generally choose oxidation of methionine and acetylation of the protein N-terminus.

    h. *Mass spectrometry parameters*: MALDI-TOF instrument, peptide monoisotopic masses with a tolerance of ±30 ppm.

    i. *Minimum number of peptides required to match*: 4 is a good starting point.

2. Under reported hits, don't expect all the masses that you put into the search engine to be tryptic peptides from the protein spot, as some of them will be contaminants. It is not only the number of hits, i.e., the number of matched peptides, that is important. There is also a MOWSE score that uses larger fragments, which are statistically more significant when measuring probability. The protein recovery percentage from the matched peptides is also a useful parameter.

3.5.4. Postsource Decay MALDI–MS

When the confidence of a PMF search is too low (**Fig. 3**), additional sequence information on the observed peptides can be provided from PSD spectra (**Fig. 4**). Our MALDI-TOF instrument is fitted with a variable voltage reflector, which involves a long and fastidious recording of the spectra (as the reflector has to be scanned at different voltage values), as well as the different spectra being added and then reconstructed by the software. PSD has other drawbacks with regard to ESI–MS/MS techniques: ion selection is not very specific and is made over a relatively large mass range ±20 Dalton, and there is no way to control or improve the fragmentation. We only consider very abundant parent ions $[M + H]^+$ for PSD analysis.

PSD MALDI–MS spectra are generally very complicated, as all the classical peptide ion fragments containing both N- and C-termini are observed (for nomenclature, *see* ref. *23*) as well as internal fragments. We use instrument software (a protein fragmentation calculator) to interpret PSD spectra. Starting with the supposed sequence, the software calculates all possible fragmentations, and then the theoretical ion fragments are compared with those observed on the PSD MALDI–MS spectrum (*see* **Note 15**).

4. Notes

1. Prepare the appropriate volume just before cell extraction or cartilage digestion, as enzyme solutions are less effective after the freeze-thaw step.

A

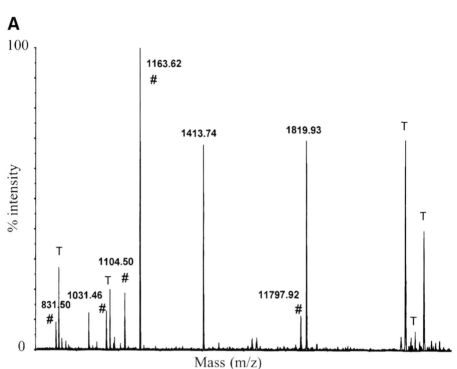

Fig. 3. (A) MALDI-TOF mass spectrum of a tryptic digest of a 2D gel separated protein. (B) *(opposite page)* The MS-Fit search results show only five matched peptides (labeled # on the mass spectrum) for the 27-kDa heat shock protein (SwissProt accession number P42929) from *Canis familiaris* (CANFA). The abundant ions at m/z 1413.74 and 1819.93 are not identified. Protein identification is completed using a post source decay mass spectrum (*see* **Fig. 4**).

2. As the goal of the separating steps is to be able to identify the proteins present in the different samples using mass spectrometry analysis, it is recommended to wear gloves (powder-free or nitrile) at each stage, first to eliminate contamination with keratin and second, to be able to use silver staining methods safely (*see* ref. *22* for details) when a higher sensitivity than Coomassie blue is desired.
3. Make sure to run the gels from corresponding experiments in a similar way so as to be able to compare gel patterns by image analysis, if necessary.
4. When the purpose of the study is to compare different chondrocyte culture conditions, scan the wet gels (e.g., with the Personal Densitometer SI and Image Quant software from Amersham Biosciences) in order to make significant comparisons and qualitative and quantitative analyses of the proteins of interest.

B

MS-Fit Search Results

Parameters

Database searched : **SwissProt. 10.25.2002**
Digest Used : **Trypsin**
Max. # Missed Cleavages : **1**
Peptide N terminus : **Hydrogen**
Peptide C terminus : **Free Acid**
Cysteine Modification : **carbamidomethylation**
Instrument Name : **MALDI-TOF**
Sample ID (comment) : **T462 digest**
Minimum Matches : **4**
Sort Type : **Score Sort**
Considered modifications : **Oxidation of M**
Min Parent Ion Matches : 1
MOWSE On : 1
MOWSE P Factor : **0.4**

MS-Fit search selects 5 entries.

Pre Search Results

Number of entries in the database : **116819**
Molecular weight search (**10000-100000 Da**) selects 99526 entries.
Full pI range : **116819** entries.
Species search (**MAMMALS**) selects 21366 entries
Combined molecular weight, pI and species searches select 18117 entries.
Pre searches select **18117** entries.

Data Set 1 Results

Results Summary

	MOWSE Score	#/16(%) Masses Matched	% Cov	Mean Err ppm	Data Tol ppm	MS-Digest Index #	Protein MW (Da)/pI	Accession #	Species	Protein Name
1	994	5 (31)	23.0	-6.06	7.65	30070	22939/6.2	P42929	CANFA	Heat shock 27 kDa protein (HSP 27)
2	308	4 (25)	19.0	-7.14	6.85	8489	22893/6.1	P42930	RAT	Heat shock 27 kDa protein (HSP 27)
3	306	4 (25)	19.0	-7.14	6.85	38653	23014/6.1	P14602	MOUSE	Heat shock 27 kDa protein (HSP 27) (Growth-Related 25 kDa protein) (P25) (HSP25)
4	149	4 (25)	16.0	-4.60	9.21	31927	22783/6.0	P04792	HUMAN	Heat shock 27 kDa protein (HSP 27) (Stress-Responsive protein 27) (SRP27) (28 Kda heat shock protein)
5	100	4 (25)	4.0	1.03	18.5	62854	80612/6.7	O99797	HUMAN	Mitochondrial intermediate peptidase, mitochondrial precursor (MIP)

Detailed Results

1. 5/16 matches (31 %).
Acc. # : P42929 **Species** : CANFA **Name** : heat shock 27kDa protein (HSP 27)
Index : 30070 **MW**: 22939 Da **pI** : 6.2

m/z Submitted	MH⁺ Matched	Delta ppm	Modifications	Start	End	Missed Cleavages	Database Sequence
831.4998	831.5092	-11		6	12	0	(R)VPFSLLR (S)
1031.4645	1031.4699	-5.2		21	28	0	(R)DWYPAHSR (L)
1104.5034	1104.5074	-3.6		132	140	0	(R)QDEHGYISR (R)
1163.6193	1163.6213	-1.7		29	38	0	(R)LFDQAFGLPR(L)
1797.9237	1797.9387	-8.3		101	116	0	(R)VSLDVNHFAPEELTVK(T)

The matched peptides cover **23%** (50/209AA's) of the protein.
Coverage Map for This Hit (MS-Digest index #) : 30070

5. One of the main problems encountered is keratin contamination of samples. You must wear a lab coat and gloves to avoid any contact with gel electrophoresis samples, reagents, and in-gel digestion equipment by skin, fingers, or any keratin source (woolen sweater, and so).

6. When excising the spot, try to include only the protein-containing gel by cutting close to the edge of the spot. Excise another piece of roughly the same size in a gel region without protein spots (to be used as a blank control).

7. In cases of silver-stained gels, destaining is carried out as described in ref. *24*.

8. Make sure that the lyophilized trypsin powder is at the bottom of the vial, as it sometimes sticks under the vial cap.

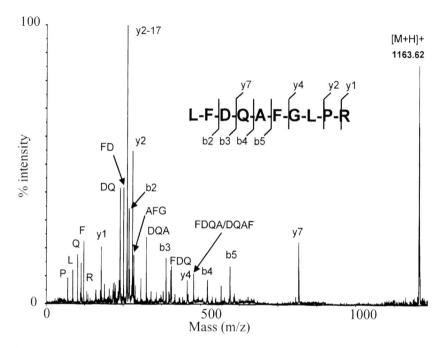

Fig. 4. Post source decay (PSD) mass spectrum of the peptide at m/z 1163.62 from the tryptic digest shown in **Fig. 3**. The immonium ions (P, L, Q, F, and R), C-terminal ions y2, y4, and y7, N-terminal ions b2, b3, b4, and b5 and internal fragment ions confirm the sequence LFDQAFGLPR. This peptide belongs to the 27-kDa heat shock protein family (*see* MS-Fit results in **Fig. 3**). As the bovine form of this protein has probably not been fully sequenced, the peptides at m/z 1413.74 and 1819.93 in **Fig. 3A** might be attributed to as yet uncharacterized sequences.

9. Lack of buffer leads to the gel pieces drying if left above the liquid surface, and an excess of buffer means a dilution of trypsin outside the gel. In both cases this could lead to the incomplete digestion of in-gel proteins.

10. Information and technical services concerning ZipTip$_{SCX}$ are available at www.millipore.com/ziptip.

11. Carry out each movement slowly, to give enough contact time between the sample and the ZipTip$_{SCX}$ packing. Avoid passing air through the tip.

12. General information on MALDI-TOF–MS can be found on the following Website: http://www.srsmaldi.com.

13. Gel contaminants can easily be detected by comparison with a blank spot gel (*see* **Note 6**). The corresponding ions appear with a mass default on the first decimal: m/z 855.03, 871.03, 1060.05, and so on.

14. Do not be too accurate in the initial estimation of protein MW because, if it is slightly out, you may exclude the protein from the search parameters. MW of a

protein parameter in Mascot is not really a cutoff value, as in MS-Fit, for searching in the SwissProt database. In this case, the input value must not be greater than the sum of the peptide masses listed.

15. It is also possible to match ion fragments from the PSD MALDI–MS spectrum to MS/MS databases using a customized search engine such as MS-Tag (ProteinProspector).

References

1. Hunziker, E. B. (2002) Articular cartilage repair: basic science and clinical progress. A review of the current status and prospects. *Osteoarthritis Cartilage* **10,** 432–463.
2. Benya, P. D. and Brown, P. D. (1986) Modulation of the chondrocyte phenotype in vitro, in *Articular Cartilage Biochemistry* (Kuettner, K. E., Schleyerbach, R., and Hascall, V. C., eds.), Raven, New York, NY, pp. 219–233.
3. Ronzière, M. C., Farjanel, J., Freyria, A. M., Hartmann, D. J., and Herbage, D. (1997) Analysis of types I, II, III, IX and XI collagens synthesized by fetal bovine chondrocytes in high-density culture. *Osteoarthritis Cartilage* **5,** 205–214.
4. Roche, S., Ronzière, M. C., Herbage, D., and Freyria, A. M. (2001) Native and DPPA cross-linked collagen sponges seeded with fetal bovine epiphyseal chondrocytes used for cartilage tissue engineering. *Biomaterials* **22,** 9–18.
5. Freyria, A. M., Ronziere, M. C., Boutillon, M. M., and Herbage, D. (1995) Two-dimensional electrophoresis of intracellular and secreted protein synthesized by fetal bovine chondrocytes in high-density culture. *Electrophoresis* **16,** 1268–1272.
6. Freyria, A. M., Ronziere, M. C., Boutillon, M. M., and Herbage, D. (1995) Effect of retinoic acid on protein synthesis by foetal bovine chondrocytes in high-density culture: down-regulation of the glucose-regulated protein, GRP-78, and type II collagen. *Biochem. J.* **305,** 391–396.
7. Freyria, A. M., Ronzière, M. C., Roche, S., Rousseau, C. F., and Herbage, D. (1999) Regulation of growth, protein synthesis and maturation of foetal bovine chondrocytes grown in high-density culture in the presence of ascorbic acid, retinoic acid and dihydrocytochalasin B. *J. Cell. Biochem.* **76,** 84–98.
8. Hermansson, M., Bolton, M., Alexander, S., and Wait, R. (2002) Application of proteomics to analysis of chondrocyte gene expression in normal and osteoarthritis cartilage, in *XVIIIth Federation of European Connective Tissue Societies Meeting Abstracts,* Brighton, England, p. 46.
9. Sinz, A., Bantscheff, M., Mikkat, S., et al. (2002) Mass spectrometric proteome analyses of synovial fluids and plasmas from patients suffering from rheumatoid arthritis and comparison to reactive arthritis or osteoarthritis. *Electrophoresis* **23,** 3445–3456.
10. Karas, M. and Hillenkamp, F. (1988) Laser desorption ionisation of proteins with molecular masses exeeding 10,000 daltons. *Anal. Chem.* **60,** 2299–3201.
11. Fenn, J. B., Mann, M., Meng, C. K., Wong, S. F., and Whitehouse, C. M. (1989) Electrospray ionisation for mass spectrometry of large biomolecules. *Science* **246,** 64–71.

12. Yates, J. R. III (1998) Mass spectrometry and the age of the proteome. *J. Mass Spectrom.* **33,** 1–19.

13. Mann, M., Hendrickson, R. C., and Pandey, A. (2001) Analysis of proteins and proteomes by mass spectrometry. *Ann. Rev. Biochem.* **70,** 437–473.

14. Shevchenko, A., Wilm, M., Vorm, O., and Mann, M. (1996) Mass spectrometric sequencing of proteins from silver-stained polyacrylamide gel. *Anal. Chem.* **68,** 850–858.

15. Jungblut, P. and Thiede, B. (1997) Protein identification from 2-D gels by MALDI mass spectrometry. *Mass Spectrom. Rev.* **16,** 145–162.

16. Jensen, O. N., Wilm, M., Shevchenko, A., and Mann, M. (1999) Sample preparation methods for mass spectrometric peptide mapping directly from 2-DE gels, in *Methods in Molecular Biology: 2-D Proteome Analysis Protocols* (Link, A. J., ed.), Humana, Totowa, NJ, pp. 513–530.

17. Henzel, W. J., Billeci, T. M., Stults, J. T., Wong, S. C., Grimley, C., and Watanabe, C. (1993) Identifying proteins from two-dimensional gels by molecular mass searching of peptide fragments in protein sequence databases. *Proc. Natl. Acad. Sci. USA* **90,** 5011–5015.

18. Beavis, R. C. and Fenyö, D. (2000) Data base searching with mass spectrometric information. *Trends Biochem. Sci. Suppl. Proteomics: A Trends Guide,* pp. 22–27.

19. Kinter, M., and Sherman, N. E. (eds.) (2001) *Protein Sequencing And Identification Using Tandem Mass Spectrometry.* John Wiley & Sons, New York, NY.

20. Spengler, B. (1997) Post-source decay analysis in matrix-assisted laser desorption/ ionization mass spectrometry of biomolecules. *J. Mass Spectrom.* **32,** 1019–1036.

21. Courschesne, P. L. and Patterson, S. D. (1999) Identification of proteins by matrix-assisted laser desorption/ionization mass spectrometry using peptide and fragment ion masses, in *Methods in Molecular Biology: 2-D Proteome Analysis Protocols* (Link, A. J., ed.), Humana, Totowa, NJ, pp. 487–511.

22. Rabilloud, T. (1999) Silver staining of 2-D electrophoresis gels, in *Methods in Molecular Biology: 2-D Proteome Analysis Protocols* (Link, A. J., ed.), Humana, Totowa, NJ, pp. 297–305.

23. Biemann, K. (1990) Appendix 5. Nomenclature for peptide fragment ions (positive ions). *Methods Enzymol.* **193,** 886–887.

24. Gharahdaghi, F., Weinberg, C. R., Meagher, D. A., Imai, B. S., and Mische, S. M. (1999) Mass spectrometric identification of proteins from silver-stained polyacrylamide gel: a method for the removal of silver ions to enhance sensitivity. *Electrophoresis* **20,** 601–605.

14

Analysis of Chondrocyte Functional Markers and Pericellular Matrix Components by Flow Cytometry

Gust Verbruggen, Jun Wang, Lai Wang, Dirk Elewaut, and Eric M. Veys

Summary

Flow cytometry has been used as a procedure to characterize the phenotype and function of human articular cartilage cells cultured as monolayers or in gelled artificial matrices. Procedures allowing intact cells with their cell-associated matrix, to be obtained have been described. Appropriate monoclonal antibodies have allowed plasma membrane-associated proteins, e.g., growth factors and cytokine receptors, as well as the cell-associated extracellular matrix macromolecules, to be studied. Intracellular compounds have been traced in permeabilized cells after blocking of their intracellular transport and secretion mechanisms. We report the use of fluorescent dye-labeled monoclonal antibodies or specific binding proteins against extracellular matrix compounds such as hyaluronan, aggrecan, types I and II collagen, and fibronectin. The autocrine and paracrine growth factor and cytokine pathways considered include the insulin-like growth factor-1 (IGF-1)/IGF receptor I (IGFRI), and the transforming growth factor-β1 (TGF-β1)/TGF-β receptor II (TGF-βRII) cascades, as well as the interleukin-1α/β (IL-1α/β)/interleukin-1 receptors I and II (IL-1RI and II) systems. Catabolic enzymes that mediate extracellular matrix turnover, e.g., some matrix metalloproteinases and their natural inhibitors, were also studied. Finally, flow cytometry was used to assess the results of some pharmacological interventions on the aforementioned variables in cultured chondrocytes.

Key Words: Flow cytometry; chondrocyte culture; agarose; alginate; monoclonal antibodies; IGF; IGFRI; IL-1; IL-1RI; IL-1RII; TGF; TGFRII; MMP; TIMP; hyaluronan; aggrecan; type I collagen; type II collagen; fibronectin.

1. Introduction

Flow cytometry is used as a standard procedure to characterize the phenotype of circulating lymphomyeloid cells. The deleterious effect of any proteolytic digestion procedure on plasma membrane antigens limits application of this method to cells isolated from tissues or cultures. When articular chondrocytes are considered, the availability of fluorescent agents has enabled

From: *Methods in Molecular Medicine, Vol. 100: Cartilage and Osteoarthritis, Vol. 1: Cellular and Molecular Tools*
Edited by: M. Sabatini, P. Pastoureau, and F. De Ceuninck © Humana Press Inc., Totowa, NJ

researchers to use flow cytometry mainly to study cell viability *(1)*, proliferation and cell cycle characteristics *(2,3)*, respiratory activities, and free radical production *(4)*. The availability of specific monoclonal antibodies (MAbs) and the development of nonproteolytic procedures of cell release has allowed flow cytometry to be used for study of some plasma membrane-associated antigens, e.g., cytokine receptors *(5,6)*, cellular adhesion molecules *(7,8)*, HLA classes I and II antigens *(9)*, membrane-bound peptidases *(10)*, and intracellular cytokines *(11)*. Flow cytometry has also been used to study the synthesis of extracellular matrix (ECM) molecules *(12)*.

Articular cartilage is composed of a hydrated extensive ECM in which chondrocytes are embedded. The intercellular matrix of cartilage is composed of two compartments: the cell-associated matrix (CAM) lying close to the chondrocyte and, adjacent to this, the interterritorial matrix (ITM) *(13)*. The CAM is a constant part of the ECM *(14,15)* in which the macromolecular compounds are metabolized or turned over in a particular way *(16)*. Newly synthesized aggrecans have been shown to reside in the CAM for short periods with a higher rate of aggrecan turnover than in the ITM *(17)*. The neosynthesized CAM macromolecules leave the territorial matrix in a later stage, to diffuse to the ITM *(16)*. The ITM forms the largest domain of the intercellular matrix. One of the advantages of chondrocyte culture in alginate or agarose is the reversibility of the gelled condition of these matrices, allowing the study of the different intercellular compartments surrounding the chondrocyte in vitro. Our studies on the homeostasis of the ECM of articular cartilage have been conducted on chondrocytes that maintained their original phenotype in vitro when cultured in 3D culture systems, e.g., in gelled alginate or agarose.

In 3D culture, isolated chondrocytes resynthesize their CAM and ECM within 1–2 wk *(18)*. The CAM is characterized by a high content of large proteoglycan aggregates, bound to the cell via the interaction of hyaluronan with CD44-like receptors *(19)*. Chondrocyte cell membranes also exhibit several proteins with binding affinity for collagen, including anchorin CII *(20)*, heparan sulfate proteoglycan *(20,21)*, and chondronectin *(22)*. This enables the use of flow cytometry to study the expression of the ECM macromolecules belonging to the pericellular domain of the chondrocytes. The presence or absence of chondrocyte-specific aggrecan and collagens could then be used as phenotypic markers of cartilage cells maintained in different in vitro conditions.

Other possible targets in flow cytometry studies are the autocrine and paracrine growth factor and cytokine pathways that control ECM metabolism, which have been successfully studied by flow cytometric methods. The receptor systems have been assessed on intact cells, whereas the cytokine or growth factor levels have been assayed inside permeabilized cells *(18,23)*.

This chapter presents procedures for the isolation and culture of human chondrocytes as a monolayer or in gelled matrices, along with approaches for flow cytometric analysis of a series of markers, pericellular components, and effector molecules. Also presented is an overview of the investigations performed on chondrocytes by flow cytometric analysis.

2. Materials

Chondrocytes are cultured in an incubator set at 37°C in water-saturated air at 5% CO_2.

2.1. Chondrocyte Isolation

1. Dulbecco's modified Eagle's medium (DMEM) with Na-pyruvate and low (1 g/L) glucose (Gibco).
2. Stock solution of 10^4 U/mL penicillin, 10 mg/mL streptomycin and 0.025 mg/mL fungizone (PSF; Gibco).
3. Fetal bovine serum (FBS; Gibco)
4. Solution of 0.25% hyaluronidase (from sheep testes; Sigma) in DMEM with 1% PSF. Filter-sterilize through a 0.22-μm membrane.
5. Solution of 0.25% pronase E (from *Streptomyces griseus*; Sigma) in DMEM with 1% PSF. Filter-sterilize through a 0.22-μm membrane.
6. Solution of 0.25% collagenase (from *Clostridium histolyticum*; Sigma) in DMEM with 1% PSF and 10% FBS. Filter-sterilize through a 0.22-μm membrane.

2.2. Chondrocyte Culture

2.2.1. Culture in Monolayer

1. DMEM with 1% PSF and 10% FBS.
2. Tissue culture flasks (25-cm² surface area; Nunc) or 50-mm-diameter culture dishes (6-well culture plates; Nunc).

2.2.2. Culture in Agarose Gel

1. Ultralow-gelling-temperature agarose, type IX, gelling at <15°C and remelting at >50°C (Sigma). Prepare a solution of 3% agarose in distilled water, and then autoclave it twice at 120°C for 15 min. This solution can be stored at 4–8°C before use.
2. Nunc cryotubes (3.8-mL capacity). Coat each cryotube with 100 μL of melted 3% agarose, and then allow to gel at 4–8°C for 15 min.
3. Double concentrated (2X) DMEM: one package of DMEM in powder (Gibco), normally used for 1 L of medium, is solubilized in 450 mL of distilled water. Add 3.7 g of $NaHCO_3$, check the pH, bring to 500 mL, and filter-sterilize through a 0.22-μm membrane. Add ascorbic acid (Sigma) and FBS at twice the desired final concentration.
4. Nutrient medium: DMEM plus 1% PSF, 10% FBS, and 50 μg/mL ascorbic acid.

2.2.3. Culture in Alginate Gel

1. 2X Hanks' balanced salts solution (HBSS): one package of HBSS in powder without calcium and magnesium (Sigma), normally used for preparation of 1 L, is solubilized in 450 mL of distilled water. Add 0.35 g of $NaHCO_3$, check the pH, bring to 500 mL and filter-sterilize through a 0.22-μm membrane.
2. Alginate, low viscosity, from *Macrocystis pyrifera* (Sigma). Prepare a 4% solution in distilled water, and then sterilize by autoclaving at 120°C for 15 min. This solution can be stored at 4°C and brought to 37°C before use.
3. Calcium chloride solution, 102 mM in distilled water. Filter sterilize through a 0.22-μm membrane.
4. Isotonic saline solution: 0.15 M sodium chloride in distilled water. Filter sterilize through a 0.22-μm membrane.
5. Nutrient medium: DMEM plus 1% PSF, 10% FBS, and 50 μg/mL ascorbic acid.
6. 6-Well plates.

2.3. Chondrocyte Collection for Flow Cytometry

1. Monensin (GolgiStop™, BD Biosciences Pharmingen).
2. Cytofix/Cytoperm Plus™ Kit (BD Biosciences Pharmingen).

2.3.1. Chondrocytes in Monolayers

1. EDTA solution: 1 mmol/L EDTA in HBSS without Ca^{2+}/Mg^{2+}.
2. Cell scraper.

2.3.2. Harvesting From Agarose Gel

1. Agarase solution: 50 U/mL of agarase (agarose 3-glycanohydrolase from *Pseudomonas atlantica*; Sigma) in phosphate buffered saline (PBS). Prepare fresh on the day of use.

2.3.3. Harvesting From Alginate Gel

1. Sodium citrate solution: 55 mM tri-sodium citrate dihydrate, pH 6.8, 0.15 M NaCl.

2.4. Flow Cytometry

1. Antibodies: all the antibodies are conjugated with fluorescein isothiocyanate (FITC). They can be prepared as previously described (*24*), or by using commercial kits such as the FluoroTag™ FITC conjugation kit (Sigma Aldrich).
   a. The optical density of the FITC-conjugated antibodies is measured at 495 nm (FITC) and 280 nm (protein) by spectrophotometry.
   b. The degree of conjugation is calculated according to the following equation: antibody/FITC = $(2.87 \times A_{495})/(A_{280} - 0.35 \times A_{495})$. Optimal conjugation requires a ratio between three and five.
   c. Antibodies can be alternatively conjugated with phycoerythrin (PE) as previously described (*25*), or by using the Phycolink® phycoerythrin conjugation kits by Prozyme.
   d. The conjugated monoclonal antibodies (MAbs) are used in a direct immunofluorescent staining protocol for flow cytometry. Appropriate FITC- or PE-labeled isotype-matched mouse or rabbit IgG_1 or IgG $_{2\alpha}$ can be used as a negative control.

e. The different monoclonal and polyclonal antibodies, or specific reporter proteins used thus far in our flow cytometry protocols are given in **Table 1** (*see* also refs. *26–28*).

2. Propidium iodide (PI): solution of 5 µg/mL in PBS.
3. PBS containing 0.1% sodium azide and 0.2% bovine serum albumin (BSA).
4. Quantum Simply Cellular Microbead Kit (Sigma).
5. Cell fluorimeter: FACSort, (Becton Dickinson) with CELLQuest software, or equivalent apparatus.

3. Methods

3.1. Isolation of Chondrocytes

Human articular chondrocytes are isolated as described elsewhere *(29,30)*, with a few modifications. For studies on healthy cartilage cells, only donors who have died after a short illness are selected. Cartilage samples from people who have received corticosteroids or cytostatic drugs are not used.

1. Sample visually intact cartilage from the femur condyles, and dice it in small (1-mm^3) fragments.
2. Liberate the cells from their extracellular matrix through sequential enzymatic digestion at 37°C. First add to the tissue the solution of 0.25% hyaluronidase in DMEM with 1% PSF for 120 min.
3. Replace the hyaluronidase solution with 0.25% pronase in DMEM with 1% PSF and incubate for 90 min.
4. Wash the tissue twice with DMEM with 1% PSF and 10% FBS and incubate overnight in the same medium (*see* **Note 1**).
5. Aspirate the medium, and then solubilize the tissue matrix by incubating for 3–6 h in 0.25% collagenase in DMEM 1% PSF plus 10% FBS (*see* **Note 2**).
6. Centrifuge the cells at 500*g* for 10 min and wash the pellet with DMEM 1% PSF plus 10% FBS. Repeat this steps two more times. Count the viable cells on a hemocytometer by the trypan blue exclusion test. Usually, 150×10^6 chondrocytes can be obtained from the femoral condyles of one adult individual and more than 95% of the cells are viable after isolation.

3.2. Culture of Chondrocytes

Cells can be cultured in monolayers or in gelled artificial matrices.

3.2.1. Culture in Monolayer

To prepare chondrocytes in monolayer for flow cytometry, seed 5×10^4 cells in 0.5 mL of DMEM with 1% PSF and 10% FBS as nutrient medium per 1 cm^2 of culture dish. Allow the cells to attach for 48 h (*see* **Note 3**). Medium is replaced every 2–3 d. Chondrocytes are seeded in low-density cultures and phenotypic analysis by flow cytometry must be done when cells are still subconfluent, usually after 4 d. This culture procedure makes possible to obtain single cells embedded in their CAM.

Table 1
Antibodies or Protein-Specific Reporter Molecules [a]

	MAb clone	Isotype		Source
Aggrecan	AD11-2A9	IgG_1	Mouse	Biosource Europe, Nivelles, Belgium
Type I collagen	I-8H5	IgG_{2a}	Mouse	ICN Biochemicals, Aurora, OH
Type II collagen	II-4C11	IgG_1	mouse	ICN Biochemicals
Fibronectin	polyclonal	IgG	Rabbit	Chemicon International, Harrow, UK
IGFRI	33255.111	IgG_1	Mouse	R&D Systems, Abingdon, UK
IL-1RI	35730.111	IgG_1	Mouse	R&D Systems
IL-1RII	34141.11	IgG_1	Mouse	R&D Systems
TGF-βRII	polyclonal	IgG	Rabbit	Santa Cruz Biotechnology,Santa Cruz, CA
IGF-1	AHG0014	IgG_1	Mouse	Biosource Europe, Nivelles, Belgium
IL-1α	624B3F2	IgG_1	Mouse	Biosource Europe
IL-1β	8516.311	IgG_1	Mouse	R&D Systems
TGF-β1	9016.2	IgG	Rabbit	R&D Systems
MMP-1	36665.111	IgG	Rabbit	R&D Systems
MMP-3	55-2A4	IgG_1	Mouse	Oncogene Research Products, Boston, MA

MMP-13	181-15A12	IgG_1	Mouse	Oncogene Research Products
TIMP-1	7-6C1	IgG_1	Mouse	Oncogene Research Products
TIMP-3	136-13H4	IgG_1	Mouse	Oncogene Research Products
Hyaluronan				$bHABP^{b}$
IgG_1 negative control		IgG_1	Mouse	R&D Systems
				Becton Dickinson, San Jose, CA
IgG negative control		IgG	Rabbit	Santa Cruz Biotechnology
IgG_{2a} negative control		IgG_{2a}	Mouse	R&D Systems

[a] The antihuman chondrocyte-specific aggrecan MAb was shown to react specifically with the G1-domain of the invariable hyaluronan-binding region of the human aggrecan molecule. No crossreactivity with other known matrix components could be detected (34,35). Antihuman type I and II collagen MAbs were raised in BALB/c mice after immunization with human placental type I collagen and type II collagen from human costal cartilage, respectively. On Western blots antitype I collagen was shown to react specifically with the α-chains and the triple helix molecular form of type I collagen, and the antitype II collagen MAb specifically reacted with the α2(II) chain of type II collagen (36). Matrix metalloproteinase (MMP)-1 antibody was against both pro- and active form of MMP-1. MMP-3 antibody recognized latent and active MMP-3 and reacted with MMP-3/tissue inhibitor of metalloproteinase (TIMP)-1 complexes. MMP-13 MAb recognized both latent and active MMP-13. TIMP-1 antibody reacted with free TIMP-1 and MMP/TIMP-1 complexes. Anti-TIMP-3 recognized both glycosylated and unglycosylated TIMP-3 (23). IGF, insulin-like growth factor; IGFRI, IGF receptor I; IL, interleukin; IL-R, IL receptor; TGF, transforming growth factor.

[b] Biotinylated hyaluronic acid binding protein (bHABP) was a kind gift from Dr. J. Melrose (Raymond Purves Research Laboratories, University of Sidney, Australia) and was used to trace hyaluronan in the CAM. Binding of bHABP to hyaluronan in the CAM was followed by a second-step avidin-FITC (Becton Dickinson) staining.

3.2.2. Culture in Agarose Gel

Chondrocytes are cultured in gelled agarose as previously described *(31)* with some modifications *(32,33)*. Chondrocyte suspension cultures are established in 1.5% agarose in Nunc cryotubes (*see* **Note 4**).

1. Melt 3% (double concentrated) agarose gel and keep it at 37°C.
2. Mix equal volumes of melted 3% agarose and 2X DMEM supplemented with 20% FBS and 100 µg/mL of ascorbic acid.
3. Adjust the density of the chondrocyte suspension to 5×10^7 cells/mL in DMEM supplemented with 1% PSF and 10% FBS.
4. Mix 10 vol of agarose in DMEM with 1 vol of the chondrocyte suspension, then pipet 300-µL aliquots in coated cryotubes, and allow to gel at 4–8°C for 15 min. The final cell density is around 1.5×10^6 chondrocytes per culture.
5. Add 3 mL of culture of nutrient medium (DMEM plus 1% PSF, 10% FBS, and 50 mg/mL ascorbic acid).
6. Incubate the cultures for 2 wk, replacing the nutrient medium three times a wk (*see* **Note 5**).

3.2.3. Culture in Alginate Gel

Chondrocyte cultures in alginate beads are prepared as described elsewhere *(34)* with some modifications.

1. Adjust the density of the chondrocyte suspension to 1×10^7 cells/mL in 2X HBSS without calcium and magnesium.
2. Carefully mix 1 vol of chondrocyte suspension with an equal vol of 4% alginate. Chondrocyte concentration is 5×10^6 cells/mL in 2% alginate.
3. Slowly drip the suspension through a 23-gage needle into a 102 m*M* calcium chloride solution. The tip of the needle should be positioned about 1 cm above the surface of the CaCl solution. Allow complete polymerization of the beads for 10 min at room temperature.
4. Aspirate the calcium chloride solution, and wash the beads three times with isotonic saline solution.
5. Transfer the beads to a six-well plate in 4 mL/well of nutrient medium (DMEM plus 1% PSF, 10% FBS, and 50 µg/mL of ascorbic acid). A culture of 20 beads consists of about 1×10^6 chondrocytes. Replace the nutrient medium twice weekly for 7–14 d (*see* **Note 5**).

3.3. Collection of Chondrocytes for Flow Cytometry

If the aim of the study is to evaluate the expression of proteins inside the cells (cytokines, growth factors, matrix metalloproteinases (MMPs) and their tissue inhibitors of metalloproteinases (TIMPs), and others, chondrocyte cultures must be ended by incubation with 0.67 µL of monensin (GolgiStop)/mL of medium for 5 h, in order to block protein transport from the Golgi apparatus *(18,23,35)*. No monensin treatment will be needed if the aim of the study is to evaluate the expression of protein-epitopes located on the cell membrane or in the CAM (e.g., receptors for growth factors and cytokines; integrins and other receptors of CAM components; CAM macromolecules such as aggrecan, type II collagen, and fibronectin).

3.3.1. Chondrocytes in Monolayer

Chondrocytes cultured on dishes are detached by EDTA treatment. The limitation of EDTA treatment is the difficulty of dissociating confluent monolayer-cultured chondrocytes embedded in a dense matrix. This procedure is therefore applied to subconfluent cultures and makes it possible to obtain single chondrocytes embedded in their CAM *(35)*.

1. Aspirate the medium from the culture dish, replace with 20 mL of EDTA solution, and incubate at 37°C for 30 min.
2. If necessary, help cell detachment using a cell scraper, and collect the suspension in a tube. Wash the dish with 10 mL of PBS, and add to the tube. For further processing, *see* **Subheading 3.4.**

3.3.2. Chondrocytes in Agarose

Chondrocytes cultured in agarose are released by digestion of the gel with agarase *(36)* (*see* **Note 6**).

1. Aspirate the medium from each cryotube, add 2 mL of agarase solution, and incubate at 37°C for 1 h.
2. Collect the suspension in a tube. Wash the cryotube with 1 mL of PBS, and add the wash to the tube. For further processing, *see* **Subheading 3.4.**

3.3.3. Chondrocytes in Alginate

Chondrocytes cultured in alginate are released by solubilization of the gel by a Ca^{2+}-chelating agent (*see* **Note 6**) *(18)*.

1. Aspirate the medium from each culture well, wash the beads once with PBS without Ca^{2+} and Mg^{2+}, then add 3 mL of sodium citrate solution, and incubate for 10 min at 25°C.
2. Collect the suspension in a 10-mL tube. Wash the dish with 3 mL of PBS, and add the wash to the tube. For further processing, *see* **Subheading 3.4.**

3.4. Preparation of Chondrocytes for Flow Cytometry

The chondrocytes harvested from the different culture systems are prepared for further processing with antibodies. If the aim of the study is to evaluate the expression of intracellular proteins, monensin-treated chondrocytes are fixed and permeabilized using the Cytofix/Cytoperm Plus Kit, according to the manufacturer's instruction.

Cells (either in native form, or fixed and permeabilized) are then prepared for incubation with MAbs *(18,23,35)*, as follows:

1. Centrifuge the cells at 800–1500*g* for 10 min.

2. Wash the pellets with the chondrocytes and their CAM with PBS.
3. Resuspend about 2×10^5 chondrocytes in 100 μL of PBS containing 0.1% sodium azide and 0.2% BSA prior to further use.
4. Add 20 μL of 50 μg/mL FITC- or phycoerythin (PE)-labeled antibodies and incubate for 30 min in the dark at 4°C.
5. When epitopes on the membrane or in the CAM are analyzed *(35,37)*, PI, which binds to DNA in dead cells with an unintact plasma membrane, is added to recognize and exclude dead cells. For DNA labeling, add 5 μL of PI solution/300 μL cell suspension.
6. Wash cells with PBS before flow cytometer analysis.

3.5. Flow Cytometric Analysis

1. Stained cells are analyzed on a flow cytometer.
2. For each sample, 15,000–20,000 events are analyzed.
3. Cells are gated on forward and side scatter to exclude dead cells, debris, and aggregates. Propidium iodide was additionally used to exclude dead cells when the epitopes outside the cells and cell-associated ECM molecules were analyzed.
4. The mean fluorescence intensity (MFI) of the positive cell population, which is owing to the binding of the conjugated antibodies to the specific antigen, is used to quantify the presence of plasma membrane-associated epitopes, e.g., the receptors for biological mediator proteins, the accumulation of the ECM molecules in the CAM, and the levels of growth factors and cytokines, or distinct enzymes and their natural inhibitors inside the cells (*see* **Note 7**).
5. MFI values are obtained by subtraction of the MFI of the negative control population from the MFI of the positive stained population.
6. For comparison between experiments, Quantum Simply Cellular Microbead Kit is used to calibrate the fluorescence scale of the flow cytometer *(23)*.
7. The microbeads are stained and processed in parallel with the cell samples using the same amount of FITC-labeled antibodies and incubation time.
8. The fluorescence scale of the cytometer is adapted before every experiment in order to keep identical MFIs for the four peaks of the calibration beads.
9. The MFI of cell samples is then analyzed without changing any instrument settings. The reproducibility and reliability of the whole procedure have been demonstrated previously *(35,37)*.
10. Classically, flow cytometry is used to define percentages of cells staining with antigen-specific monoclonal antibodies. The interface channel for positivity is arbitrarily set at the point at which less than 2% of the control fluorescence (cells exposed to isotype-matched FITC-mouse IgG) is positive.

3.5.1. Reproducibility and Reliability Tests

To evaluate the reproducibility of the flow cytometry assays, the method was tested on aliquots of cells obtained from the same culture. To study the reliability of the whole procedure, cells from the same donor were cultured separately in four cultures. Coefficients of variation were calculated to estimate the reliability of the values obtained for the presence of the respective cell-bound epitopes *(35)*, by the formula:

$$\text{Coefficient of variation} = 1\ SD \times 100/X$$

where SD is standard deviation, and X is the mean of the values.

3.5.2. Influence of Isolation Procedures on Detection of Cell-Bound Molecules

1. In order to exclude the effects of the isolation methods on the presence of cell-bound ECM molecules, isolated chondrocytes were analyzed by flow cytometry before and after exposure to EDTA, Na-citrate, or agarase.
2. To test the effect of agarase, subconfluent monolayer cultured cells were detached after 4 d of culture with 1 mmol/L EDTA in HBSS without Ca^{2+}/Mg^{2+} and harvested.
3. The expression of aggrecan and types I and II collagen was tested on the isolated cells before and after exposure to 50 U/mL of agarase at 37°C for 1 h.
4. To test the effect of EDTA, chondrocytes were obtained from 1-wk-old agarose cultures after digestion of the agarose gel with agarase.
5. The expression of aggrecan and types I and II collagen was then tested on the isolated cells before and after exposure to EDTA in HBSS without Ca^{2+}/Mg^{2+} *(37)*.

3.6. Results and Discussion

3.6.1. Flow Cytometric Analysis

A typical flow cytometry dot plot is shown in **Fig. 1**. The chondrocytes in this experiment were harvested after 1 wk of primary culture in agarose. A two-parameter dot plot of the cells was performed following PI staining to exclude the dead cells. According to their size (forward scatter) and their PI staining, the cells separated on these two-dimensional plots into three groups: PI-positive dead cells, PI-negative debris, and PI-negative living cells. The population of single living cells was analyzed for their expression of the ECM compounds. Flow cytometry histograms representing the proportions of chondrocytes staining for aggrecan and types I and II collagen are shown in **Fig. 1** *(35)*.

3.6.2. Reproducibility and Reliability of Flow Cytometry

To evaluate the reproducibility of the method, subconfluent monolayer cultured cells were dissociated with EDTA and tested fourfold for the presence of cell-bound ECM molecules. Coefficients of variation of the assay for aggrecan and types I and II collagen were in between 2.5 and 13.2% *(35)*. The same procedure was repeated with a sample of third-passage monolayer-cultured chondrocytes that were subcultured in agarose. Coefficients of variation of the assay for the CAM ECM molecules were from 2.6 to 11.0% *(35)* (**Table 2**).

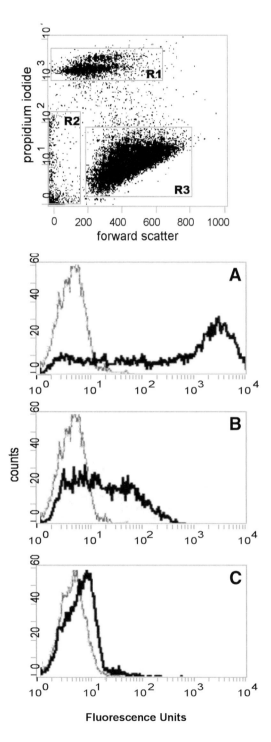

Table 2
Reproducibility (Interassay Variability)
of Flow Cytometric Analysis of Human Cartilage
Chondrocytes in Monolayer and in Agarose Culture [a]

	X ± SD	CV (%)
Monolayer		
Aggrecan	66.2 ± 2.5	3.8
Type II collagen	14.4 ± 1.9	13.2
Type I collagen	25.9 ± 0.6	2.5
Agarose		
Aggrecan	14.7 ± 0.9	6.1
Type II collagen	37.2 ± 4.1	11.0
Type I collagen	53.2 ± 1.2	2.6

[a] Percentages of cells positive for a given epitope are represented.
$X \pm SD$, mean ± 1 SD; CV, coefficient of variation = 1 SD × 100/X.

The reliability of the whole procedure was also tested on aliquots of four chondrocyte monolayers originating from the same donor but cultured separately *(35)*. After 1 wk in culture, the subconfluent cells were dissociated with EDTA and tested for the presence of cell-bound ECM molecules. Coefficients of variation of the assay for aggrecan and types I and II collagen were 2.2, 18.8, and 9.0%, respectively. The same procedure was repeated with a sample of second-passage monolayer-cultured chondrocytes that were subcultured in four separate agarose cultures. After 1 wk, the agarose matrix was digested with agarase to isolate the cells, which were tested for the presence of cell-bound ECM epitopes. Coefficients of variation of the assay for aggrecan and types I and II collagen ranged from 6.3 to 10.2% *(35)* (**Table 3**).

Fig. 1. *(opposite page)* Flow cytometric analysis of human chondrocytes harvested after 1 wk of primary culture in gelled agarose. Top: Dot plot of human chondrocytes after propidium iodide staining. R1, region 1 (PI-positive, dead cells); R2, region 2 (PI-negative, debris); R3, region 3 (PI-negative, living cells). Bottom: Histograms showing the expression of (**A**) aggrecan, (**B**) type II collagen, (**C**) type I collagen. Gray curves, negative controls; black curves, MAb FITC-labeled cells. In **A**, **B**, and **C**, ordinates are cell counts, and abscissae are fluorescence intensity units.

Table 3
Reliability (Interculture Variability)
of Flow Cytometric Analysis of Human Cartilage
Chondrocytes in Monolayer and in Agarose Culture [a]

	X ± SD	CV (%)
Monolayer		
Aggrecan	66.5 ± 1.5	2.2
Type II collagen	14.4 ± 2.7	18.8
Type I collagen	24.5 ± 2.2	9.0
Agarose		
Aggrecan	21.6 ± 2.2	10.2
Type II collagen	22.4 ± 1.4	6.3
Type I collagen	26.1 ± 2.1	8.0

[a] Percentages of cells positive for a given epitope are represented.
$X ± SD$, mean $± 1$ SD; CV, coefficient of variation $= 1$ SD $× 100/X$.

3.6.3. Influence of Isolation Methods on the Detection of Cell-Bound ECM Molecules

To test whether or not treatment of the cells with EDTA altered the presence of the cell-bound matrix antigens, chondrocytes cultured in agarose were released from the gel with agarase. Proportions of cells recognized by anti-aggrecan and antitypes I and II collagen MAbs did not change significantly after 30 min of exposure to 1 mmol/L EDTA in HBSS without Ca^{2+}/Mg^{2+} *(35)* (**Table 4**). To test whether or not treatment of the cells with agarase altered the expression of the cell-bound matrix antigens, monolayer-cultured chondrocytes were released from the culture dishes with 1 mmol/L EDTA in HBSS without Ca^{2+}/Mg^{2+} and then treated with agarase at 37°C for 1 h. Proportions of cells recognised by anti-aggrecan and antitypes I and II collagen MAbs did not change after exposure to agarase *(35)* (**Table 5**).

3.6.4. Quantifying the Molecular Contents of the CAM

The availability of MAbs directed specifically against cell proteins has enabled us to quantify numbers of intracellular and cell-associated molecules, e.g., cytokines and growth factors, MMPs and their natural inhibitors inside cells, and ECM proteins in the CAM *(18,23,37,38)*. The fluorescence intensity of the positive cell population, which is owing to the binding of FITC-MAb with equimolar amounts of intracellular or cellbound molecules, can be used to compare the quantities of these biologically active compounds, or to quantify their absolute amounts in the cell or in the CAM (**Table 6**). When

Table 4
Chondrocyte Phenotype Before
and After Treatment With EDTA [a]

| | % Change of positive cells after EDTA | | |
	Aggrecan	Collagen II	Collagen I
M40	− 4.1	− 2.3	− 24.5
M25	− 3.6	+ 0.3	+ 26.2
F28	− 5.9	+ 12.8	+ 21.0

[a] Sex (M/F) and age (yr) of the donors are given. Primary cultures were established in agarose, and the cells were harvested after 1 wk to test the effects of EDTA.

Table 5
Detection of Cell-Bound ECM Molecules
Before and After Digestion With Agarase [a]

| | % Change of positive cells after agarase | | |
	Aggrecan	Collagen II	Collagen I
M65	− 5.4	+ 2.7	+ 5.4
M40	+ 7.1	+ 4.2	− 1.3
M25	− 23.1	+ 1.0	+ 3.2

[a] Sex (M/F) and age (yr) of the donors are given. Third-passage monolayer cultures were established, and the cells were harvested after 4 d to test the effects of agarase.

flow cytometry and enzyme-linked immunosorbent assay (ELISA) were used to measure the aggrecan content in the CAM of a chondrocyte population, both methods yielded equal results (**Fig. 2**) *(37)*.

3.6.5. Chondrocyte Phenotype in the Monolayer Condition and in Suspension Culture

The percentages of cells staining positively with MAbs against chondrocyte-specific aggrecan and type II collagen in primary cultures in the monolayer condition have been reported previously *(35)*. The percentage of cells staining for aggrecan and type II collagen decreased significantly during prolonged monolayer culture, whereas the expression of type I collagen (which is a marker of chondrocyte dedifferentiation) increased in the same culture condition in primary cultures (**Fig. 3A**). This loss of the original phenotype became irreversible when secondary and tertiary cultures were investigated *(35)*.

Table 6
Expression of IGFRI, IGF-1, IL-1RI, and IL-β
by Chondrocytes From Intact Cartilage From Healthy Joints [a]

Sex/age	IGFRI	IGF-1	IL-1RI	IL-1β
M44	2.36 ± 0.05	40.27 ± 6.10	1.86 ± 0.11	44.00 ± 7.10
M47	4.25 ± 0.15	42.20 ± 0.55	2.55 ± 0.18	60.64 ± 1.98
M56	1.96 ± 0.19	19.86 ± 2.81	1.53 ± 0.07	5.60 ± 0.25
M59'	2.50 ± 0.32	27.90 ± 1.70	2.11 ± 0.08	56.48 ± 7.41
F40	5.41 ± 0.15	44.50 ± 3.85	1.57 ± 0.08	36.27 ± 3.20
M38	4.36 ± 0.08	39.15 ± 0.94	1.63 ± 0.14	30.06 ± 0.52
M18	2.64 ± 0.10	27.03 ± 0.26	1.75 ± 0.05	56.05 ± 0.05
M59''	1.82 ± 0.05	21.96 ± 4.30	2.98 ± 0.48	72.90 ± 4.56
M57	2.77 ± 0.08	40.60 ± 1.21	1.51 ± 0.06	50.16 ± 3.00
M18	0.95 ± 0.09	21.03 ± 3.00	0.91 ± 0.21	6.39 ± 0.56
F67	0.46 ± 0.02	21.80 ± 1.03	0.39 ± 0.06	5.10 ± 0.48
F73	0.47 ± 0.03	32.10 ± 0.47	0.24 ± 0.03	12.20 ± 0.84
Mean ± 1 SD [b]	2.50 ± 1.55	31.53 ± 9.47	1.59 ± 0.80	36.32 ± 24.1

[a] Sex (M/F) and age (yr) of the donors are given. Mean ± 1 SD MFI values for ligands and their receptors are represented. As MAbs are used to stain protein epitopes, and equimolar amounts of MAb and the targeted epitopes bind each other, MFI values stand for absolute amounts of cell-associated proteins. The ligands outnumber their receptors by a factor of 10. IGF, insulin-like growth factor; IGFRI, IGF receptor I; IL, interleukin; IL-1RI, IL-1 receptor I.
[b] Mean ± 1 SD MFI value recorded for the whole population ($n = 12$).

Re-expression of aggrecan and type II collagen by primary chondrocytes in suspension culture in agarose was obvious when these cells were followed over a 14-d period. However, synthesis of unusual type I collagen accompanies differentiation of the articular cartilage cell in gelled agarose (**Fig. 3B**).

3.6.6. The Chondrocyte CAM Reflects the ECM of Articular Cartilage

Flow cytometry allowed homeostasis of the ECM to be studied. For instance, exactly the same depression of aggrecan was obtained in the CAM and in the interterritorial matrix (ITM) of the ECM, when chondrocytes had been exposed to interleukin-1β (IL-1β). An equal recovery in CAM and ITM contents was observed after the incubation media of these chondrocytes had been supplemented with increasing doses of IGF (**Fig. 4**) *(18)*. Suppression of aggrecan in the CAM and in the ITM was assayed by flow cytometry on the isolated chondrocytes and by ELISA on the extract of the surrounding artificial matrix.

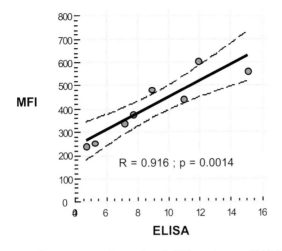

Fig. 2. Mean fluorescence intensity (MFI) owing to CAM aggrecan and ELISA for aggrecan in the CAM was carried out after chondrocytes of two donors had been exposed to IL-1. An identical procedure was used to prepare chondrocytes for flow cytometry and for ELISA to quantify the CAM aggrecans. The anti-aggrecan MAb used in flow cytometry was the same as the detection MAb used in the ELISA procedure (Biosource). Analysis of the IL-1β-induced changes in CAM content of the chondrocytes obtained in these two donors showed a close agreement between the two methods, and a significant correlation was observed when the aggrecan MFI (flow cytometry) and aggrecan absolute contents (ELISA) were compared under different doses of IL-1β.

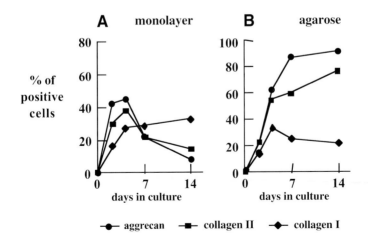

Fig. 3. Re-expression of cell membrane-bound extracellular matrix antigens by chondrocytes in secondary culture. **(A)** Monolayer-cultured chondrocytes, **(B)** chondrocytes in gelled agarose. Ordinates, % of positive cells; abscissae, culture time in days.

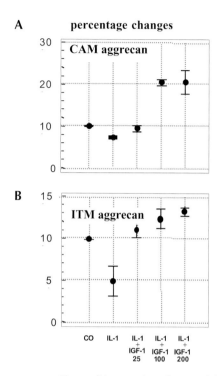

Fig. 4. Dose-response effect of increasing doses of insulin-like growth factor-1 (IGF-1) on the accumulation of aggrecan in the cell-associated matrix (CAM) **(A)** and interterritorial matrix (ITM) **(B)** of IL-1β-depressed chondrocytes. co, control cells not exposed to IL-1. Mean values ± 1 SD for percentage changes of three experiments in one chondrocyte population are shown.

3.6.7. Homeostasis of the ECM by Chondrocytes From Normal Cartilage

When addressing the homeostasis of the ECM by chondrocytes in normal articular cartilage, our flow cytometry studies were focused on the accumulation of aggrecan and type II collagen in the CAM of phenotypically stable articular cartilage chondrocytes cultured in alginate.

Immediately after their isolation and after the initiation of the culture procedure, the chondrocytes showed high levels of intracellular growth factors and cytokines *(18)*. Mechanical stress, sustained by the cells during the process of their isolation, is thought to have initiated these metabolic changes. Similar processes of activation of cells by mechanical forces, known as mechanotransduction, have been described for different cells, e.g., skeletal muscle cells *(39)*, chondrocytes *(40,41)*, and endothelial cells *(42)*. However, elevated val-

Table 7
**Correlations Among the Expression of IGFRI, IL-1RI, and IL-1RII
on the Cell Membrane, of IGF-1 and IL-1α and β Intracellularly
and of Aggrecan and Type II Collagen in the CAM** [a]

	IGFRI	IGF-1	IL-1RI	IL-1RII	IL-1α	IL-1β
IGF-1	S					
IL-1RI	—	—				
IL-1RII	S	S	—			
IL-1α	—	—	S	—		
IL-1β	—	—	S	—	S	
Coll II	S	S	—	S	—	—
Aggr	S	S	—	S	—	—

[a] S, significant correlation; Coll II, type II collagen; Aggr, aggrecan; IGF-1, insulin-like growth factor-1; IGFRI, IGF receptor I; IL, interleukin; IL-1R, IL-1 receptor.

ues of insulin-like growth factor-1 (IGF-1) and of IL-1α and -β inside the cells decreased and stabilized within the first 2 wk in culture. The cells were thus allowed to recover from the isolation procedure, to restore their repertoire of plasma membrane receptor proteins, and to rebuild the cell-associated ECM that had been lost during the isolation procedure. The new equilibriums were reached after 1–2 wk in culture *(18)*.

After 1 wk in culture, the cellular levels of both parts of the IGF receptor I (IGFRI)/IGF-1 pathway significantly correlated with the amounts of aggrecan and type II collagen that had accumulated in the CAM. In addition, there was a significant correlation between IGFRI/IGF-1 and the presence of the decoy receptor for IL-1:IL-1RII. Additionally, the same extent of correlation was found between IL-1RII and the ECM molecules in the CAM. Levels of CAM ECM molecules did not correlate with the agonists of the IL-1 pathway (**Table 7**) *(18)*.

Cause/effect relation experiments were then performed to explore the effects of IGF on synthesis and turnover of the ECM. IGF-1 was shown to dose-dependently enhance the accumulation of aggrecan and of type II collagen in the chondrocyte CAM *(18)*. These results supported the observations of others who have shown that growth factors, especially IGF, direct the production and accumulation of ECM by chondrocytes in normal and diseased cartilage *(43–47)*. Furthermore, exogenous IGF-1 was shown to induce the expression of IL-1RII on the chondrocyte plasma membrane. IL-1RII binds and neutralizes IL-1β, but does not, or barely, bind or neutralize IL-1α in bioassays *(48,49)*.

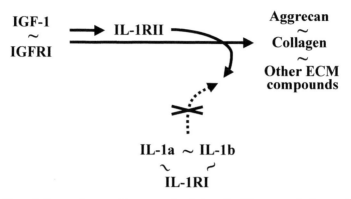

Fig. 5. Correlations observed between both insulin-like growth factor-1 (IGF-1)/ IGF receptor I (IGFRI) and interleukin-1 (IL-1)/IL-1 receptor (IL-1R) auto/paracrine pathways and accumulated CAM compounds, and the results of a number of additional cause/effect experiments allowed us to conclude that IGF-1-induced IL-1RII overrides IL-1 activity and controls the homeostasis of the extracellular matrix.

IL-1RII acts as a molecular trap for the IL-1 agonist without participating in its signaling. Through the upregulation of IL-1RII, IGF-1 can protect cartilage cell ECM against IL-1-induced destruction (**Fig. 5**). This was illustrated in our in vitro experiments in which IGF-1 countered the action of IL-1β, e.g., the deficient synthesis, degradation, and inadequate deposition of aggrecan in the CAM and in the ECM of IL-1β-depressed chondrocytes (**Fig. 4**). This protective effect was shown to be modulated through the upregulation of plasma membrane IL-1RII levels, since an IL-1RII-neutralizing IgG abolished the supporting activity of IGF-1 *(18)*. A decrease in both the basal and the cytokine-stimulated degradation of proteoglycan by IGF-1 in cartilage explant cultures, demonstrated earlier *(47)*, is consistent with these findings.

3.6.8. Homeostasis of the ECM by Chondrocytes From Osteoarthritic Cartilage

Although chondrocytes from degenerated tissues—when compared with those from unaffected tissues from osteoarthritic (OA) joints—showed a significantly increased expression of IGFR1 and IGF-1, equally significant increases of intracellular IL-1α, IL-1β, and plasma membrane IL-1RI were observed in these cartilage cells. On the other hand, chondrocytes derived from degenerated tissue of OA joints expressed less membrane-bound IL-1RII than cells isolated from unaffected cartilage of the same knee. It was anticipated that IL-1 activity around chondrocytes from degenerated tissue was not neutralized by IL-1RII and, therefore, mean chondrocyte MFI values for CAM aggrecan, type II collagen, and fibronectin significantly decreased in these cells *(50)*.

3.6.9. Use of Flow Cytometry to Assess the Results of Pharmacological Interventions on Chondrocytes

Our studies have shown that chondrocytes treated with 0.05 µg/mL hydrocortisone showed a significantly increased accumulation of CAM aggrecan, type II collagen, and fibronectin *(38)*. This increased accumulation of CAM macromolecules obviously resulted from a decrease in the activity of the catabolic pathways, since the intracellular levels of both IL-1 isoforms were depressed in chondrocytes after the exposure to hydrocortisone. The intracellular growth factors and cytokines represent a reservoir of biologically active agents, of which variable amounts are secreted following various stimuli. It can be anticipated that the intracellular amounts of these bioactive molecules predict their extracellular function. Further suppression of the IL-1 catabolic pathway was observed as the expression of the signaling IL-1RI receptor decreased, and as the plasma membrane IL-1RII decoy receptor levels raised concomitantly on the cells exposed to hydrocortisone. The decreased activity of the IL-1–mediated catabolic pathways in hydrocortisone-treated chondrocytes—as reported by others *(51)*—explains the well-documented reduction of neutral protease activities in steroid-treated OA cartilage samples *(52–55)*.

3.7. Summary

Flow cytometry offers a technique to study intracellular and extracellular cell-associated proteins. As far as the cells under investigation have survived their isolation procedure without any degradation of their CAM- or plasma membrane-associated molecular components, they can react with mono- or polyclonal antibodies and be subjected to flow cytometry. The presence and levels of intracellular proteins can be investigated in permeabilized cells.

Isolation of the chondrocytes from different culture conditions, e.g., monolayer culture or suspension culture in agarose or alginate gel, did not affect their surrounding cell-bound matrix since treatment of the cells with EDTA, agarase, or Na-citrate did not alter the expression of the cell-bound matrix antigens. The flow cytometry technique was reproducible, and the whole procedure was shown to be reliable. Finally, assessment of the MFI of the chondrocytes offered a precise quantification of the synthesis and accumulation of the ECM molecules studied.

Flow cytometry thus allows the composition of the CAM to be studied. The biochemical composition of the CAM realistically reflects the instant phenotype of chondrocytes cultured in different culture conditions.

As the CAM represents a constant part of the ECM, the changes in the composition of the CAM closely reflect the ongoing metabolic processes in the ECM. This methodology allows the influence of growth and differentiation factors and cytokine cascades on the synthesis and degradation of a variety of extracellular matrix components to be investigated. These investigations have been done in cartilage cells obtained from normal and from OA tissues and have allowed therapeutic targets in this disease to be defined.

The possibilities of pharmacological interventions, e.g., corticosteroids, have been investigated.

4. Notes

1. In between the hyaluronidase/pronase and the collagenase digestion steps, it is essential to build in an overnight recovery period for the chondrocytes in the presence of serum. This improves viability of the cells during the entire 48-h isolation procedure.

2. Adult human articular cartilage is particularly difficult to digest. The first chondrocytes appear after 2–3 h of collagenase treatment. After 6 h, part of the cartilage still remains undigested. If an attempt is made to digest these remaining parts, additional exposure to collagenase will kill the cells that were liberated after the initial 2–3 h.

3. Attachment and growth of the chondrocytes is better in Ham's F12 with 1% PSF and 10–20% FBS. For studies on synthesis and turnover of the ECM, DMEM with 1% PSF and 10% FBS is preferred.

4. Proliferation of chondrocytes occurs at lower concentrations of the gel. At 1.5% agarose, chondrocyte numbers during culture are fairly stable.

5. Culture media should be added with extreme care as the agarose gel is easily disrupted when the nutrient media are added. As alginate beads are much more stable in culture, replacement of the culture media can be done in no time.

6. Agarase, used to liberate chondrocytes from the agarose gel, is much more expensive than the Na-citrate that is used to isolate chondrocytes from an alginate bead.

7. Mean or median fluorescence intensity (MFI) values characterize a chondrocyte population much better than does the classically used % of positive cells on a scattergram.

References

1. Bell, R. S., Bouret, L. A., Bell, D. F., Gebhardt, M. C., Rosenberg, A., and Berrey, H. B. *et al.* (1988) Evaluation of fluorescein diacetate for flow cytometric determination of cell viability in orthopaedic research. *J. Orthop. Res.* **6**, 467–74.

2. Vincent, F., Brun, H., Clain, E., Ronot, X., and Adolphe, M. (1989) Effects of oxygen-free radicals on proliferation kinetics of cultured rabbit articular chondrocytes. *J. Cell Physiol.* **141**, 262–266.

3. Jaffray, P., Ronot, X., Adolphe, M., Fontagne, J., and Lechat, P. (1984) Effects of D-penicillamine on growth and cell cycle kinetics of cultured rabbit articular chondrocytes. *Ann. Rheum. Dis.* **43**, 333–338.

4. Thuong-Guyot, M., Domarle, O., Pocidalo, J. J., and Hayem, G. (1994) Effects of fluoroquinolones on cultured articular chondrocytes flow cytometric analysis of free radical production. *J. Pharmacol. Exp. Ther.* **271**, 1544–1549.

5. Westacott, C. I., Atkins, R. M., Dieppe, P. A., and Elson, C. J. (1994) Tumor

necrosis factor-alpha receptor expression on chondrocytes isolated from human articular cartilage. *J. Rheumatol.* **21,** 1710–1715.

6. Martel-Pelletier, J., McCollum, R., DiBattista, J., et al. (1992) The interleukin-1 receptor in normal and osteoarthritic human articular chondrocytes. Identification as the type I receptor and analysis of binding kinetics and biologic function. *Arthritis Rheum.* **35,** 530–340.

7. Lapadula, G., Iannione, F., Zuccaro, C., et al. (1998) Chondrocyte phenotyping in human osteoarthritis. *Clin. Rheumatol.* **17,** 99–104

8. Bujia, J., Behrends, U., Rotter, N., Pitzke, P., Wilmes, E., and Hammer, C. (1996) Expression of ICAM-1 on intact cartilage and isolated chondrocytes. *In Vitro Cell. Dev. Biol. Anim.* **32,** 116–122.

9. Lance, E. M., Kimura, L. H., and Manibog, C. N. (1993) The expression of major histocompatibility antigens on human articular chondrocytes. *Clin. Orthop.* **291,** 266–282

10. Lapadula, G., Iannione, F., Zuccaro, C., et al. (1995) Expression of membrane-bound peptidases (CD10 and CD26) on human articular chondrocytes. Possible role of neuropeptidases in the pathogenesis of osteoarthritis. *Clin. Exp. Rheumatol.* **13,** 143–148.

11. Vivien, D., Boumedienne, K., Galera, P., Lebrun, E., and Pujol, J. P. (1992) Flow cytometric detection of transforming growth factor-β expression in rabbit articular chondrocytes (RAC) in culture–association with S-phase traverse. *Exp. Cell. Res.* **203,** 56–61.

12. Adolphe, M., Froger, B., Ronot, X., Corvol, M. T., and Forest, N. (1984) Cell multiplication and type II collagen production by rabbit articular chondrocytes cultivated in a defined medium. *Exp. Cell. Res.* **155,** 527–536.

13. Mok, S. S., Masuda, K., Häuselmann, H. J., Aydelotte, M.B., and Thonar, E. J.-M. A. (1994) Aggrecan synthesized by mature bovine chondrocytes suspended in alginate. *J. Biol. Chem.* **269,** 33,021–33,027.

14. Malfait, A. M. (1994) Development of an in vitro model to study cytokine-mediated interactions between inflammatory cells and human chondrocytes. *Ghent University Thesis*: pp. 45.

15. Almqvist, K.F., Wang, L., Wang, J., et al. (2001) Culture of chondrocytes in alginate surrounded by fibrin gel: characteristics of the cells over a period of 8 weeks. *Ann. Rheum. Dis.* **60,** 781–790.

16. Platt, D., Wells, T., and Bayliss, M. T. (1997) Proteoglycan metabolism of equine articular chondrocytes cultured in alginate beads. *Res. Vet. Sci.* **62,** 39–47.

17. Bayliss, M. T. (1992) Metabolism of animal and human osteoarthritic cartilage, in *Articular Cartilage and Osteoarthritis.* (Kuettner, K. E., Schleyerbach, R., Peyron, J. G., Hascall, V. C., eds.), Raven, New York, NY, pp. 487–500.

18. Wang, J., Elewaut, D., Veys, E. M., and Verbruggen, G. (2003) IGF-1-induced IL-1RII overrules IL-1 activity and controls the homeostasis of the extracellular matrix of cartilage. *Arthritis Rheum.* **48,** 1281–1291.

19. Knudson, C. B. and Knudson, W. (1993) Hyaluronan-binding proteins in development, tissue homeostasis, and disease. *FASEB J.* **7,** 1231–1241.

20. Von der Mark, K., Mollenhauer, J., Pfaeffle, M., van Menxel, M., and Mueller, P. K. (1986) Role of anchorin CII in the interaction of chondrocytes with extracellular collagen, in *Articular Cartilage Biochemistry.* (Kuettner, K.E., Schleyerbach, R., and Hascall, V.C., eds.) Raven, New York, NY, pp.125–141.

21. Repraeger, A. and Bernfield, M. (1982) An integral membrane proteoglycan can bind the extracellular matrix directly to the cytoskeleton. *J. Cell Biol.* **95(Abstract),** A125.

22. Hewitt, A. T., Varner, H. H., Silver, M. H., Dessau, W., Wilkes, C. M., and Martin, G.R. (1982) The isolation and partial characterization of chondronectin, an attachment factor for chondrocytes. *J. Biol. Chem.* **257,** 2330–2334.

23. Wang, L., Almqvist, K. F., Veys, E. M., and Verbruggen, G. (2002) Control of extracellular matrix homeostasis of normal cartilage by a TGFβ autocrine pathway. Validation of flow cytometry as a tool to study chondrocyte metabolism in vitro. *Osteoarthritis Cartilage* **10,** 188–198.

24. Wood, B. T., Thompson, S. H., and Goldstein, G. (1965) Fluorescent antibody staining. III. Preparation of fluorescein-isothiocyanate-labeled antibodies. *J. Immunol.* **95,** 225–229.

25. Kronick, M. N. and Grossman, P. D. (1983) Immunoassay techniques with fluorescent phycobiliprotein conjugates. *Clin. Chem.* **29,** 1582–1586.

26. Gysen, P. and Franchimont, P. (1984) Radioimmunoassay of proteoglycan. *J. Immunoassay* **5,** 221–243.

27. Heinegård, D., and Oldberg, A. (1989) Structure and biology of cartilage and bone matrix noncollagenous macromolecules. *FASEB J.* **3,** 2042–2051.

28. Kumagai, J., Sarkar, K., Uhthoff, H. K., Okawara, Y., and Coshima, A. (1994) Immunohistochemical distribution of type I, II and III collagen in the rabbit supraspinous tendon insertion. *J. Anat.* **185,** 279–284.

29. Green, W. T. (1971) Behavior of articular chondrocytes in cell culture. *Clin. Orthop.* **75,** 248–260.

30. Kuettner, K. E., Pauli, B. U., Gall, G., McMemoli, V. A., and Schenk, R. K. (1982) Synthesis of cartilage matrix by mammalian chondrocytes in vitro. Isolation, culture characteristics and morphology. *J. Cell Biol.* **93,** 743–750.

31. Benya, P. D. and Shaffer, J.D. (1982) Dedifferentiated chondrocytes reexpress the differentiated collagen phenotype when cultured in agarose gels. *Cell* **30,** 215–224.

32. Cornelissen, M., Verbruggen, G., Malfait, A. M., Veys, E. M., Broddelez, C., and De Ridder, L. (1993) The study of representative populations of native aggrecan aggregates synthesized by human chondrocytes in vitro. *J. Tissue Culture Methods* **15,** 139–146.

33. Verbruggen, G., Veys, E. M., Wieme, N., et al. (1990) The synthesis and immobilisation of cartilage-specific proteoglycan by human chondrocytes in different concentrations of agarose. *Clin. Exp. Rheumatol.* **8,** 371–378.

34. Guo, J., Jourdian, G.W., and MacCallum, D.K. (1989) Culture and growth charecteristics of chondrocytes encapsulated in alginate beads. *Connect. Tissue Res.* **9,** 277–297.

35. Wang, L., Verbruggen, G., Almqvist, K. F., Elewaut, D., Broddelez, C., and Veys, E. M. (2001) Flow cytometric analysis of the human articular chondrocyte phenotype in vitro. *Osteoarthritis Cartilage* **9**, 73–84.
36. Cornelissen, M., Dewulf, M., Verbruggen, G., et al. (1993) Size distribution of native aggrecan aggregates of human articular chondrocytes in agarose. *In Vitro Cell. Dev. Biol. Anim.* **29A**, 356–358.
37. Wang, L., Almqvist, K. F., Broddelez, C., Veys, E. M., and Verbruggen, G. (2001) Evaluation of chondrocyte cell-associated matrix metabolism by flow cytometry. *Osteoarthritis Cartilage* **9**, 454–462.
38. Wang, L., Wang, J., Almqvist, K. F., Veys, E. M., and Verbruggen, G. (2002) Influence of polysulphated polysaccharides and hydrocortisone on the extracellular matrix metabolism of human articular chondrocytes in vitro. *Clin. Exp. Rheumatol.* **20**, 669–676.
39. Martineau, L. C. and Gardiner, P. F. (2001) Insight into skeletal muscle mechanotransduction: MAPK activation is quantitatively related to tension. *J. Appl. Physiol.* **91**, 693–702.
40. Hung, C. T., Henshaw, D. R., Wang, C. C., et al. (2000) Mitogen-activated protein kinase signaling in bovine articular chondrocytes in response to fluid flow does not require calcium mobilization. *J. Biomech.* **33**, 73–80.
41. Honda, K., Ohno, S., Tanimoto, K., et al. (2000) The effects of high magnitude cyclic tensile load on cartilage matrix metabolism in cultured chondrocytes. *Eur. J. Cell Biol.* **79**, 601–609.
42. Fujiwara, K., Masuda, M., Osawa, M., Kano, Y., and Katoh, K. (2001) Is PECAM-1 a mechanoresponsive molecule? *Cell. Struct. Funct.* **26**, 11–17.
43. Verschure, P. J., van Marle, J., Joosten, L. A., and van den Berg, W. B. (1995) Chondrocyte IGF-1 receptor expression and responsiveness to IGF-1 stimulation in mouse articular cartilage during various phases of experimentally induced arthritis. Ann. Rheum. Dis. **54**, 645–653.
44. Guenther, H. L., Guenther, H. E., Froesch, E. R., and Fleisch, H. (1982) Effect of insulin-like growth factor on collagen and glycosaminoglycan synthesis by rabbit articular chondrocytes in culture. *Experientia* **38**, 979–981.
45. McQuillan, D. L., Handley, C. J., Campbell, M. A., Bolis, S., Milway, V. E., and Herington, A. C. (1986) Stimulation of proteoglycan synthesis by serum and insulin-like growth factor-1 in cultured bovine articular cartilage. *Biochem. J.* **240**, 423–430.
46. Tesch, G. H., Handley, C. J., Cornell, H. J., and Herington, A. C. (1992) Effects of free and bound insulin-like growth factors on proteoglycan metabolism in articular cartilage explants. *J. Orthop. Res.* **10**, 14–22.
47. Tyler, J. A. (1989) Insulin-like growth factor 1 can decrease degradation and promote synthesis of proteoglycan in cartilage exposed to cytokines. Biochem. J. **260**, 543–548.
48. Kollewe, C., Neumann, D., and Martin, M. U. (2000) The first two N-terminal immunoglobulin-like domains of soluble human IL-1 receptor type II are sufficient to bind and neutralize IL-1β. *FEBS Lett.* **487**, 189–193.

49. Colotta, F., Saccani, S., Giri, J. G., et al. (1996) Regulated expression and release of the IL-1 decoy receptor in human mononuclear phagocytes. *J. Immunol.* **156,** 2534–2541.

50. Wang, J., Verdonk, P., Elewaut, D., Veys, E. M., and Verbruggen, G. (2003) Homeostasis of the extracellular matrix of normal and osteoarthritic human articular cartilage chondrocytes in vitro. *Osteoarthritis Cartilage* **11,** 801–809.

51. Lee, S. W., Tsou, A. P., Chan, H., et al. (1988) Glucocorticoids selectively inhibit the transcription of the interleukin 1β gene and decrease the stability of interleukin 1β mRNA. *Proc. Natl. Acad. Sci. USA* **85,** 1204–1208.

52. Pelletier, J. P., Mineau, F., Raynauld, J. P., Woessner, J. F., Gunja-Smith, Z., and Martel-Pelletier, J. (1994) Intraarticular injections with methylprednisolone acetate reduce osteoarthritic lesions in parallel with chondrocyte stromelysin synthesis in experimental osteoarthritis. *Arthritis Rheum.* **37,** 414–423.

53. Pelletier, J. P., Martel-Pelletier, J., Cloutier, J. M., and Woessner, J. F. (1987) Proteoglycan-degrading acid metalloproteinase activity in human osteoarthritic cartilage, and the effects of intraarticular steroid injections. *Arthritis Rheum.* **30,** 541–548.

54. Pelletier, J. P. and Martel-Pelletier, J. (1985) Cartilage degradation by neutral proteoglycanases in experimental osteoarthritis. Suppression by steroids. *Arthritis Rheum.* **28,** 1393–1401.

55. McGuire, M. B., Murhy, M., Reynolds, J. J., and Russel, R. G. G. (1981) Production of collagenase and inhibitor (TIMP) by normal, rheumatoid and osteoarthritic synovium in vitro: effects of hydrocortisone and indomethacine. *Clin. Biol.* **61,** 703–710.

15

A Simple and Reliable Assay of Proteoglycan Synthesis by Cultured Chondrocytes

Frédéric De Ceuninck and Audrey Caliez

Summary

A simple and reliable method to measure proteoglycan synthesis by chondrocytes in culture is described. Confluent chondrocytes in 24-well plates are labeled for 24–72 h with $^{35}SO_4^{2-}$ in the presence of stimulating agents. At the end of treatment, the secretion medium containing radiolabeled neosynthesized secreted proteoglycans (SP) is harvested, and cell-associated proteoglycans (CAP) are extracted with guanidine hydrochloride for 48 h. Aliquots of medium and cell extracts are distributed on Whatman paper and left to dry. SP and CAP are trapped by precipitation with the cationic detergent cetyl pyridinium chloride (CPC), whereas nonincorporated $^{35}SO_4^{2-}$ remains in solution. After drying, each spot corresponding to one well in the plate is cut, and its radioactivity is measured. Counts are proportional to the amount of neosynthesized proteoglycans. In a representative experiment using rabbit chondrocytes, total proteoglycan synthesis (SP plus CAP) was increased 3.5-fold after the addition of 1.34 nM insulin-like growth factor-1 (IGF-1) compared with nonstimulated cells. Further addition of a fourfold molar ratio of IGF binding protein-3 completely abolished this effect. This method can be used to measure proteoglycan synthesis by chondrocytes from many species, including human osteoarthritic chondrocytes, as well as guinea pig, rabbit, and rat chondrocytes.

Key Words: Chondrocyte; proteoglycan synthesis; glycosaminoglycan; anabolism; osteoarthritis; assay; cell culture; cetyl pyridinium chloride; precipitation, guanidine hydrochloride.

1. Introduction

Proteoglycans are, after collagens, the main solid components of articular cartilage. Cartilage proteoglycans are made of structurally different core proteins bearing polysulfated glycosaminoglycan chains, which give cartilage its hydrophilic nature and the osmotic pressure necessary to resist compressive loads. By working on osteoarthritic chondrocytes, with impaired anabolic responses, or more generally, on anabolic processes in cultured chondrocytes from different

From: *Methods in Molecular Medicine, Vol. 100: Cartilage and Osteoarthritis, Vol. 1: Cellular and Molecular Tools*
Edited by: M. Sabatini, P. Pastoureau, and F. De Ceuninck © Humana Press Inc., Totowa, NJ

species, it is important to have an accurate measure of the overall anabolism. For this, proteoglycans are a good choice since in addition to their biological importance in cartilage, their abundance totally eliminates potential problems of method sensitivity.

The most abundant cartilage proteoglycan, aggrecan, contains a 250-kDa core protein substituted with chondroitin sulfate and keratan sulfate chains and forms a macromolecular complex of about 3000 kDa *(1)*. The presence of the chondroitin sulfate proteoglycan versican has also been found in articular cartilage, although its expression level is much lower than that of aggrecan *(2)*. Besides these two large aggregating proteoglycans, some smaller proteoglycans belonging to the family of leucine-rich repeat (LRR) proteins are found in articular cartilage. They include decorin and biglycan, which possess dermatan/chondroitin sulfate chains *(3)*, fibromodulin *(4)*, and lumican *(5)*, which possess keratan sulfate chains. These molecules have the ability to interact with fibrillar collagens and are important for creating a functional network within cartilage. A large variety of proteoglycans bearing heparan sulfate chains are also synthesized by chondrocytes. These heparan sulfate proteoglycans include, among others, the basement membrane heparan sulfate proteoglycan (HSPG) perlecan *(6,7)*, syndecans -1, -3, and -4 *(8–10)*, the endocytic receptor for hyaluronan, CD44 *(11)*, and fibroglycan, glypican, and betaglycan *(8)*. Some methods designed to measure some of these proteoglycans specifically have been developed. Generally, these assays use antibodies directed against the core protein, which implies prior digestion of the glycosaminoglycan chains to facilitate antibody accessibility. Alternatively, some dyes of varying degree of specificity for glycosaminoglycan chains of proteoglycans have been used to develop colorimetric assays. This chapter describes an assay that measures neosynthesized proteoglycans in their whole, irrespective of their structural diversity.

The method takes advantage of the fact that cartilage proteoglycans have a high molar ratio of the sulphur atom per glycosaminoglycan chain, so that labeling of chondrocytes with $^{35}SO_4^{2-}$ leads to quite exclusive incorporation of the radioactive atom in neosynthesized proteoglycans. It is estimated that ^{35}S incorporated in cysteine and methionine of proteins is negligible, being less than 5% of the total ^{35}S taken by the cells. In the method, two pools consisting of cell-associated and secreted neosynthesized ^{35}S-labeled proteoglycans are precipitated with the cationic detergent cetyl pyridinium chloride (CPC), whereas free nonincorporated $^{35}SO_4^{2-}$ is eliminated by successive washes. Simple counting in scintillation fluid gives an accurate measure of proteoglycan synthesis by chondrocytes. Our routine method, originally developed in the laboratory of Dr. M. Corvol in Paris, is described here in details, with tips to improve sensitivity and accuracy.

2. Materials

2.1. Cell Culture and Treatment

1. Articular cartilage explants from guinea pigs, rabbits, or rats (for preparation, *see* Chapter 16) or from human osteoarthritic cartilage obtained after surgery for total knee joint replacement (femoral condyles and tibial plateaus) or total hip replacement (femoral head).
2. Hanks' balanced salt solution (HBSS; Gibco).
3. Ham's F-12 culture medium with Glutamax (Gibco).
4. Fetal calf serum (FCS).
5. Penicillin (10,000 U/mL)/streptomycin (10,000 µg/mL) stock solution (PS; Gibco).
6. Enzyme solutions: prepare a solution of 3 mg/mL of collagenase (type I, Worthington) and 2 mg/mL of dispase (from *Bacillus polymixa*, Gibco) in either:
   a. HBSS for digestion of cartilage from guinea pig, rabbit, or rat.
   b. Ham's F-12 supplemented with 10% FCS and 1% PS for digestion of human cartilage.
7. Cell culture equipment including: 10-mm-diameter Petri dishes, pipets, multipipets, and appropriate tips or combitips.
8. 24-Well culture plate, flat bottomed (Nunc).
9. Bovine serum albumin (BSA), IgG-free, protease-free (Jackson Immuno Research). Prepare a stock solution of 10% BSA (w/v) in deionized water and filter through disposable units fitted with 0.22-µm filters. Freeze in aliquots of 1 mL until use.
10. Insulin-like growth factor-1 (IGF-1); insulin-like growth factor binding protein-3 (IGFBP-3; Sigma).
11. Sulphur-35, sulfate, 100 µCi (3.7 MBq) in aqueous solution ($^{35}SO_4^{2-}$; Amersham).

2.2. Proteoglycan Precipitation and Extraction

1. Dulbecco's phosphate-buffered saline without calcium and magnesium (DPBS; Gibco).
2. Guanidine hydrochloride (Fluka).
3. Cetyl pyridinium chloride (CPC; Sigma).
4. Proteoglycan extraction solution: 3 *M* guanidine hydrochloride, 50 m*M* Tris-HCl, pH 7.4. Store at 4°C.
5. Whatman chromatography paper, 3 MM. For one culture plate in the experiment, cut two rectangles of exactly 12 × 18 cm. One will be used for secreted proteoglycans and the other for cell-associated proteoglycans. On each rectangle, draw 24 squares of 9 cm^2 with a lead pencil, reproducing the pattern of a 24-well plate. Number each square in one of its angles (*see* **Note 1**).
6. Trays of 15 × 21 cm (ideally) or more.
7. Precipitating solution: 1% (w/v) CPC containing 0.3 *M* NaCl. Do not adjust pH (*see* **Notes 2** and **3**). Prepare fresh just before use.
8. Rocking platform.

9. Mixer, of Vortexer type.
10. Safe-lock microtubes of 1.5 mL (Eppendorf or equivalent).
11. Scintillation fluid.
12. Safety equipment for radioactive material.
13. Additional tools: gloves, scissors, lead pencil.

3. Methods

3.1. Chondrocyte Culture and Treatment

3.1.1. Chondrocyte Culture

Chondrocytes from any species can be isolated and cultured as described in Chapter 1 (*see* **Note 4**). This alternative method is routinely used in our laboratory:

1. Finely mince the cartilage isolated from animals (guinea pig, rat, or rabbit) or humans down to fragments of 1-mm size.
2. Transfer the fragments to a Petri dish containing 20 mL of the appropriate enzyme solution, as described in **Subheading 2.1., item 6**.
3. Incubate at 37°C under a 5% CO_2 atmosphere. For cartilage from guinea pig, rat, or rabbit, digestion time is 5–6 h. For human cartilage, digestion time is 16 h (*see* **Note 5**).
4. Collect cells by centrifugation (3 min at 900*g*). Resuspend in Ham's F-12 medium containing Glutamax plus 10% FCS and 1% PS. Count cells and dispense in 24-well plates at 10^5 cells/mL/well (*see* **Note 6**).
5. Change medium every 2–3 d until chondrocytes are confluent (*see* **Note 7**).
6. Replace culture medium with 1.2 mL/well of serum-free Ham's F-12 medium containing BSA at a final concentration of 0.1% (w/v; stock solution diluted 1:100) for 24 h.

3.1.2. Treatment (see **Note 4**)

1. Replace medium with 400 µL (treated wells) or 450 µL (control wells) of fresh serum-free medium containing 0.1% BSA. In treated wells, add 50 µL of growth factor or cytokine to be studied at the desired concentration. Finally, add in every well 50 µL of a $^{35}SO_4^{2-}$ solution at 15 µCi/mL (final concentration 1.5 µCi/mL). Each condition should have at least four replicates to ensure reproducibility and to allow statistical analysis of the results.
2. Treatments may last for 24, 48, or 72 h, as required (*see* **Note 8**).

3.2. Measure of Proteoglycan Synthesis

The overall method is depicted in **Fig. 1** and described here in detail.

1. At the end of treatment, harvest the secretion media in 1.5-mL-safe-lock microtubes and centrifuge for 5 min at 900g at 4°C to pellet floating cells. For further processing of media, go to **step 5**.
2. Wash the cells three times with 1 mL of DPBS to eliminate residual $^{35}SO_4^{2-}$ not specifically associated to chondrocytes.

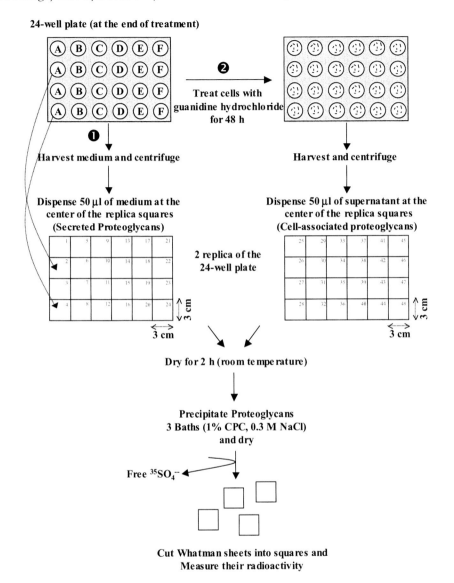

Fig 1. Schematic representation of the method for measuring proteoglycan synthesis by chondrocytes. CPC, cetyl pyridinium chloride.

3. Dispense 0.5 mL of proteoglycan extraction solution in each well and rock the plates gently for 48 h at 4°C to ensure complete extraction of cell-associated proteoglycans (CAP).
4. Harvest extraction mixtures in 1.5-mL safe-lock microtubes and centrifuge for 10 min at 10,000g. The supernatant contains CAP.

5. The supernatant (collected as in step 1) containing secreted proteoglycans (SP) and the fraction containing CAP (as collected in step 4) are then processed in a similar way.

6. Take 50 μL of the solution of either SP or CAP from the microtube and lay exactly at the center of a 9-cm^2 square in Whatman 3MM predrawn sheets (*see* **Note 9**). Perform this operation on separate sheets, one for SP and one for CAP.

7. Let dry for at least 2 h at room temperature.

8. Plunge the dry sheets into 15×21 cm trays (one sheet per tray) containing 100 mL of precipitating solution (*see* **Note 3**) and shake gently for 30 min at room temperature. Repeat three times by renewing with fresh precipitating solution. During this step, precipitated $^{35}SO_4^{2-}$ radiolabeled proteoglycans are trapped within the Whatman sheets, whereas free unincorporated $^{35}SO_4^{2-}$ stays in solution.

9. Let dry for 24 h at room temperature, or 5 h at 37°C (ensure that the sheets are completely dry).

10. Cut each 9-cm^2 square, roll it (*see* **Note 2**) and put it into a scintillation vial.

11. Add scintillation fluid and count (*see* **Note 10**).

3.3. Expression of Results

3.3.1. Total Proteoglycan Synthesis

1. Assuming that in **Fig. 1** (upper left), A are four controls (untreated wells), and B are four treated wells, the effect of treatment in terms of percent total proteoglycan synthesis compared with controls can be expressed as [(mean dpm of SP + mean dpm of CAP) in B]/[(mean dpm of SP + mean dpm of CAP) in A] × 100.

2. A typical experiment is depicted in **Fig. 2**, where IGF-I at 1.34 n*M* stimulated the basal synthesis of proteoglycans by rabbit chondrocytes approx 3.5 times after a 24-h treatment. Cotreatment of chondrocytes with IGF-I and a fourfold molar excess of IGFBP-3, one of the binding proteins that captures IGF-I and neutralizes its biological effects, brought back proteoglycan synthesis to the control value. Note that the high level of precision of the method leads to very low intra-assay variation, with standard errors typically being around 2% of the means.

3. The basal incorporation of $^{35}SO_4^{2-}$ by chondrocytes depends on the species studied. **Table 1** shows that, with 1.66×10^6 dpm added at T_0, about seven times higher amounts of $^{35}SO_4^{2-}$ were incorporated into proteoglycans neosynthesized by rabbit chondrocytes than by human osteoarthritic chondrocytes. According to this observation, the counting time should be adjusted to obtain maximum accuracy (*see* **Note 10**).

3.3.2. Cell-Associated Proteoglycans

1. Depending on the conditions, some factors may affect the distribution of neosynthesized proteoglycans between the cells and the culture medium. In this case, the percentage of cell-associated proteoglycans/total proteoglycans for treated cells compared with control cells is calculated as: [mean dpm of CAP/(mean dpm of SP + mean dpm of CAP) in B]/[mean dpm of CAP/(mean dpm of SP + mean dpm of CAP) in A] × 100.

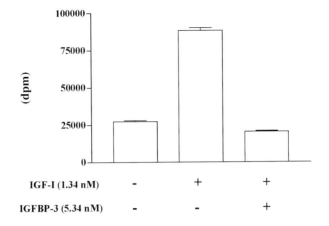

IGF-I (1.34 nM)   -   +   +

IGFBP-3 (5.34 nM)   -   -   +

Fig 2. Regulation of total proteoglycan synthesis (SP + CAP) by actors of the IGF system in cultured rabbit chondrocytes. Shown is one representative experiment out of six. Bars are means ± SEM of four replicates for each condition. Statistical differences: insulin-like growth factor-1 (IGF-1) vs control, $p < 0.001$; IGF binding protein-3 (IGFBP-3) vs IGF-1, $p < 0.001$.

Table 1
Relative Proteoglycan Synthesis by Chondrocytes
From Different Species After 24 h of Incubation With $^{35}SO_4^{2-}$

Species of chondrocytes	No. of experiments	dpm (mean ± SEM)
Human	6	4120 ± 883
Rabbit	6	28,300 ± 7360
Guinea pig	3	11,100 ± 2980
Rat	1	13,000

2. The proportion of CAP may vary when working with chondrocytes isolated from different species. For example, the percentage of CAP in nonstimulated rabbit chondrocytes after 24 h of incubation with $^{35}SO_4^{2-}$ was 32.4 ± 3.2% (mean ± SEM of six independent experiments), and was only 10.9 ± 0.5% (mean ± SEM of five independent experiments) in human osteoarthritic chondrocytes in similar conditions.

4. Notes

1. Lines and numbers should be drawn exclusively with a lead pencil. Any other tools such as ball-point pens or felt pens should be avoided, since the writing will disappear when the sheets are plunged into the precipitation baths.

families involved in cartilage loss made possible simple adjustments of already existing culture protocols, in order to separately analyze the degradative activities of aggrecanases and MMPs.

We present here a simple assay system, based on culture of rabbit cartilage explants, that allows study of the effects of protease inhibitors on the three major aspects of cartilage loss, namely, aggrecanase- and MMP-mediated proteoglycan degradation, and collagen degradation.

1.1. Degradation of Proteoglycan

Aggrecan, the most abundant cartilage proteoglycan, is a large macromolecule (about 2500 kDa) made up of a core protein (about 250 kDa) to which keratan and chondroitin sulfate glycosaminoglycans (GAGs) are linked (2). Aggrecan core protein can be degraded by both aggrecanases and MMPs. Two aggrecanases were recently identified as members of the ADAMTS family (a disintegrin and metalloproteinase with thrombospondin domain), namely, aggrecanase-1/ADAMTS-4 and aggrecanase-2/ADAMTS-5 (3,4). The effects of aggrecanases and MMPs on aggrecan can be classically distinguished on the basis of different cleavage sites in the interglobular domain. Whereas aggrecanases cleave at $NITEGE_{373}$—$_{374}ARGSVIL$, MMPs cleave at $VDIPEN_{341}$ —$_{342}FFGV$. The different terminal neoepitopes can be recognized using specific antibodies, allowing discrimination of aggrecan degradative activity (**Fig. 1**) (5).

We previously determined in rat cartilage explants, using Western blot analysis of NITEGE and VDIPEN in tissue extracts, the conditions under which proteoglycans are degraded in vitro by either aggrecanases or MMPs (6). Proteoglycan degradation was quantified as percent release of radioactivity from cartilage explants previously labeled with $^{35}SO_4^{2-}$. We tried the same protocol with rabbit cartilage explants and found a stronger response to interleukin-1 (IL-1), in terms of both aggrecanase and MMP degradative activities, coupled with lower dispersion of the data, and easier collection of the tissue from larger joints.

The assay is based on the ability of IL-1 to stimulate both aggrecanase activity and pro-MMP production. Since no endogenous activation of pro-MMPs takes place in rabbit cartilage explants, IL-1-induced proteoglycan degradation depends on aggrecanases only, as shown by increased levels of NITEGE, but not VDIPEN (**Fig. 2A**). If, instead, IL-1-induced pro-MMPs are activated by p-aminophenylmercuric acetate (APMA), then the breakdown of aggrecan is mediated by MMPs, as shown by a strong increase of VDIPEN (**Fig. 2B**).

To confirm the specificity of aggrecan degradation caused by aggrecanases or MMPs, we used AG-3340 (prinomastat), which inhibits several MMPs with K_i values around 10^{-10} M (7), and also inhibits aggrecanases at concentrations

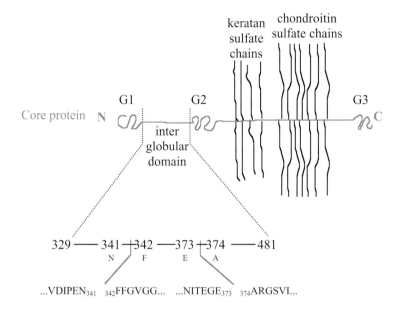

Fig. 1. General structure of the aggrecan molecule and cleavage sites in the G1–G2 interglobular domain of the core protein.

around 10^{-6} *M (8)*. In IL-1-stimulated cartilage explants, 10^{-5} *M* AG-3340 blocked the increase of NITEGE levels in tissue extracts (**Fig. 2A**), as well as proteoglycan degradation, measured as radioactivity release, with a mean inhibitory concentration (IC_{50}) of 7×10^{-7} *M* (**Fig. 2C**). In the case of proteoglycan degradation induced by IL-1 followed by APMA, 10^{-7} *M* AG-3340 was sufficient to block both the increase of VDIPEN (**Fig. 2B**) and proteoglycan release, with an IC_{50} of 2×10^{-9} *M* (**Fig. 2D**). Different sensitivities to AG-3340 confirm that proteoglycan degradation owing to IL-1, or IL-1 followed by APMA, is caused by different types of enzyme.

1.2. Degradation of Collagen

Type II collagen represents 90–95% of the total collagen content of the cartilage, and is found in fibrils made of type II collagen molecules stabilized by collagen IX and XI. Each type II collagen molecule is composed of a triple helix of three identical α-chains covalently linked at their ends *(9)*. Native fibrillar collagen is known to be highly resistant to proteases, and its initial cleavage must be collagenase-mediated. Three collagenases have been identified, MMP-1, MMP-8, and MMP-13, which cleave type II collagen at a single point, three-fourths of the distance from the N terminus (**Fig. 3**).

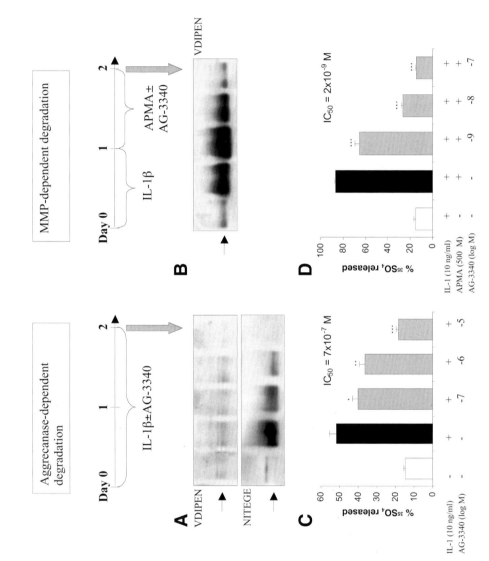

Aggrecanase-dependent degradation

MMP-dependent degradation

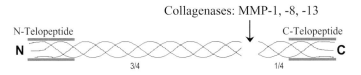

Collagenases: MMP-1, -8, -13

N-Telopeptide ↓ C-Telopeptide

N 3/4 1/4 **C**

Fig. 3. Schematic representation of type II collagen and matrix metalloproteinase (MMP) cleavage site.

Once denatured by collagenases, type II collagen is further degraded by gelatinases (MMP-2 and MMP-9) and stromelysin (MMP-3) *(10)*. Collagen degradation in cultures of rabbit cartilage explants can be stimulated by the addition of IL-1 and plasminogen *(11)*. The cytokine increases both plasminogen activation and the production of pro-MMPs, which are in turn activated by plasmin. Plasminogen probably plays an important role in pathological activation of pro-MMPs, since it is present in the synovial fluid of patients with osteoarthritis and rheumatoid arthritis *(12)*. Here we describe a modification of the assay by Saito et al. *(11)*, which allows for a more rapid MMP activation and ECM degradation, mainly by the replacement of plasminogen with plasmin.

Collagen degradation is calculated as percent release of collagen, measured by colorimetric assay of hydroxyproline (OH-pro) in medium and tissue hydrolysates, using a modification of Grant's method *(13)*. Using this protocol, the MMP inhibitor blocked collagen degradation at 10^{-7} *M* with an IC_{50} of 4×10^{-8} *M* (**Fig. 4**).

Fig. 2. *(opposite page)* Effects of interleukin-1 (IL-1) alone and IL-1 followed by *p*-aminophenylmercuric acetate (APMA) on NITEGE and VDIPEN levels (**A,B**) and proteoglycan degradation (**C,D**) in the absence and presence of AG-3340 in rabbit cartilage explant cultures. Plans of the experiments are shown at the top of the figure. (**A**) Effect of IL-1 on NITEGE and VDIPEN levels, analyzed by Western blot, in the absence and presence of AG-3340. (**B**) Effect of IL-1 followed by APMA, on VDIPEN levels, analyzed by Western blot, in the absence and presence of AG-3340. (**C**) Effect of IL-1 on proteoglycan degradation in the absence and presence of AG-3340. Proteoglycan degradation was measured as % release of radiolabeled material between d 0 and 2. Asterisks indicate a significant difference between IL-1 alone and IL-1 plus AG-3340: ***, $p < 0.001$, **, $p < 0.01$, *, $p < 0.5$; data are averages ± Sem; $n = 8$. (**D**) Effect of IL-1 followed by APMA on proteoglycan degradation in the absence and presence of AG-3340. Proteoglycan degradation was measured as % release of radiolabeled material between d 1 and 2. Asterisks indicate a significant difference between APMA alone and APMA plus AG-3340: ***, $p < 0.001$; data are averages ± Sem; $n = 8$.

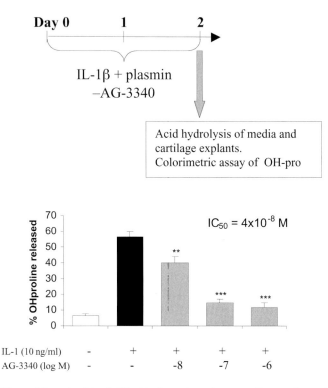

Fig. 4. Effect of interleukin-1 (IL-1) plus plasmin on collagen degradation in the absence and presence of AG-3340 after 2 d of treatment. Collagen degradation was measured as % release of OH-pro. Asterisks indicate a significant difference between IL-1/plasmin alone and IL-1/plasmin plus AG-3340: ***, $p < 0.001$, **, $p < 0.01$; data are averages ± Sem; $n = 8$.

2. Materials

2.1. Cartilage Explant Preparation and Culture

1. Cartilage source: male New Zealand albino rabbits weighing 500–600 g.
2. Sterile surgical instruments: large (16 cm) and small (12 cm) scissors, large and small tissue forceps, fine, curved pliers.
3. Sterile disposable scalpels with straight (no. 11) and curved (no. 23) blades (Feather).
4. Dulbecco's phosphate-buffered saline without calcium and magnesium (PBS; Gibco).
5. Dulbecco's minimal essential medium/Ham's F12 medium, 50/50 mixture with Glutamax™ (DMEM/F12; Gibco).

6. Penicillin (10,000 U/mL) plus streptomycin (10 mg/mL), 100X concentrated stock solution (PS; Gibco).
7. Fetal bovine serum (FBS), previously decomplemented by heating for 30 min at 56°C (Gibco).
8. Bovine serum albumin (BSA), 35%, fraction V solution (Sigma).
9. Recombinant mouse IL-1β (Sigma): make up a stock solution at 5 µg/mL in PBS containing 0.1% BSA, aliquot and store at –20°C.
10. APMA (Sigma): make up a 100X concentrated solution at 0.05 M in 0.05 M sodium hydroxide. Prepare fresh on day of use (*see* **Note 1**).
11. Dimethyl sulfoxide (DMSO): used as solvent for tested compounds.
12. Cell culture dish, 100 × 20 mm (Becton Dickinson).
13. Sterile 5-mL polypropylene round-bottomed test tubes (Becton Dickinson).
14. 96-Well culture plate, flat bottomed (Becton Dickinson).
15. Sterile laminar flow hood for tissue culture.
16. Tissue culture incubator, with humidified atmosphere of 5% CO_2/air at 37°C.

2.2. Cartilage Degradation (Aggrecan; $^{35}SO_4^{2-}$)

1. DMEM/F12 medium supplemented with 10% FBS and 1% PS: to 500 mL of DMEM/F12 add 55 mL of FBS and 5 mL of PS (10% FBS DMEM/F12).
2. DMEM/F12 medium supplemented with 0.1% BSA and 1% PS: to 500 mL of DMEM/F12 add 1.43 mL of BSA 35% and 5 mL of PS (0.1% BSA DMEM/F12).
3. Sulphur 35, sulfate, in aqueous solution ($^{35}SO_4^{2-}$); (Amersham): use at a final activity of 3.7 MBq (100 µCi) for explant labeling. Use appropriate protective equipment (gloves, goggles, and plexiglass screen) when handling the source and labeled culture material.
4. DL-Dithiothreitol (DTT; Sigma).
5. EDTA (Sigma).
6. 20 mM Phosphate buffer: 2.76 g/L $NaH_2PO_4·H_2O$, 0.38 g/L EDTA (1 mM), pH 6.8.
7. Papain (Sigma): make up at 0.6 mg/mL (w/v) in 20 mM phosphate buffer plus 0.25 mg/mL (w/v) DTT. Prepare fresh on day of use.
8. Miniature 6-mL vial (Pony Vial™; Packard).
9. Cocktail for liquid scintillation (LSC; Ultima Gold; Packard).
10. Liquid scintillation analyzer (Tri Carb 2900 TR; Packard).
11. Oven, set at 56°C, with timer.

2.3. Cartilage Degradation (Collagen; OH-pro)

In the following steps, handle the corrosive solutions (hydrochloric acid, perchloric acid and sodium hydroxide) under a hood, with appropriate protective equipment (gloves, goggles).

1. DMEM/F12 medium supplemented with 0.1% BSA and 1% PS: to 500 mL of DMEM/F12 add 1.43 mL of BSA 35% and 5 mL of PS 100X concentrated (0.1% BSA DMEM/F12).

2. Plasmin, ε-aminocaproic acid (EACA)- and lysine-free from human plasma (Calbiochem): make up a stock solution at 10 U/mL in sterile deionized water, aliquot, and store at –20°C.

3. Hydrochloric acid fuming 37% (HCl 12 *M*; Merck).

4. Perchloric acid 70–72% (Merck).

5. 6 *M* Sodium hydroxide solution (NaOH 6 *M*): 60 g/250 mL final vol, in deionized water. Solution heats strongly during solubilization.

6. OH-pro (Merck): for standard curve preparation, prepare a stock solution at 5 m*M* in deionized water, aliquot and store at –20°C.

7. OH-pro buffer: 30 g citric acid monohydrate, 15 g sodium hydroxide, 90 g sodium acetate anhydrous; adjust to pH 6.0 and complete to 1000 mL with deionized water.

8. Chloramine T trihydrate (CT; Merck): 96 mg of CT, 6.2 mL OH-pro buffer, 13.8 mL deionized water (sufficient for one 96-well plate). Prepare fresh on day of use.

9. 4-(Dimethylamino)benzaldehyde (pDAB; Merck): to 1.47 g of pDAB, add 7.4 mL deionized water and 2.6 mL perchloric acid (sufficient for one 96-well plate). Prepare fresh on day of use.

10. Borosilicate vials, 2 mL with cap (Wheaton).

11. 96-Well deep plate, 1.2 mL/well capacity (Costar).

12. 96-Well microtiter plate, flat bottomed (Costar).

13. Photometric microplate reader with 540-nm filter and calculation software (Labsystems iEMS reader and Genesis™ software).

14. Oven, set at 110°C, with timer.

15. Water thermostated bath, set at 70°C.

3. Methods

3.1. Cartilage Explant Preparation

3.1.1. Animal Sacrifice

Anesthetize rabbits with isoflurane (Forene®, Abbott) using standard veterinary equipment (Minerve®, France) (**Fig. 5A**), then sacrifice by rupture of the cervical vertebrae, and exsanguinate by carotid section. The use of animals must conform to ethical guidelines. This procedure can only be used after acceptance by the local Ethics Committee on animal experimentation.

3.1.2. Sampling of the Knee Joint

Prepare one culture dish filled with 20 mL of PBS. Use ethanol 70% (v/v) to disinfect and wet the rabbit's fur all over the hind limbs, then cut the skin around the ankle, pull the skin off the leg and the thigh, and roughly remove the muscles with the scissors. Cut the femur and the tibia 2–3 cm away from the knee, and then put the joint in the cell culture dish and transfer to a sterile tissue culture hood (**Fig. 5B**).

A

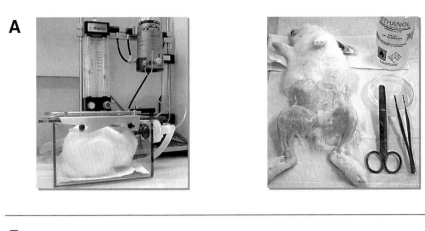

B

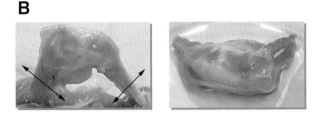

C

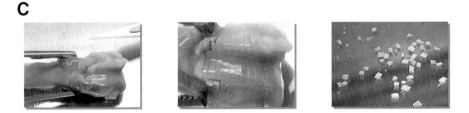

Fig. 5. Animal sacrifice and cartilage collection. (**A**) Rabbit anesthesia using Minerve apparatus and animal preparation before knee isolation. (**B**) Knee isolation; arrows show dissection points. (**C**) Isolated femur; grid incision in the cartilage between the condylar ridges; explants collected in the culture dish.

3.1.3. Cartilage Explant Preparation

All the following steps of explant preparation and culture are performed under sterile conditions. Have ready two more culture dishes, one for tissue dissection, and the other for collection of cartilage explants (*see* **Note 2**).

Prepare the DMEM/F12 for collection of isolated cartilage explants. Two alternative supplements are used, depending on whether the explants are used for proteoglycan or collagen degradation.

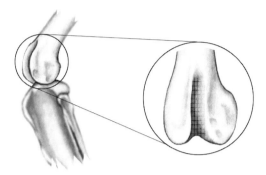

Fig. 6. Location of the sampling zone in the articular cartilage of the distal femur.

1. Proteoglycan degradation: 10% FBS DMEM/F12.
2. Collagen degradation: 0.1% BSA DMEM/F12.

Add 25 mL of the appropriate medium to one culture dish.

1. Remove the muscles around the joint, and cut the capsule and the ligaments to separate the femur from the tibia. Transfer the femur into a clean culture dish and cover with PBS. Repeat the operation for each knee.
2. With the no. 11 scalpel, incise a grid in the cartilage between the condylar ridges, of squares of approx 1 mm per side (**Figs. 5C** and **6**), reaching with the tip of the blade the underlying hard tissue (*see* **Note 3**).
3. Gently shave the cartilage as close as possible to the underlying hard tissue and place the explants into the culture dish containing the appropriate medium. Repeat the operation until all the cartilage in the gridded zone has been collected.
4. Use the no. 23 scalpel to trim the largest explants already collected in the culture dish (*see* **Note 4**).

3.2. Cartilage Explant Culture

3.2.1. Proteoglycan Degradation (Aggrecan; $^{35}SO_4^{2-}$)

Two procedures for proteoglycan degradation assays are described, the first for aggrecanase-, and the second for MMP-dependent release of radiolabeled material. The different steps of the two procedures are outlined as a flow chart in **Fig. 7**.

3.2.1.1. EXPLANT LABELING, COMMON TO BOTH PROCEDURES

1. Add 3.7 MBq (100 µCi) of $^{35}SO_4^{2-}$ to the culture dish containing the explants in 10% FBS DMEM/F12, usually before the weekend, and put in the tissue culture incubator.
2. After 3 days in culture, remove the unincorporated radioactivity by six media changes, each with 30 mL of medium, over 24 h using 0.1% BSA DMEM/F12.

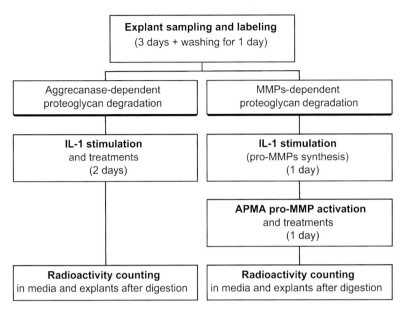

Fig. 7. Assay procedures for aggrecanase- and matrix metalloproteinase (MMP)-dependent proteoglycan degradation. APMA, *p*-aminophenylmercuric acetate; IL-1, interleukin-1.

3.2.1.2. AGGRECANASE-DEPENDENT PROTEOGLYCAN DEGRADATION

1. Prepare treatments in 5-mL tubes. For each group, prepare 2.5 mL of 0.1% BSA DMEM/F12, with or without treatments. The assay pattern is as follows:
    a. One basal control group of medium plus vehicle at the same concentration as in the treated groups.
    b. One stimulated control group with IL-1β at a final concentration of 10 ng/mL plus vehicle at the same concentration as in the treated groups.
    c. Several treatment groups with IL-1β at a final concentration of 10 ng/mL plus treatment. The concentration of the vehicle (usually DMSO) is made the same for all treatment groups (*see* **Note 5**).

    Each group is made up of eight wells. Distribute treatments from tubes to 96-well plates, 250 µL/well (**Fig. 8**).

2. Transfer the fragments into the 96-well plate, at one fragment per well, and put in the tissue culture incubator.

3. After 2 d of culture, stop the incubation and transfer each fragment into 500 µL of papain solution/Pony Vial, then cover, and digest in the oven at 56°C for 16 h (*see* **Note 6**). Then add 5 mL of LSC per vial and measure the radioactivity.

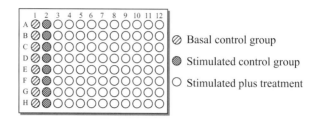

Fig. 8. 96-Well plate format for proteoglycan or collagen degradation.

4. Pipet an aliquot of 200 μL of culture media from each well into counting vials and then add 5 mL of LSC. Measure the radioactivity, and multiply the dpm result of counting by 1.25 to obtain the total radioactivity in the media per well.
5. Express proteoglycan degradation in each fragment as the percentage of released radioactivity by the formula:

$$\text{degradation} = \frac{\text{media radioactivity}}{\left(\text{media radioactivity} + \text{tissue radioactivity}\right)} \times 100$$

3.2.1.3. MMP-Dependent Proteoglycan Degradation

1. After labeling and washing the explants, add 20 mL of 0.1% BSA, DMEM/F12 to the culture dish plus IL-1β at a final concentration of 10 ng/mL.
2. Incubate for 1 d and then wash one time with 25 mL of 0.1% BSA, DMEM/F12.
3. Prepare treatments in 5-mL tubes. For each group, prepare 2.5 mL of 0.1% BSA, DMEM/F12, with or without treatments. The assay pattern is as follows:
   a. One basal control group of medium plus vehicle at the same concentration as in the treated groups.
   b. One stimulated control group with APMA at a final concentration of 500 μ*M* plus vehicle at the same concentration as in the treated groups.
   c. Several treatment groups with APMA at a final concentration of 500 μ*M* plus treatment. The concentration of the vehicle (usually DMSO) is made the same for all treatment groups (*see* **Note 5**).

   Each group is made up of eight wells. Distribute treatments from tubes to 96-well plates, 250 μL/well.

4. Transfer the fragments into the 96-well plate, at one fragment per well (**Fig. 8**), and put in the tissue culture incubator.
5. After 1 d of culture, stop the incubation and transfer each fragment into 500 μL of papain solution/Pony Vial, and then cover and digest in the oven at 56°C for 16 h (*see* **Note 6**). Then add 5 mL of LSC per vial and measure the radioactivity.
6. Pipet an aliquot of 200 μL of culture media from each well into counting vials and then add 5 mL of LSC. Measure the radioactivity, and multiply the dpm result of the media aliquot by 1.25 to obtain the total radioactivity in the media per well.

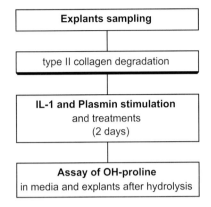

Fig. 9. Procedure for collagen degradation assay. IL-1, interleukin-1.

7. Express proteoglycan degradation in each fragment as the percentage of released radioactivity by the formula:

$$\text{degradation} = \frac{\text{media radioactivity}}{\left(\text{media radioactivity} + \text{tissue radioactivity}\right)} \times 100$$

3.2.2. Collagen Degradation (Collagen; OH-pro)

The different steps of the procedure are presented as a flow chart in **Fig. 9**.

3.2.2.1. TYPE II COLLAGEN DEGRADATION

1. Prepare treatments in 5-mL tubes. For each group, prepare 1.2 mL of 0.1% BSA, DMEM/F12, with or without treatments. The assay pattern is as follows:
   a. One basal control group of medium plus vehicle at the same concentration as in the treated groups.
   b. One stimulated control group with IL-1β and plasmin, respectively, at a final concentrations of 10 ng/mL and 0.1 U/mL plus vehicle at the same concentration as in the treated groups.
   c. Several treatment groups with IL-1β and plasmin, at final concentrations, of 10 ng/mL and 0.1 U/mL respectively, plus treatment. The concentration of the vehicle (usually DMSO) is the same for all treatment groups (*see* **Note 5**).

   Each group is made up of eight wells. Distribute treatments from tubes to 96-well plates, 120 μL/well.
2. Transfer the fragments into the 96-well plate, at two fragments per well (**Fig. 8**), and put in the tissue culture incubator.
3. After 2 d of culture, stop the incubation and collect media and fragments for hydrolysis.
   a. For media, mix 100 μL of culture medium from each well with 100 μL of 37% HCl in a borosilicate vial.

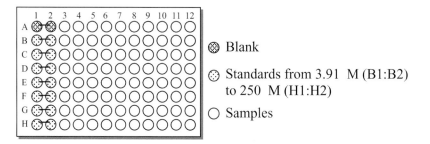

Fig. 10. 96-well plate format for hydroproline (OH-pro) colorimetric assay.

b. For explants, put both fragments from each well into a borosilicated vial containing 100 μL of deionized water, and then add 100 μL of 37% HCl.

Close the vials tightly with the appropriate caps and hydrolyze in the oven at 110°C for 12 h.

3.2.2.2. Assay of Hydroxyproline: Modified Grant's Method

1. Transfer 100 μL from each vial into a 96-well plate, and add 75 μL NaOH, 6 *M* to take the sample close to neutrality. Mix energetically with an orbital plate shaker for 5 min. at 1000 rpm (*see* **Note 7**).
2. Standard curve preparation: add 500 μL of deionized water to eight tubes numbered from 0 (blank) to 7. Dilute 100 μL of 5 m*M* OH-pro stock solution into 900 μL of deionized water, then transfer 500 μL of this solution into tube 1, and mix thoroughly. Transfer 500 μL from tube 1 into tube 2 and mix thoroughly. Repeat this procedure to tube 7. You obtain a 7-point standard curve plus a blank with a concentration range from 250 to 3.91 μ*M* by 1:2 dilutions. Prepare a standard curve each time the assay is performed.
3. For the reaction setup, use a 1.2-mL 96-well deep plate; assay each standard point in duplicate. Add 50 μL of standard or neutralized sample per well following the pattern depicted in **Fig. 10**.
4. Add 185 μL of CT solution and mix gently on an orbital shaker for 5 min at 600 rpm.
5. Add 75 μL of pDAB solution and mix energetically on an orbital shaker for 2 min at 1000 rpm.
6. Cover the plate and incubate for 5 min at 70°C in a water thermostated bath.
7. Let the plate cool down at room temperature and transfer, using a multichannel pipet, 250 μL from each well into a 96-well microtiter plate.
8. Read the plate at 540 nm within 15 min.

3.2.2.3. Calculating the Results

1. Plot OD_{540} vs concentration of standards. Read unknowns from the standard curve (**Fig. 11**).

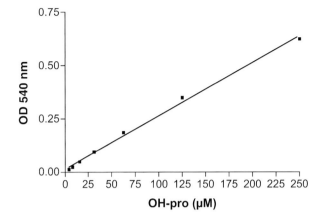

Fig. 11. Standard curve for hydroproline (OH-pro) assay. OD_{540} corrected from blank.

2. To obtain the total content of OH-pro per well, multiply each value from media and fragments by the appropriate factor; *see* the following formulas:

$$F_{medium} = \frac{V_T \times V_H \times V_N}{V_M \times 10^3 \times 10^2} = 0.42$$

$$F_{explant} = \frac{V_H \times V_N}{10^3 \times 10^2} = 0.35$$

V_T = treatment volume = 120 µL.
V_H = hydrolyzed solution volume = 200 µL.
V_N = volume of neutralized solution = 175 µL.
V_M = volume of hydrolyzed medium = 100 µL.

3. Collagen degradation in each fragment is expressed as the percentage of released OH-pro by the formula:

$$degradation = \frac{media\ OH\text{-}pro}{\left(media\ OH\text{-}pro + tissue\ OH\text{-}pro\right)} \times 100$$

3.3. Statistical Analysis

For all degradation protocols, namely, aggrecanase- and MMP-dependent proteoglycan degradation and collagen degradation, the data are treated in the same way.

1. Calculate mean and standard error of degradation for each group.

2. Validate the assay by verifying the stimulation of degradation by comparing the mean of the basal control with that of the stimulated group without treatment. For these two groups calculate the percentage of variation using the formula:

$$\%_{variation} = \frac{\left(\bar{y}_{stimulated} - \bar{x}_{control}\right)}{\bar{x}_{control}} \times 100$$

where $\bar{x}$ and $\bar{y}$ are, respectively, the degradation means of the control and stimulated-without-treatment groups (*see* **Note 8**).

3. For treated groups, calculate the percentage of inhibition in each group using the formula:

$$\%_{inhibition} = \frac{\left(\bar{y}_{stimulated} - \bar{z}_{treated}\right)}{\left(\bar{y}_{stimulated} - \bar{x}_{control}\right)} \times 100$$

where $\bar{z}$ is the degradation mean of the treated group.

4. Compare basal control and stimulated-without-treatment group by unpaired *t*-test. Compare stimulated-without-treatment and treated groups by analysis of variance followed by a Dunnett's multiple comparison test.

4. Notes

1. Solubilize APMA by fast stirring using a magnetic bar, or by sonication.
2. Always keep cartilage sample in PBS buffer or medium, thus avoiding tissue drying.
3. In preliminary experiments (data not shown), it was observed that the cartilage fragments from this region expressed a stronger response to degradative agents such as retinoic acid and IL-1 than tissue fragments from femoral condyles, or from femoral or humeral heads. Even if cartilage from different regions can be used, it is strongly recommended not to mix tissue fragments collected from different locations in the same assay.
4. It is important that cartilage samples be homogenous in size and shape in order to limit variability, especially for collagen degradation.
5. All groups are matched for concentration of vehicle (i.e., DMSO), generally not more than 1% at final concentration.
6. During digestion of cartilage fragments, put a container filled with water in the oven, thus reducing evaporation of papain solution.
7. For the assay of OH-pro, a precipitate may occur during the neutralization step, which usually disappears during stirring and has no effect on the final result.
8. Typical values for degradation in all protocols are given below (data are mean ± standard error of seven experiments):
   a. *Aggrecanase dependent proteoglycan degradation*: results expressed as the percentage of released radioactivity.
      i. Basal control = 13.33 ± 0.71

      ii. Stimulated group without treatment = 44.00 ± 1.82
     iii. Percentage of stimulation = 235 ± 19

  b. *MMP-dependent proteoglycan degradation*: results expressed as the percentage of released radioactivity.

       i. Basal control = 11.90 ± 1.17
      ii. Stimulated group without treatment = 75.24 ± 3.07
     iii. Percentage of stimulation = 567 ± 68

  c. *Type II collagen degradation*: results expressed as the percentage of released OH-pro.

       i. Basal control = 8.86 ± 0.44
      ii. Stimulated group without treatment = 46.24 ± 2.93
     iii. Percentage of stimulation = 428 ± 39

References

1. Goldring, M. B. (2000) The role of chondrocyte in osteoarthritis. *Arthritis Rheum.* **43,** 1916–1926.
2. Hascall, V. C. and Kimura, J. H. (1992) Proteoglycans: isolation and characterization. *Methods Enzymol.* **82,** 769–800.
3. Tortorella, M. D., Burn, T. C., Pratta, M. A., et al. (1999) Purification and cloning of aggrecanase-1: a member of the ADAMTS family of proteins. *Science* **284,** 1664–1666.
4. Abbaszade, I, Liu, R. Q., Yang, F., et al. (1999) Cloning and characterization of ADAMTS11, an aggrecanase from the ADAMTS family. *J. Biol. Chem.* **274,** 23,443–23,450.
5. Caterson, B., Flannery, C. R., Hughes, C. E., and Little, C. B. (2000) Mechanisms involved in cartilage proteoglycan catabolism. *Matrix Biol.* **19,** 333–344.
6. Sabatini, M., Bardiot, A., Lesur, C., et al. (2002) Effects of agonists of peroxisome proliferator-activated receptor γ on proteoglycan degradation and matrix metalloproteinase production in rat cartilage in vitro. *Osteoarthritis Cartilage* **10,** 673–679.
7. Sorbera, L. A. and Castaner, J. (2000) Prinomastat. *Drugs Fut.* **25,** 150–158.
8. Sugimoto, K., Takahashi, M., Yamamoto, Y., Shimada, K., and Tanzawa, K. (1999) Identification of aggrecanase activity in medium of cartilage culture. *J. Biochem.* **126,** 449–455.
9. Cremer, M. A., Rosloniec, E. F., and Kang, H. A. (1998) The cartilage collagens; a review of their structure, organization, and role in the pathogenesis of experimental arthritis in animals and in human disease. *J. Mol. Med.* **76,** 275–288.
10. Billinghurst, R. C., Dahlberg, L., Iionescu, M., et al. (1997) Enhanced cleavage of type II collagen by collagenases in osteoarthritic articular cartilage. *J. Clin. Invest.* **99,** 1534–1545.
11. Saito, S., Katoh, M., Masumoto, M., Matsumoto S.-I., and Masuho Y. (1997) Collagen degradation induced by the combination of IL-1α and plasminogen in rabbit articular cartilage explant culture. *J. Biochem.* **122,** 49–54.

12. Kummer, J. A., Abbink, J. J., Deboer, J. P., et al. (1992) Analysis of intraarticular fibrinolytic pathways in patients with inflammatory and non inflammatory joint diseases. *Arthritis Rheum.* **36,** 884–893.

13. Grant, R. A. (1964) Estimation of OH-proline by the autoanalyser. *J. Clinical Pathol.* **17,** 685–686.

17

Production of Antibodies Against Degradative Neoepitopes in Aggrecan

John S. Mort and Peter J. Roughley

Summary

The use of synthetic peptides to generate rabbit polyclonal anticatabolic neoepitope antibodies that can be used to study the presence of defined proteolytic cleavage sites in aggrecan is described. Principles of peptide design and methods for preparation and characterization of ovalbumin conjugates are presented along with approaches for the characterization and affinity purification of the resulting antisera. Limitations associated with the use of antipeptide antibodies to study authentic protein neoepitopes are discussed.

Key Words: Peptide synthesis; affinity purification; coupling; bifunctional reagent; ELISA; SDS-PAGE; HPLC; peptide sequencing.

1. Introduction

Antibodies with the ability to recognize specific epitopes generated following the cleavage of proteoglycans by different proteolytic enzymes (anticatabolic neoepitope antibodies) have played an important role in the characterization of the proteases active within cartilage during normal development *(1)* and degeneration of this tissue in arthritis *(2)*. These antibodies appear to bind the terminal residues of the epitope into a pocket in the antigen binding site and are thus unable to recognize uncleaved proteoglycans *(3,4)*.

For the production of antineoepitope antibodies, synthetic peptides representing the appropriate sequence upstream or downstream of the cleavage site are prepared with an additional spacer sequence and a terminal cysteine residue to allow coupling to a protein carrier using a bifunctional reagent *(5)*. Although other strategies can be used, we have had good success using peptide-ovalbumin conjugates coupled using the bifunctional reagent *N*-succinimidyl bromoacetate (**Fig. 1**). Ovalbumin has several advantages as the carrier protein.

From: *Methods in Molecular Medicine, Vol. 100: Cartilage and Osteoarthritis, Vol. 1: Cellular and Molecular Tools*
Edited by: M. Sabatini, P. Pastoureau, and F. De Ceuninck © Humana Press Inc., Totowa, NJ

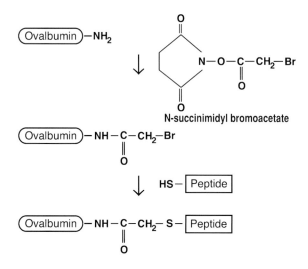

Fig. 1. Schematic representation of the steps in the coupling of peptides to ovalbumin using the bifunctional reagent *N*-succinimidyl bromoacetate.

It is highly soluble, even following derivatization, and it runs as a discrete band on sodium dodecyl sulfate–polyacrylamide gel electrophoresis (SDS-PAGE), making it easy to characterize the conjugated products. It contains 20 lysine residues for derivatization by a coupling reagent, no free sulfhydryl groups, and its N-terminus is blocked by acetylation. Reaction with *N*-succinimidyl bromoacetate results in a well-derivatized protein ready to bind free sulfhydryl groups in a peptide with the introduction of a minimal amount of nonpeptide material (a methylene group), thus decreasing the potential for antibody production against physiologically irrelevant epitopes.

Two approaches have been used for neoepitope antibody generation. Mouse monoclonal antibodies have the advantage of being unique immunoglobulins that can, in principle, be produced in unlimited quantities. Effective monoclonal antibodies have been produced to aggrecan cleavage epitopes *(6,7)*. However, considerable time and effort must be invested to generate the required hybridoma clones. In contrast, rabbit polyclonal antibodies are much easier to produce, but the resulting sera of necessity contain a heterogeneous population of immunoglobulins. This can result in polyclonal antisera being less specific for the neoepitope than monoclonal antibodies. Affinity purification, using the immobilized immunizing peptide, removes antibodies to ovalbumin and other serum components contributing to high background reactivity on Western blotting and immunohistochemistry.

In this chapter, principles of peptide design and methods for preparation and characterization of ovalbumin conjugates are outlined, along with approaches for the production, characterization, and affinity purification of the resulting rabbit immunoglobulins. In addition, some possible pitfalls associated with the use of these antibodies are discussed.

2. Materials

1. Peptides can be obtained either commercially or by synthesizing in-house. Purification by high-performance liquid chromatography (HPLC) and characterization by mass spectrometry or peptide sequencing is required.
2. DL-Cysteine (Sigma, cat. no. C 4022).
3. Ellman's reagent *(8):* 5,5'-dithiobis (2-dinitrobenzoic acid) (Sigma, cat. no. D 8130). Make a stock solution of 4 mg/mL in 0.1 M potassium phosphate, pH 7.0, containing 0.05% sodium azide, and (store at 4°C).
4. Ellman's reaction buffer: 0.1 M potassium phosphate, pH 8.0, containing 1 mM EDTA and 0.05% sodium azide. (Store at room temperature.)
5. Ellman's reaction mix: 4 mL Ellman's reaction buffer and 0.12 mL Ellman's reagent solution. Make up to 14 mL with water.
6. Dithiothreitol (Sigma, cat. no. D 9163).
7. Ovalbumin (Sigma, cat. no. A 5503; albumin from chicken egg white), stored at 4°C.
8. Coupling reagent: the bifunctional reagent *N*-succinimidyl bromoacetate is available from Sigma-Aldrich (cat. no. B8271, bromoacetic acid *N*-hydroxy-succinimide ester) or can be synthesized with little difficulty *(9)*. It is extremely important that this compound be stored under dry conditions. Before use, the bifunctional reagent is dissolved in dimethylformamide. This should be stored over molecular sieves (3 Å) to prevent decomposition resulting in the formation of ammonia, which would react with the coupling reagent.
9. Coupling buffer and column buffer: 0.1 M potassium phosphate, pH 7.5, containing 1 mM EDTA. (Adjust with 10% potassium hydroxide.) Filter and de-gas.
10. Phosphate-buffered saline (PBS): 6 mM Na$_2$HPO$_4$, 4 mM KH$_2$PO$_4$, 145 mM NaCl, pH 7.2.
11. SDS-PAGE equipment.
12. Electrophoretic transfer equipment.
13. PVDF (polyvinylidenedifluoride) and nitrocellulose membranes (Bio-Rad).
14. Sephadex G10 and G25 columns, (Amersham Biosciences).
15. New Zealand white rabbits (female, 2.5–3.0 kg).
16. Freund's complete and incomplete adjuvants (Difco).
17. Immunlon 2 flat-bottomed 96-well ELISA plates.
18. PBS-T: PBS containing 0.05% Tween-20.
19. Blocking buffer: PBS-T containing 1% bovine serum albumin.
20. Alkaline phosphate-conjugated goat anti-rabbit immunoglobulins (Sigma, cat. no. A-3812).

21. Alkaline phosphatase substrate (p-nitrophenylphosphate: Sigma Diagnostics, cat. no. 104-105). Dissolve 1 tablet in 10 mL diethanolamine buffer (9.6% v/v diethanolamine in 0.26 mM MgCl$_2$, pH 9.8).

22. TBS-T: Tris-buffered saline (10 mM Tris-HCl, pH 8.0, 150 mM NaCl) containing 0.05% Tween-20.

23. Alkaline phosphatase blot development solution: add 66 μL of nitroblue tetrazolium (50 mg/mL in dimethylformamide) and 33 μL of 5-bromo-4-chloro-3-indolyl phosphate (50 mg/mL in dimethylformamide) in 10 mL of alkaline phosphatase buffer (100 mM Tris-HCl, pH 9.5, 100 mM NaCl, 5 mM MgCl$_2$).

24. Sulfolink coupling gel (Pierce)

25. Affinity column equibration buffer: 50 mM Tris-HCl, pH 8.5, containing 5 mM EDTA.

3. Methods

3.1. Peptide Design

As a general rule, peptides are prepared consisting of five to seven amino acid residues representing the sequence immediately upstream, or downstream, of the target cleavage site, as appropriate. Two glycine residues are then routinely added as a spacer to facilitate accessibility of the epitope, followed by a cysteine residue to allow coupling through the sulfhydryl group on the side chain. Hydrophobic residues may predominate in the target sequence and this would result in peptides with low water solubility. In such cases the addition of arginine and lysine residues to the spacer sequence has proved helpful. GKG, AKKG, and GKARAKG linkers have been used successfully *(10)* (**Fig. 2**). A basic linker region may also help solubilize acidic peptides for reverse-phase HPLC purification using trifluoroacetic acid/acetonitrile (*see* **Note 1**).

To characterize fully the specificity of the antipeptide antisera, additional peptides representing a one-residue truncation and a one-residue extension of the neoepitope sequence are synthesized together with the immunizing peptide for use in a competitive ELISA.

Success of peptide coupling depends on the status of the cysteine sulfhydryl group. Often peptides are partially, or occasionally completely, oxidized. The sulfhydryl content of the peptide can be determined. In some cases a reduced peptide can be regenerated from the oxidized form by treatment with a reducing agent such as dithiothreitol.

3.2. Testing for Free Sulfhydryl Content of Peptides

3.2.1. Standard Curve

1. Prepare a fresh 4 mM solution of cysteine in water and make a working solution of 0.4 mM in water.

2. Prepare 0.3 mL serial dilutions of cysteine in water from 0 to 0.4 mM in increments of 40 μM.

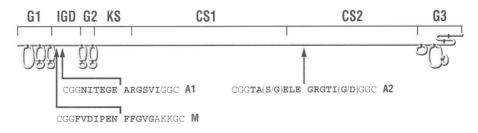

Fig. 2. Schematic representation of the aggrecan core protein and peptides designed for production of anti-neoepitopes for well-characterized metalloproteinase cleavage sites. The aggrecan core protein is depicted as an N-terminal globular region (G1) separated from a second globular region (G2) by an interglobular domain (IGD). The IGD is susceptible to cleavage by many proteolytic enzymes. Shown are the aggrecanase (A1) and matrix metalloproteinase (M) cleavage sites. Although some keratan sulfate substitution is present in the G1 and IGD, the predominant sites of attachment are in a region (KS) immediately following the G2 region. This is followed by two extended regions of chondroitin sulfate substitution (CS1 and CS2). Four aggrecanase cleavage sites are located in the CS2 domain, of which only one is shown for convenience (A2). The aggrecan core protein is terminated with a third globular region (G3). Peptides designed for production of antibodies to detect the products of aggrecanase cleavage in the IGD (A1) followed the general principle of including the six residues bordering the cleavage site (bold font), followed by the standard linker region (normal font). For the most N-terminal cleavage site in the CS2 region (A2), redundant peptides were used in order to produce antisera that would recognize both human (first alternative) and bovine (second alternative) aggrecan cleavage products. In both cases a single peptide synthesis was carried out, and at cycle six an equimolar mixture of appropriately blocked serine and glycine or glycine and aspartic acid was used. No effort was made to purify the resulting peptides after cleavage from the resin. The new N-terminus generated by matrix metalloproteinases in the IGD (M) mostly consists of hydrophobic residues. In this case, positively charged amino acids were added to the linker region to assist solubility of the peptide.

3. To each tube add 0.7 mL of Ellman's reaction mix.
4. Read absorbance at 412 nm and plot standard curve.

3.2.2. Sulfhydryl Estimation

1. Accurately weigh 1–2 mg of peptide and dissolve in water to a final concentration of 3 mM (*see* **Note 2**).
2. Prepare a 1:10 dilution and assay as in **Subheading 3.2.1.**
3. Estimate free sulfhydryl content from standard curve.

3.3. Reduction of Sulfhydryl Groups on Peptides

3.3.1. Gel Filtration Column

1. Swell approx 10 g of Sephadex G10 in 1% acetic acid overnight and pack a 30 × 1 cm column. (Bio-Rad Econo columns are good.)
2. Equilibrate the column with 1% acetic acid at a flow rate of 1 mL/min.

3.3.2. Peptide Reduction

1. Dissolve the peptide at 2 mg/mL in 25 mM Tris-HCl, pH 7.5.
2. Add solid dithiothreitol to give a final concentration of 10 mM.
3. Purge solution for 2–3 min with nitrogen and leave at room temperature for at least 1 h.
4. Apply the reduced peptide sample to the Sephadex G10 column (*see* **Subheading 3.3.1.**), and elute with 1% acetic acid, collecting 1-mL fractions.
5. Assay the fractions for free sulfhydryl as in **Subheading 3.2.2.**
6. Pool the first peak and freeze-dry the reduced peptide.

3.4. Ovalbumin Activation and Peptide Coupling

3.4.1. Gel Filtration Column

1. Swell Sephadex G25 (medium) in water for at least 4 h. One gram of resin gives 4–6 mL of gel.
2. At room temperature, pack a 30 × 1-cm column. (Bio-Rad Econo columns are good.) This requires about 25 mL of resin. Equilibrate the column with coupling buffer using a flow rate of 2–3 mL/min.
3. After use the column should be washed with at least 2 bed vol of coupling buffer containing 0.05% sodium azide for storage. For future use, at least 2 column vol of coupling buffer should be passed through the column to remove the sodium azide.

3.4.2. Preparation of Activated Ovalbumin

1. Prepare an ice bath for use on a magnetic stirrer.
2. Weigh out 50 mg of ovalbumin into an 8-mL Wheaton vial, and add 2.25 mL of coupling buffer and a small magnetic stirring bar. Place the Wheaton vial in the ice bath and stir slowly to dissolve the ovalbumin.
3. Cool 1 mL dimethylformamide in a borosilicate tube. Make at least 0.2 mL of a 65 mg/mL solution of *N*-succinimidyl bromoacetate in the cold dimethylformamide.
4. Over the course of about 1 min add, dropwise, 0.2 mL of the *N*-succinimidyl bromoacetate solution to the dissolved ovalbumin with moderate stirring. Allow the reaction to incubate in the ice bath for 5 min. Lift the vial out of the ice bath and allow the vial to warm to room temperature over the course of 25 min.
5. Apply the solution of activated ovalbumin to the Sephadex G25 column and collect 25 1.5-mL fractions at a flow rate of about 1.5-mL/min.
6. Read the absorbance at 280 nm of 1:10 or 1:20 dilutions in water of the column fractions. The profile will consist of two peaks. The first peak is the derivatized ovalbumin.

7. Pool the major fractions of the first peak (usually two or three), making sure not to include any trace of the second peak.
8. The activated ovalbumin is best used immediately, but it can be stored for up to 1 wk at 4°C in the dark.

3.4.3. Coupling of Peptides to Activated Ovalbumin (see **Note 2**)

1. Dissolve 3 mg of the peptide for coupling in 0.4 mL of water (*see* **Note 3**) in a 4-mL Wheaton vial.
2. As a control, 0.4 mL of 6 mM cysteine (0.73 mg/mL) in water is used.
3. Add 0.4 mL of the activated ovalbumin to each peptide or the cysteine solution. Immediately purge the vials with nitrogen for about 30 s and allow the coupling to proceed at room temperature for 2 h on a rocking platform with the vials lying on their sides. Subsequently leave the vials on the rocking platform overnight at 4°C.
4. Then add 2-mercaptoethanol (1 µL) and leave the solution for 1 h to block unreacted sites on the ovalbumin.
5. Estimate the efficiency of coupling by SDS-PAGE (*see* **Subheading 3.5.**)
6. Dialyze conjugate solutions, against three changes of PBS-azide and keep at 4°C for immediate use or at –20°C for long-term storage.

3.5. Estimation of Coupling Efficiency

Before using conjugates for immunization, it is advisable to check that good peptide substitution has been obtained. Decreased mobility on SDS-PAGE relative to an ovalbumin-cysteine control conjugate represents a simple qualitative demonstration that substantial coupling has occurred (**Fig. 3**).

Although a substantial retardation on SDS-PAGE is a good indication that coupling has occurred, some conjugates that exhibit minimal retardation have produced good antibodies. Before writing off apparently failed conjugates, it can be worth checking for bound peptide by N-terminal sequencing of the conjugate. To ensure complete removal of free peptide prior to sequencing, conjugates are separated by SDS-PAGE, blotted to a PVDF membrane, and stained briefly with Coomassie blue. The target bands are excised and subjected to N-terminal sequencing. Since the N-terminus of ovalbumin is blocked (acetylated), only the sequence of the peptide should be observed. A rough estimate of the amount of peptide bound can be made from the yield of several cycles. In the case of peptides coupled through an N-terminal cysteine residue, the first cycle will be blank, but subsequent cycles give a good representation of the expected signal.

3.5.1. Mobility Shift on SDS-PAGE

1. Prepare 10% SDS-PAGE gels (*11*).
2. Run 5 µL of peptide and cysteine conjugate solutions.
3. Stain with Coomassie blue (*12*). Compare mobility of peptide conjugates relative to that to of the cysteine-ovalbumin control.

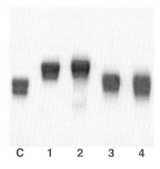

Fig. 3. Evaluation of coupling efficiency by SDS-PAGE. Activated ovalbumin was coupled to cysteine (C, control) and to four different peptides (1–4). A clear shift in mobility was seen for peptides 1 and 2 indicating extensive derivatization. In the case of peptides 3 and 4 little difference in mobility was seen relative to the cysteine control, although a slight difference in the appearance of the bands is discernable. In such instances more detailed analysis of the putative conjugates is in order, for example by N-terminal sequencing, to determine whether any peptide is coupled. In these particular examples enough peptide was in fact present to yield useful antisera. However, in most cases where the migration pattern of the reacted ovalbumin closely resembles the cysteine control, failure of coupling should be suspected.

3.6. Antibody Production

Although immunization of one rabbit per conjugate can be successful, it is often wise to use several animals to increase the odds of producing an antibody with the required properties.

3.6.1. Immunization

1. Obtain a preimmune bleed (5 mL) from each rabbit to be used as control serum later.
2. In a 1.5-mL Eppendorf tube, add peptide conjugate and enough PBS to result in 0.75 mg of peptide conjugate in 0.375 mL. Add 0.375 mL of Freund's complete adjuvant. Cap the tube and agitate violently on a vortex mixer to produce a stiff emulsion. It should be possible to draw enough emulsion into a syringe to inject the rabbit intramuscularly on each flank with 0.25 mL of emulsion (total 0.5 mg of antigen).
3. After 2 wk, boost the rabbits with a similar mixture produced using Freund's incomplete adjuvant.
4. After a further 10 d, take a test bleed and assess the antigenic response. If this is judged to be adequate, bleed out the animal. (Up to 150 mL of blood should obtainable.) The use of 50 mL non-anticoagulant centrifuge tubes is recommended. Allow the blood to clot and store at 4°C overnight to allow the clot to

contract. Remove the serum and centrifuge at low speed to remove any contaminating red blood cells. Store serum frozen in aliquots.
5. Alternatively, if the antigenic response is not adequate administer, a second boost with emulsion containing Freund's incomplete adjuvant and bleed out the animal after a further 10 d.

3.7. Antibody Characterization

The antigenic response of the different rabbits can be determined by direct enzyme-linked immunosorbent assay (ELISA) using adsorbed peptide. Neoepitope specificity can be demonstrated by competitive ELISA, using peptides representing truncated or extended versions of the true epitope. Lack of reaction to a peptide spanning the cleavage site is also a good demonstration of specificity *(13)*. However, it is critical that reactivity of the antibody with the authentic protein cleavage site epitope also be demonstrated, as the same antibodies may react well with the immunizing peptide but not with the native protein (*see* **Subheading 3.9.**).

3.7.1. Direct ELISA

1. Coat ELISA plate wells with 50 ng of peptide in 50 µL of 0.01 M sodium bicarbonate, pH 9.6, overnight at 4°C.
2. Wash wells with PBS-T.
3. Block wells for 1 h at room temperature with 100 µL of blocking buffer.
4. Add serial antiserum dilutions (50 µL) from 1:10 to 1:100,000 in blocking buffer and incubate at 37°C for 60 min.
5. Wash wells with PBS-T.
6. Add 50 µL of alkaline phosphatase-conjugated goat anti-rabbit IgG (1:1000 dilution) and incubate at 37°C for 60 min.
7. Wash wells with PBS-T.
8. Add 50 µL of alkaline phosphatase substrate and allow color to develop for 15 min at 37°C.
9. Read absorbance at 405 nm on a plate reader.

3.7.2. Competitive ELISA to Demonstrate Neoepitope Specificity

1. Coat plates and block wells as in **steps 1–3** in **Subheading 3.7.1.**
2. Use a constant dilution of antiserum (previously demonstrated to give 50% of maximum binding) and make serial dilutions of competing peptide ranging from 25 to 150,000 ng/mL in this antibody dilution. Incubate for 1 h at room temperature.
3. Add the antibody/peptide complexes to the wells.
4. Develop as in **steps 5–9** in **Subheading 3.7.1.**
5. Plot results and calculate the mean inhiting concentration (IC_{50}) value for inhibition (**Fig. 4**).

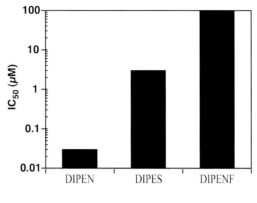

Competing Peptide

Fig. 4. Competitive ELISA analysis to demonstrate antibody selectivity. An antibody to the matrix metalloproteinase cleavage epitope ...DIPEN was produced as described in this chapter. Its specificity was investigated by competitive ELISA using CGGVDIPEN as the bound peptide. When used as a competitive antigen, this sequence gave a median inhibitory concentration (IC_{50}) of 0.03 μM. In contrast, extension of the epitope by one residue to ..DIPENF resulted in a greater than three orders of magnitude increase in IC_{50}, indicating the specificity of the antibody for the terminal epitope. In contrast, when the homologous cleavage sequence for bovine aggrecan ..DIPES was used, the IC_{50} was 3 μM, indicating that some flexibility can be tolerated, albeit at decreased reactivity.

3.7.3. Western Blotting of Authentic Protein Cleavage Product

1. Run samples of tissue extract or in vitro digest on SDS-PAGE as duplicate sets.
2. Electroblot onto nitrocellulose or PVDF membranes *(14)*.
3. Block the membrane in blocking solution for 1 h.
4. Wash membrane in TBS-T.
5. Cut membrane into separate sample sets.
6. Dilute anti-neoepitope antibody in blocking solution (1:500 is usually a good dilution) and incubate with one membrane for 1 h at room temperature.
7. To determine antibody specificity, repeat **step 6** on the membrane from the duplicate sample set using a 1:500 dilution of antibody containing 1 mg of epitope peptide for every mL of serum (2 μg/mL peptide in a 1:500 serum dilution). This mixture should be left for 1 h before use.
8. Wash membranes in TBS-T.
9. Incubate membranes in alkaline phosphatase-conjugated goat anti-rabbit immunoglobulin 1:7500 in blocking solution for 30 min at room temperature.
10. Wash the membranes in TBS-T.
11. Add alkaline phosphatase blot development solution and allow bands to develop.
12. Wash blots with water.

3.8. Affinity Purification

To reduce background staining, it is often advisable to purify the antineo-epitope antibodies by affinity chromatography on a resin containing the peptide used for immunization.

3.8.1. Affinity Column Preparation

1. Allow the Sulfolink gel to equilibrate to room temperature.
2. Pack a 10-mL disposable column with 1.5 mL of gel slurry.
3. Equilibrate the column with 10 mL of affinity column equilibration buffer and allow excess buffer to drain. Close the end of the column.
4. Add 1.5 mL of 2 mg/mL peptide in water to the gel. Cap the column and mix by inverting frequently over the course of 15 min. Leave at room temperature for a further 30 min.
5. Drain and wash the column with 5 mL of equilibration buffer.
6. To block unreacted sites on the resin, add 1.5 mL of 50 mM cysteine in equilibration buffer and mix as above.
7. Drain and wash the column with equilibration buffer.
8. After use, the column should be washed with 20 mL of 1 M NaCl and then stored in water containing 0.05% sodium azide at 4°C.

3.8.2. Affinity Purification

1. Equilibrate appropriate Sulfolink column with affinity column equilibration buffer.
2. Centrifuge serum (10 mL) at medium speed to remove any particulates and apply clarified serum to column.
3. Collect the flowthrough of the serum. (This may still contain useful antibody.)
4. Wash column with 25 mL of PBS-azide.
5. Apply 15 mL of 0.1 M glycine, pH 2.8, and collect 1 mL fractions into tubes containing 50 µL of 1 M Tris-HCl, pH 9.5, to neutralize the eluted immunoglobulin.
6. Read the absorbance of the fractions at 280 nm.
7. Dialyze the peak fractions against PBS overnight at 4°C.
8. Wash the column for storage as described in **Subheading 3.7.1.**

3.9. Pitfalls

The generation of antipeptide anti-neoepitope antibodies has several potential limitations that may interfere with their use for the analysis of physiologically and pathologically relevant protein products.

1. The epitope may not be readily accessible to the antibody owing to steric blocking by an adjacent protein substituent such as a glycosaminoglycan chain of aggrecan (**Fig. 2**). This can be overcome by chondroitinase treatment.

2. The amino acids within the epitope may themselves be amenable to post-translational modification. Such a scenario occurs within the carboxy-terminal neoepitope generated by aggrecanases in the IGD. Here asparagine and threonine residues in the sequence ...NITEGE may act as sites for *N*-linked and *O*-linked glycosylation, respectively. Glycosylation of these residues can decrease neoepitope antibody affinity for the authentic protein product *(10)*.

3. These limitations can make even semiquantitation of neoepitope abundance by visualization of antibody reaction products misleading.

4. Notes

1. An additional strategy is to substitute β-alanine for the glycine residues in the spacer region. This allows the peptide content of the final conjugate to be determined by amino acid analysis.

2. It is useful to include a peptide that from previous experience is known to couple well, as a positive control.

3. Given the diversity of possible amino acid sequences, solubility problems can be encountered with some peptides. In our experience, most peptides dissolve in water. Acidic peptides that have not been provided with a basic linker region can be rendered soluble by the addition of an organic base such as *N*-ethylmorpholine. We have also had success with dissolving peptides in dimethylformamide or dimethylsulfoxide so that the final concentration of organic solvent in the coupling reaction is no more than 20 or 50%, respectively.

Acknowledgments

This work was supported by the Shriners of North America, the Canadian Institutes of Health Research, and the Arthritis Society of Canada.

References

1. Lee, E. R., Lamplugh, L., Leblond, C. P., Mordier, S., Magny, M.-C., and Mort, J. S. (1998) Immunolocalization of the cleavage of the aggrecan core protein at the Asn^{341}-Phe^{342} bond, as an indicator of the location of the metalloproteinases active in the lysis of the rat growth plate. *Anat. Rec.* **252,** 117–132.

2. Lark, M. W., Bayne, E. K., Flanagan, J., et al. (1997) Aggrecan degradation in human cartilage. Evidence for both matrix metalloproteinase and aggrecanase activity in normal, osteoarthritic, and rheumatoid joints. *J. Clin. Invest.* **100,** 93–106.

3. Mort, J. S., Flannery, C. R., Makkerh, J., Krupa, J. C., and Lee, E. R. (2003) The use of anti-neoepitope antibodies for the analysis of degradative events in cartilage and the molecular basis for neoepitope specificity. *Biochem. Soc. Symp.* **70,** 107–114.

4. Mort, J. S. and Buttle, D. J. (1999) The use of cleavage site specific antibodies to delineate protein processing and breakdown pathways. *J. Clin. Pathol. Mol. Pathol.* **52,** 11–18.

5. Hughes, C. E., Caterson, B., White, R. J., Roughley, P. J., and Mort, J. S. (1992) Monoclonal antibodies recognizing protease-generated neoepitopes from cartilage proteoglycan degradation: application to studies of human link protein cleaved by stromelysin. *J. Biol. Chem.* **267,** 16,011–16,014.

6. Hughes, C. E., Caterson, B., Fosang, A. J., Roughley, P. J., and Mort, J. S. (1995) Monoclonal antibodies that specifically recognize neoepitope sequences generated by 'aggrecanase' and matrix metalloproteinase cleavage of aggrecan: application to catabolism in situ and in vitro. *Biochem. J.* **305,** 799–804.

7. Fosang, A. J., Last, K., Gardiner, P., Jackson, D. C., and Brown, L. (1995) Development of a cleavage-site-specific monoclonal antibody for detecting metalloproteinase-derived aggrecan fragments: detection of fragments in human synovial fluid. *Biochem. J.* **310,** 337–343.

8. Ellman, G. L. (1959) Tissue sulfhydryl groups. *Arch. Biochem. Biophys.* **82,** 70–77.

9. Bernatowicz, M. S. and Matsueda, G. R. (1986) Preparation of peptide-protein immunogens using N-succinimidyl bromoacetate as a heterobifunctional crosslinking reagent. *Anal. Biochem.* **155,** 95–102.

10. Sztrolovics, R., White, R. J., Roughley, P. J., and Mort, J. S. (2002) The mechanism of aggrecan release from cartilage differs with tissue origin and the agent used to stimulate catabolism. *Biochem. J.* **362,** 465–472.

11. Gallagher, S. R. (1995) One-dimensional SDS gel electrophoresis of proteins, in *Current Protocols in Protein Science* (Coligan, J. E., Dunn, B. M., Ploegh, H. L., Speicher, D. W., and Wingfield, P. T., eds.), John Wiley & Sons, New York, NY, pp. 10.1.1–10.1.34.

12. DeSilva, T. M., Ursitti, J. A., and Speicher, D. W. (1995) Protein detection in gels using fixation, in *Current Protocols in Protein Science* (Coligan, J. E., Dunn, B. M., Ploegh, H. L., Speicher, D. W., and Wingfield, P. T., eds.), John Wiley & Sons, New York, NY, pp. 10.5.1–10.5.12.

13. Mort, J. S., Magny, M.-C., and Lee, E. R. (1998) Cathepsin B: an alternative protease for the generation of an aggrecan "metalloproteinase" cleavage neoepitope. *Biochem. J.* **335,** 491–494.

14. Ursitti, J. A., Mozdzanowsli, J., and Speicher, D. W. (1995) Electroblotting from polyacrylamide gels, in *Current Protocols in Protein Science* (Coligan, J. E., Dunn, B. M., Ploegh, H. L., Speicher, D. W., and Wingfield, P. T., eds.), John Wiley & Sons, New York, NY, pp. 10.7.1–10.7.14.

18

Immunoassays for Collagens in Chondrocyte and Cartilage Explant Cultures

R. Clark Billinghurst, Fackson Mwale,
Anthony Hollander, Mirela Ionescu, and A. Robin Poole

Summary

Quantitative immunoassays have been developed to measure the content, degradation, and synthesis of types II and IX collagens in hyaline cartilages. Some of these assays and their applications are described in this chapter. These and other assays are commercially available. The applications of these assays are discussed with examples from recent publications.

Key Words: Cartilage; type II collagen; type IX collagen; immunoassay; degradation; collagenase.

1. Introduction

Type II collagen is the major structural component of articular cartilage and provides this tissue with its tensile strength. It exists as fibrils of crosslinked helical molecules composed of three identical α chains of approx 1000 amino acids each, with nonhelical extensions called telopeptides at both ends of each chain. During turnover in health and osteoarthritis, after these fibrils are depolymerized they are degraded (at neutral pH) by the proteolytic attack of enzymes called mammalian collagenases at a specific locus within the native triple-helical structure of each collagen molecule. These collagenases belong to the matrix metalloproteinase (MMP) enzyme family and include MMP-1 (collagenase-1 or fibroblast/interstitial collagenase), MMP-8 (collagenase-2 or neutrophil collagenase), and MMP-13 (collagenase-3). All three, in addition to a membrane-type MMP (MT-MMP) designated MT1-MMP (MMP-14), cleave the type II collagen molecules to yield characteristic 3/4 (TC[A]) and 1/4 (TC[B]) fragments.

From: *Methods in Molecular Medicine, Vol. 100: Cartilage and Osteoarthritis, Vol. 1: Cellular and Molecular Tools*
Edited by: M. Sabatini, P. Pastoureau, and F. De Ceuninck © Humana Press Inc., Totowa, NJ

The newly created carboxy (C) and amino (N) termini of the 3/4 and 1/4 fragments, respectively, represent neoepitopes that allow the specific identification of collagenase-cleaved triple helical type II collagen molecules. Cleavage site neoepitopes have proved valuable in defining MMP activity in aggrecan degradation (*see also* Chap 17). This chapter describes the procedures used to develop an antibody and immunoassay for the detection and quantitation of type II collagen bearing the C-terminal neoepitope of the 3/4 α-chain fragment created by cleavage by collagenases. This will include the production and characterization of C1, 2C (formerly called COL2-3/4Cshort), a polyclonal antibody that recognizes collagenase-cleaved fragments of type I and II collagens *(1)*. A monoclonal antibody, C2C (formerly called COL2-3/4C$_{\text{long mono}}$) has also been developed to identify specifically collagenase-generated fragments of type II collagen. Immunoassays utilizing these antibodies are commercially available (www.ibex.ca; IBEX Technologies, Montreal, Quebec, Canada).

After helical cleavage, there is spontaneous denaturation (unwinding) of the α-chains, which are susceptible to further degradation by gelatinolytic proteinases, such as MMP-2 (gelatinase A) and MMP-9 (gelatinase B). A specific assay has been developed that recognizes a linear amino acid sequence from the type II collagen α-chain (CB11B), which is "hidden" within the intact helical structure but becomes exposed upon cleavage and denaturation of the triple helical collagen molecule *(2)*. The monoclonal antibody COL2-3/4m recognizes this hidden epitope in denatured type II collagen and not the native molecule. Sequential extraction of cartilage using α-chymotrypsin and proteinase K, combined with assay of the extracts by an inhibition enzyme-linked immunosorbent assay (ELISA) using the antibody COL2-3/4m, is a reliable method for assessing the proportion of denatured type II collagen in cartilage and total type II collagen content. The COL2-3/4m assay for type II collagen content and denaturation is also described in this chapter. An immunoassay is also available (CPII; IBEX) for quantitating the levels of the C-terminal propeptide of type II collagen that is cleaved from the procollagen molecule with fibrillogenesis and is thus an indicator of type II collagen synthesis. This ELISA assay was developed from the radioimmunoassay we described previously *(3)*.

The fibrillar organization of the extracellular matrix of articular cartilage involves the assembly of collagen fibrils that contain not only type II collagen but also types IX and XI collagens. Type IX collagen is a heterotrimer composed of three genetically distinct chains designated α1(IX), α2(IX), and α3(IX), forming three triple-helical domains (COL1, COL2, and COL3) alternating with noncollagenous domains (NC1, NC2, NC3, and NC4). Type IX molecules are organized in a periodic manner on the fibril surface. The α1-chain has an N-terminal extension whereby the NC4 domain of the α1 (IX) chain extends from the fibril surface into the perifibrillar space. Type IX collagen is covalently crosslinked to type II collagen in an antiparallel orientation and may also be crosslinked to other type IX collagen molecules. The amino-terminal NC4 domain is very basic. Some forms of type IX collagen may lack the NC4 domain because of the use of an alternative promoter, and the expression of this variant is thought to be tissue-specific and developmentally regulated. This chapter describes the procedures used to develop four ELISA immunoassays utilizing antibodies to the NC4 and COL2 domains of the $\alpha 1(IX)$ chain and to denatured type II collagen (COL2-3/4m) and collagenase cleaved (C1, 2C) types I and II collagens (4). This includes the validation and experimental use of the immunoassays.

2. Materials

2.1. Polyclonal Antibody Production

2.1.1. Preparation of the Immunogens

1. 0.1 M Phosphate buffer: 5.28 g/L KH_2PO_4, 16.4 g/L $Na_2HPO_4 \cdot 7H_2O$, 0.372 g/L ethylenediaminetetraacetic acid (EDTA)-Na_2, 0.2 g/L NaN_3, pH 7.0.
2. Ovalbumin (OVA): 25 mg of grade V chicken egg albumin/mL of 0.1 M phosphate buffer.
3. Coupling reagent: 56.5 mg N-hydroxy-succinimidylbromoacetate/mL of chilled N,N-dimethylformamide (Sigma).
4. Azide-free phosphate-buffered saline (PBS): 1.61 g/L $Na_2HPO_4 \cdot 7H_2O$, 8.5 g/L NaCl, 0.55 g/L KH_2PO_4.
5. Sephadex G-25 column (Amersham; 27 × 2.2 cm) with 103 mL bed volume.
6. Synthetic peptide: 5 mg/100 µL of 0.1 M phosphate buffer.
7. Ultraviolet (UV) spectrophotometer and quartz cuvets.

2.1.2. Immunization

1. Peptide-OVA conjugate prepared in **Subheading 3.1.1.**
2. Azide-free PBS.
3. 5-mL Glass syringe and 20-gage needle.
4. Complete and incomplete Freund's adjuvant (Difco).
5. Two female New Zealand white rabbits weighing 2.5–3.0 kg each.

2.1.3. Antibody Purification

1. Saturated ammonium sulfate solution: 761 g/L $(NH_4)_2SO_4$, pH 7.0.
2. PBS: azide-free PBS + 0.5 g/L NaN_3.
3. 0.8 M Sodium acetate buffer: 65.6 g/L $C_2H_3O_2Na$, 4.0 g/L NaN_3, pH 4.0.
4. 2% (w/w) Pepsin: 20 mg 2X crystallized pepsin A (Worthington Biochemical)/g IgG.
5. 0.14 M Phosphate buffer: 1.05 g/L KH_2PO_4, 35.5 g/L $Na_2HPO_4 \cdot 7H_2O$, 0.5 g/L NaN_3, pH 8.0.
6. Econo-Pac 10DG columns packed with Bio-Gel P-6 desalting gel (Bio-Rad).

7. HiTrap affinity column with 5 mL Protein A Sepharose High Performance gel (Amersham).
8. Tris buffers: 121.1 g/L for 1 M, 12.1 g/L for 100 mM, and 1.21 g/L for 10 mM of Tris(hydroxymethyl)aminomethane, pH 8.0.
9. 100 mM Glycine-HCl: 7.51 g/L, pH 3.0.
10. SulfoLink coupling gel and column (Pierce).
11. Coupling buffer: 50 mM Tris-HCl (6.06 g/L), 5 mM EDTA-Na$_2$ (1.86 g/L), pH 8.5.
12. Blocking reagent: 50 mM L-cysteine (6.1 g/L) in coupling buffer.
13. Washing solution: 58.44 g/L NaCl (1 M).
14. Dialysis tubing (molecular weight cutoff: 12–14,000).
15. UV spectrophotometer and quartz cuvets.

2.1.4. Antibody Characterization

1. 0.1 M Carbonate buffer: add 200 mL of 0.1 M Na$_2$CO$_3$ (10.6 g/L) to 0.1 M NaHCO$_3$ (8.4 g/L) until pH = 9.2.
2. PBS-Tween: PBS + 0.1% (v/v) polyoxyethylenesorbitan monolaurate (Tween-20).
3. PBS-bovine serum albumin (BSA): PBS+1% (w/v) radioimmunoassay grade BSA.
4. PBS-BSA-Tween: PBS + BSA + 0.1% (v/v) Tween-20.
5. High-binding, irradiated polystyrene, 96-well flat-bottomed, microtiter plates (Immulon 2 HB; Dynex).
6. Polystyrene, 96-well U-bottomed, microtiter plates (Dynex).
7. Photometric microplate reader with 405- and 490-nm filters and software to determine concentrations of unknowns from standard curves.
8. Secondary antibody: alkaline phosphatase-conjugated goat anti-rabbit IgG (F[ab']$_2$ fragment of goat antibody).
9. Freshly prepared substrate solution: 0.5 mg/mL disodium p-nitrophenyl phosphate (104 phosphatase substrate, 5-mg tablet; Sigma) in 10 mL of 1.0 M diethanolamine buffer (containing 24.5 mg MgCl$_2$ in 500 mL dH$_2$O, pH to 9.8). Store at room temperature in amber bottle.
10. ELISA amplification system (Gibco BRL).
11. Peptides synthesized as described in **Subheading 3.1.4.** with residues added to (+1, +2, +3), deleted from (−1, −2, −3), and bridging the cleavage site terminus of the immunizing C1, 2C peptide. For the NC4 and COL2 antibody characterizations, the NC4 and COL2 synthetic peptides are used.
12. Native, heat-denatured, and collagenase-cleaved types I, II, and III collagen from species of choice for the COL2-3/4m and C1, 2C antibodies (*see* **Note 1**). Purified native type IX collagen and NC4 domain for the COL2 and NC4 antibodies (*see* **Note 2**).

2.2. Immunoassays

2.2.1. Preparation of the Coating Peptides
for the C1, 2C, COL2, and NC4 Immunoassays

1. 0.1 M Phosphate buffer: 5.28 g/L KH$_2$PO$_4$, 16.4 g/L Na$_2$HPO$_4$ · 7H$_2$O, 0.372 g/L EDTA-Na$_2$, 0.2 g/L NaN$_3$, pH 7.0.

2. Keyhole limpet hemocyanin (KLH): 20 mg (Pierce) reconstituted with 2 mL of distilled water (dH$_2$O).
3. Coupling reagent: 56.5 mg N-hydroxy-succinimidylbromoacetate/mL of chilled N,N-dimethylformamide (Sigma).
4. Tris-buffered saline (TBS): 8.78 g/L NaCl, 6.06 g/L Tris-HCl, pH 7.5.
5. Sephadex G-25 column (27 × 2.2 cm) with 103 mL bed volume.
6. C1, 2C (formerly COL2-3/4C$_{Short}$) synthetic peptide (CGP P$_{OH}$ GPQG), COL2 (CGDTGPGVDGRDGY) synthetic peptide containing glycine spacer and N-terminal cysteine and NC4 (CRRPRFPVNSNSNGGNEY) synthetic peptide: used at 5 mg/100 µL of 0.1 M phosphate buffer.
7. Coating peptides for C1, 2C, and COL2 assays as described in **Subheading 3.2.1.** and diluted in TBS, pH 7.5.
8. UV spectrophotometer and quartz cuvets.

2.2.2. Preparation of the Coated Microtiter Plates

1. High-binding, irradiated, polystyrene, 96-well flat-bottomed, microtiter plates (Immulon 2 HB; Dynex).
   For the COL2-3/4m assay, heat-denatured type II collagen (HDC) is prepared immediately before use. Dissolve native bovine type II collagen (Sigma) in carbonate buffer (pH 9.2) to a final concentration of 1 mg/mL in a screw-capped 1.5-mL centrifuge tube. At this concentration it will be partly in suspension. Place the tube in a water bath at 80°C for 20 min, but remove it for brief periods of mixing over the first 2 min, to ensure complete dissolution of the collagen. Dilute the HDC in carbonate buffer to a final concentration of 40 µg/mL.
2. Carbonate buffer: 1 L of 0.1 M NaHCO$_3$ and 200 mL of 0.1 M Na$_2$CO$_3$. Gradually add the Na$_2$CO$_3$ to the NaHCO$_3$, with mixing, until the pH is 9.2.
3. TBS: 8.78 g/L NaCl, 6.06 g/L Tris-HCl, pH 7.5.
4. TBS-Tween: TBS + 0.1% (v/v) polyoxyethylenesorbitan monolaurate (Tween-20).
5. TBS-BSA: TBS + 1% (w/v) radioimmunoassay (RIA) grade BSA.

2.2.3. Assaying Samples

2.2.3.1. THE C1, 2C, COL2, AND NC4 ELISAS

1. C2C (for C1, 2C assay), COL2, or NC4 peptides.
2. TBS: 8.78 g/L NaCl, 6.06 g/L Tris-HCl, pH 7.5.
3. TBS-Tween: TBS + 0.1% (v/v) Tween-20.
4. TBS-BSA: TBS + 1% (w/v) RIA grade BSA.
5. TBS-BSA-Tween: TBS + 1% (w/v) BSA + 0.1% (v/v) Tween-20.
6. Polypropylene 96-well U-bottomed microtiter plates (Costar).
7. Affinity-purified C1, 2C, COL2, or NC4 antibodies: as prepared in **Subheading 3.1.3.**
8. Secondary antibody: alkaline phosphatase-conjugated goat anti-rabbit IgG (F[ab']$_2$ fragment of goat antibody; Sigma).

9. ELISA amplification system (Gibco-BRL).
10. Photometric microplate reader with 490-nm filter and software to determine concentrations of unknowns from standard curves.
11. Stop solution: 0.3 M H_2SO_4 (1 mL concentrated H_2SO_4 slowly added to 59 mL of dH_2O).

2.2.3.2. THE COL2-3/4M ELISA

1. Tris(hydroxymethyl)aminomethane (Tris): prepare a stock solution at 50 mM, including NaN_3, to a final concentration of 0.05% (w/v) and adjust the pH to 7.6 with HCl.
2. PBS: prepare a stock solution of 0.85% (w/v) NaCl, 0.16% (w/v) Na_2HPO_4, 0.054% (w/v) KH_2PO_4 and 0.05% (w/v) NaN_3. Adjust the pH to 7.4.
3. BSA: prepare a stock solution of 1% (w/v) BSA in PBS and store at 4°C.
4. PBS/Tween: add Tween-20 (Sigma) to PBS to a final concentration of 0.1% (v/v).
5. Polypropylene 96-well U-bottomed microtiter plates (Costar).
6. Antibody COL2-3/4m.
7. Peptide CB11B: GKVGPSGA P_{OH} GEDGR P_{OH} GP P_{OH} GPQ.
8. Second antibody: goat anti-mouse IgG labeled with alkaline phosphatase (available from many sources).
9. Freshly prepared substrate solution: 0.5 mg/mL disodium *p*-nitrophenyl phosphate (104 phosphatase substrate, 5-mg tablet; Sigma in 10 mL of 1.0 M diethanolamine buffer (containing 24.5 mg $MgCl_2$ in 500 mL dH_2O, pH to 9.8)). Store at room temperature in amber bottle.
10. Photometric microplate reader with 405-nm filter and software to determine concentrations of unknowns from standard curves.

2.2.4. Assay Validation

All reagents as listed in **Subheading 2.1.4.**

2.2.5. Experimental Requirements for the C1, 2C, COL2-3/4m, NC4, and COL2 ELISAs

1. Chymotrypsin digestion solution: 50 mg type VII α-chymotrypsin (Sigma) in 49.25 mL of 50 mM Tris-HCl (6.06 g/L, pH 7.6), plus the general metallo-, cysteine, and aspartic protease inhibitors added as 250 µL EDTA (76 mg/mL dH_2O), 250 µL iodoacetamide (37 mg/mL dH_2O), and 250 µL pepstatin A (2 mg/mL in 95% ethanol), respectively.
2. Proteinase K digestion solution: 50 mg proteinase K (Sigma) plus 250 µL of each of the protease inhibitors in the chymotrypsin digestion solution, made up to 50 mL with 50 mM Tris-HCl, pH 7.6.
3. TPCK (irreversible chymotrypsin inhibitor): 8 mg *N*-tosyl-L-phenylalanine-chloromethyl ketone (Sigma) in 800 µL of 95% ethanol added dropwise to 19.2 mL of 50 mM Tris-HCl, pH 7.6.

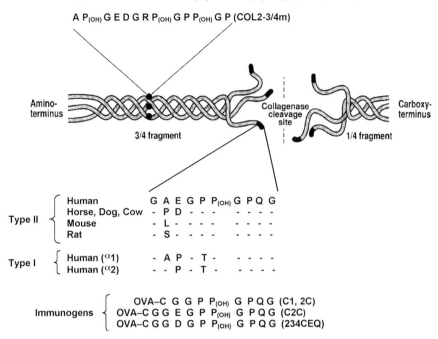

Fig. 1. Location of cleavage-site neoepitope (C1, 2C) and the hidden denaturation epitope (COL2-3/4m) in triple-helical type II collagen. Shown above the collagen molecule is the immunogen (CB11B) that was used to generate the COL2-3/4m monoclonal antibody, and below that is the 13-amino acid peptide it specifically recognizes (COL2-3/4m). Below the collagen molecule are the aligned amino acid sequences of the C termini of the collagenase-generated 3/4 α1-chain fragments of type II collagen from various species and the collagenase-generated 3/4 α_1 and α_2 fragments of human type I collagen. A dash indicates an identical amino acid to that similarly located in the human α_1(II) sequence. The peptide sequences used as immunogens for production of the C1, 2C (formerly COL2-3/4C$_{short}$), C2C, and 234CEQ antineoepitope antibodies are also shown.

3. Methods

3.1. Polyclonal Antibody Production

3.1.1. Preparation of the Immunogens

The amino acid sequence, GPP$_{(OH)}$GPQG used for the synthesis of the neoepitope peptide C1, 2C (formerly COL2-3/4C$_{short}$), which corresponds to the C-terminus of the 3/4 (TC^A) fragment of the α1-chains of collagenase-cleaved triple-helical type II collagen, was based on the published amino acid sequence for the primary MMP-1 cleavage site in human type II collagen (**Fig. 1**).

The five C-terminal amino acids in this peptide are identical to the five amino acids at the C termini of collagenase-cleaved α_1 and α_2-chain 3/4 fragments of type I collagen accounting for the crossreactivity of an antibody produced to the C1, 2C peptide for both collagenase-cleaved type I and II collagens. In an attempt to produce an antibody specific to type II collagen, a longer peptide, **GAEGPP**$_{(OH)}$GPQG, was synthesized that incorporated the three amino acids of human type II collagen (in bold) that were N-terminal to the C1, 2C peptide and designated C2C (formerly COL2-3/4C$_{long}$). It is in this region of the collagen molecule that significant differences exist between the α-chains of the different collagen types, as well as between species for type II collagen (**Fig. 1**). This latter feature was utilized in the production of the 234CEQ antibody: the peptide, GPDGPP$_{(OH)}$GPQG was synthesized to create an antibody that recognized collagenase-created 3/4 fragments of type II collagen in dogs and horses *(5)*. The assignment of the third residue in these synthetic peptides as a hydroxylated proline, P$_{(OH)}$, is based on the assumption that the prolines in the Y-position of the repeating Gly-X-Y triplets in collagen α-chains are potential hydroxylation sites.

For synthesis of the NC4 and COL2 immunogenic peptides, we chose sequences from within the noncollagenous NC4 domain so that we could monitor the long form of type IX collagen and the collagenous COL2 domain for total type IX collagen *(4)*. The cDNA sequences of two distinct forms of the human $\alpha1(IX)$ collagen chain are known. The type IX collagen COL2 domain sequence GDTGPGVDGRDG and that for the NC4 domain RRPRFPVNSNSNGGNE were identified as specific for type IX collagen by reference to the SWISS-PROT protein sequence database, using MacMolly Tetra software (Soft Gene, Berlin, FRG).

For the production of the COL2-3/4m monoclonal antibody, a peptide was identified as a hydrophilic domain within the immunogenic cyanogen bromide peptide 11 (CB11) of the $\alpha1(II)$ chain that satisfied additional criteria as a suitable immunogen *(2)*. The 21-amino acid sequence GKVGPSGAP$_{(OH)}$GEDGRP$_{(OH)}$GPP$_{(OH)}$GPQ (CB11B peptide) was synthesized for the immunization of mice (**Fig. 1**).

All peptides were synthesized at a 0.25-mmol scale, using standard Fmoc (9-fluoroenylmethoxycarbonyl) chemistry, on a solid-phase peptide synthesizer. Crude peptides were purified by reverse phase chromatography. A cysteine was added to the *N* termini of the peptides for conjugation to the carrier proteins OVA, BSA, and KLH. These proteins are commonly used in hapten-protein conjugates to improve the immunogenicity of the hapten. A tyrosine was added to the carboxy terminus of the peptide for iodination, if required. The procedure for conjugation to OVA is as follows:

1. Slowly add (dropwise) 0.2 mL of the coupling reagent to 2.0 mL of chilled OVA, with stirring, and then warm to 25°C over 30 min.

2. Centrifuge the sample and apply to a previously washed (50 mL of 0.1 *M* phosphate buffer, pH 7.0) Sephadex G-25 column, eluting with phosphate buffer at 1 mL/min and collecting 2-mL fractions.
3. Measure the absorbance at 280 nm in 1-cm quartz cuvets of each fraction, pool those containing the protein peak, and measure the absorbency of the pooled sample.
4. Determine the OVA concentration in mg/mL by dividing the absorbency value by 1.2 (the extinction coefficient of OVA at 1 mg/mL), and adjust OVA to 2–3 mg/mL.
5. Add 4 mg of the activated OVA (about 1.5 mL) to 5 mg of the synthetic peptide solution (100 µL) and leave at 25°C for 2 h, with occasional mixing, before transferring to 4°C overnight.
6. Dialyze against 1 L of phosphate buffer (pH 7.0), with three changes over 24 h, and then against 1 L azide-free PBS with one change over 24 h. Aliquot at 300 µL and store at –20°C.
7. Confirm effective incorporation by applying coupled OVA-peptide to one lane and activated OVA to another lane of a 10% sodium dodecyl sulfate-polyacrylamide gel electrophoresis (SDS-PAGE) gel and by showing a decrease in electrophoretic mobility of the OVA-peptide conjugate on SDS-PAGE relative to the activated OVA.

3.1.2. Immunization

The particular strain or breed of an animal species may affect the affinity or specificity of the antibodies produced in that animal. Young (but skeletally mature), disease-free, female rabbits are the principal source for raising polyclonal antibodies in the research laboratory. Polyclonals are easily raised against most antigens and haptens. Young (6–8 wk-old), disease-free, female Balb/C mice are the principal source of antibody-secreting B cells for producing monoclonal antibodies in the research laboratory. Monoclonal antibodies are generally produced after a successfully characterized polyclonal antibody has been identified, and this chapter will not describe the extensive procedures for monoclonal antibody production. Thus, the following is the protocol for raising C1, 2C (formerly COL2-3/4C$_{short}$), NC4, and COL2 polyclonal antibodies:

1. Thaw out one 300-µL aliquot of peptide-OVA conjugate, add 600 µL of azide-free PBS and mix (~1 mg conjugate/mL).
2. Take up the peptide-OVA conjugate into a glass syringe and emulsify in 900 µL of complete Freund's adjuvant (CFA) by forcing through a 20-gage needle several times until a drop of emulsion retains its shape when added to the surface of a beaker of water (final concentration ~0.5 mg/mL).
3. Inject two rabbits intramuscularly (in both hind limbs) with 0.5 mL of emulsion (~ 200 mg of conjugate) divided between two different sites.
4. Give booster injections of similar quantities of peptide-OVA emulsified with incomplete Freund's adjuvant (IFA) intramuscularly every 3–4 wk.

exception that the absorbance of the pooled fractions with the activated BSA is divided by 0.7 (the extinction coefficient at 1 mg/mL) to determine the BSA concentration.

2. For the coating of the NC4 and COL2 immunoassay plates, peptides are used that include a N-terminal cysteine.

3. For the coating of the COL2-3/4m immunoassay plates, HDC is used.

4. Dilute the assay peptide (C2C-BSA conjugate, NC4 or COL2) to 20 µg/mL or the HDC (COL2-3/4m assay) to 40 µg/mL in 0.1 M carbonate buffer (pH 9.2), to promote noncovalent adsorption of the conjugate, and add 50 µL to each well of Immulon-2, 96-well flat-bottomed microtiter plates.

5. After overnight incubation at 4°C, wash the plates three times with PBS-Tween, block the noncoated binding sites with 150 µL/well of PBS-BSA for 30 min at room temperature and then wash once with PBS-Tween. Plates can then be stored, covered with plastic wrap, for up to 6 mo at 4°C.

3.1.4.2. ANTIBODY TITER

1. Add serial dilutions (1:10–1:1280) of the antibody preparations as 50-µL aliquots, in duplicate, to wells of the coated plates; after a 90-min incubation at 37°C, wash the plates with PBS-Tween. Seal the plates in paraffin sheets for all incubations.

2. Dilute the secondary antibody conjugate according to the manufacturer's recommendations in PBS-BSA-Tween and add at 50 µL/well for 1 h at 37°C.

3. Wash the plates three times with PBS-Tween and once with dH₂0, and then add the alkaline phosphatase substrate at 50 µL/well for 20–30 min at 37°C. Read the absorbance at 405 nm with a microplate photometer.

3.1.4.3. ANTIBODY SPECIFICITY

1. Precoat 96-well U-bottomed microtiter plates with PBS-BSA at 100 µL/well for 30 min at room temperature and wash once with PBS-Tween.

2. To act as nonspecific binding (NSB) wells, add 50 µL of PBS-BSA and 50 µL of PBS-BSA-Tween to each of four wells. To all other wells add 50 µL of the appropriate dilution of antibody preparation (*see* **Note 3**).

3. As the immunoassays are inhibition ELISAs, add 50 µL of PBS-BSA to each of another four wells containing 50 µL antiserum, to determine maximum binding (MB) of the antibody in the absence of the inhibitory peptides.

4. To each of remaining test wells add, in duplicate, 50 µL of serial dilutions of either the C1, 2C, or C2C peptides, the addition (+1, +2, +3) and deletion (−1, −2, −3) peptides described above, the peptide bridging the collagenase cleavage site in native type II collagen α-chains, or native (triple-helical), heat-denatured (80°C for 20 min) and collagenase-cleaved type I, II, and III collagens (*see* **Note 1**). For the NC4 and COL2 immunoassays, add, in duplicate, 50-µL dilutions of NC4 or COL2 peptides, NC4 domain, or type IX collagen (*see* **Note 2**). For the COL2-3/4m ELISA, add, in duplicate, 50-µL dilutions of CB11B peptide or HDC.

5. After 1 h at 37°C, transfer 50 µL from each well to the equivalent wells of plates precoated, as described above, with the one exception that the C2C-BSA conjugate is diluted at 50 ng/well in PBS (pH 7.2) for the C1, 2C assay.
6. Incubate the plates for 30 min at 4°C, wash three times with PBS-Tween, and then add the secondary antibody conjugate, at the dilution recommended by the manufacturer in PBS-BSA-Tween, for 1 h at 37°C.
7. After a further three washes with PBS-Tween and dH$_2$0, use an ELISA amplification system kit, according to manufacturer's instructions (Gibco-BRL) or 50 µL/well of alkaline phosphatase (AP) substrate solution (Sigma).
8. Read the absorbance for each well at the appropriate wavelength (490 nm for the amplification kit and 405 nm for the AP substrate) and subtract the mean of the NSB wells from the values for each of the other wells to obtain a corrected absorbance. Calculate the percentage binding for each peptide from their corrected absorbance values relative to the mean absorbance of the four MB wells, which represent 0% inhibition.

$$\% \text{ binding} = \frac{\text{corrected absorbance (absorbance} - \text{mean absorbance of nonspecific well)} \times 100}{\text{mean absorbance of maximum binding wells}}$$

Calculate the percentage inhibition by subtracting the percentage binding from 100.

3.2. Immunoassays

3.2.1. Preparation of the Coating Peptides for the C1, 2C, and COL2 Immunoassays

To improve the sensitivity of the C1, 2C immunoassay, which is of particular importance when assaying biological fluids, the C1, 2C peptide is conjugated to KLH. A similar approach was used for the COL2 immunoassay. This is not necessary for the NC4 assay. The KLH protein is commonly used in hapten-protein conjugates to enhance the noncovalent binding of a hapten to a solid support, such as the wells of microtiter plates used in immunoassays, and to ensure that the peptide is "exposed" for antibody binding. A cysteine was added to the *N*-termini of both the C1, 2C and COL2 peptides for conjugation to the KLH carrier protein.

The procedure for conjugation of the C1, 2C and COL2 peptides to KLH for use as the coating peptide in the immunoassays is as follows:

1. Reconstitute 20 mg of KLH with 2 mL dH$_2$0 and dialyze overnight against 0.1 *M* phosphate buffer (pH 7.0).
2. Slowly add (dropwise) 0.2 mL of the coupling reagent to 2.0 mL of chilled KLH, with stirring, warm to 25°C over 30 min, and then cool on ice.
3. Repeat **step 2**, but do not cool after warming.
4. Centrifuge the sample and apply the supernatant to a previously washed (50 mL of 0.1 *M* phosphate buffer, pH 7.0) Sephadex G-25 column, eluting with phosphate buffer at 1 mL/min and collecting 2-mL fractions.

5. Measure the absorbency at 280 nm in quartz cuvets of each fraction, pool those containing the first protein peak (bluish gray color), and measure the absorbency of the pooled sample.
6. Determine the [KLH] in mg/mL by dividing the absorbency value by 1.5 (the extinction coefficient of KLH at 1 mg/mL) and adjust [KLH] to 2–3 mg/mL.
7. Add 4 mg of the activated KLH (about 1.5 mL) to 5 mg of the synthetic peptide in solution (100 μL) and leave at 25°C for 2 h, with occasional mixing, before transferring to 4°C overnight.
8. Dialyze against 1 L of phosphate buffer (pH 7.0), with three changes over 24 h, and then against 1 L TBS with one change over 24 h. Aliquot at 300 μL and store at –20°C.
9. Confirm effective incorporation by applying coupled KLH-peptide to one lane and activated KLH to another lane of a 10% SDS-PAGE gel and by showing a decrease in electrophoretic mobility of the KLH-peptide conjugate on SDS-PAGE relative to the activated KLH.

3.2.2. Preparation of the Coated Microtiter Plates

The immunoassays are inhibition ELISAs, wherein standards and samples are preincubated with the primary antibody, and the more of the epitope that is present in each, the less antibody that is left to bind to the solid phase epitope, i.e., the heat-denatured type II collagen (HDC) or the C1, 2C-KLH, COL2-KLH, and NC4 peptides that are coating the immunoassay plates. Here is the procedure for coating the microtiter plates to be used in these inhibition ELISAs:

1. Add to all but the 36 perimeter wells of 96-well flat-bottomed Immulon 2 microtiter plates, 50 μL/well (5 ng/well) of the C1, 2C-KLH conjugate or NC4 peptide diluted to 100 ng/mL in TBS (pH 7.5) and incubate overnight at 4°C. For the COL2 assay, add 50 μL/well (2 ng/well) of the COL2 peptide coupled to KLH and diluted to 40 ng/mL in TBS (pH 7.5). For the COL2-3/4m assay, add 50 μL/well (2 μg/well) of the HDC diluted to 40 μg/mL in carbonate buffer (pH 9.2). The exclusion of the outer wells is because of the potential for excessive evaporation from these wells during incubation (**Fig. 2**).
2. After washing three times with TBS-Tween, block the plates with 100 μL/well of TBS-BSA for 30 min at 25°C and then wash three times with TBS-Tween.

3.2.3. Assaying Samples

The following is the procedure for all the ELISAs, with differences between the assays noted:

1. Prepare standards for the C1, 2C ELISA by diluting a 1 mg/mL stock solution of C2C peptide to 10, 2.5, 0.63, 0.16, 0.04, 0.01 and 0.0025 μg/mL in TBS-BSA.
2. Prepare standards for the NC4 ELISA by diluting a 1 mg/mL stock solution of NC4 peptide to 100, 50, 25, 12.5, 3.12, 1.56, 0.78, and 0.39 ng/mL in TBS-BSA.

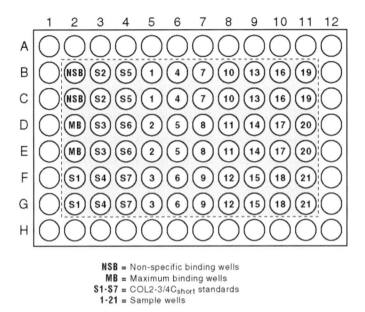

NSB = Non-specific binding wells
MB = Maximum binding wells
S1-S7 = COL2-3/4C$_{short}$ standards
1-21 = Sample wells

Fig. 2. Microtiter plate template for the C1, 2C ELISA. The perimeter wells corresponding to columns 1 and 12 and to rows A and H are not used. All blanks, standards, and samples are assayed in duplicate. Symbols shown represent nonspecific binding (NSB) wells with no C1, 2C antibody added, maximum binding (MB) wells with no inhibiting C2C peptide added, standard wells (S1–S7) with 10, 2.5, 0.63, 0.16, 0.04, 0.01, and 0.0025 μg of inhibiting C1, 2C peptide/mL of TBS-BSA, and sample wells (1–21). Similar templates are employed for the NC4, COL2, and COL2-3/4m immunoassays, with different concentrations of standards used, as indicated in **Subheading 3.2.3.**

3. Prepare standards for the COL2 ELISA by diluting a 1 mg/mL stock solution of COL2 peptide to 10000, 1000, 100, 10, 1, 0.1, and 0.01 ng/mL in TBS-BSA.
4. Prepare standards for the COL2-3/4m ELISA by diluting a 1 mg/mL stock solution of COL2 peptide to 8, 6, 4, 3, 2, 1, 0.5, and 0.25 μg/mL in TBS-BSA.
5. Add each standard at 50 μL/well, in duplicate, to 96-well U-bottomed polypropylene plates, as outlined in the template shown as **Fig. 2**, again ignoring all outside wells. The duplicate NSB wells consist of 50 μL TBS-BSA and 50 μL TBS-BSA-Tween, and the duplicate maximum binding (MB) wells contain 50 μL TBS-BSA and 50 μL of the antibody preparation, at a dilution in TBS (pH 7.5), as previously determined (*see* **Note 3**).
6. Add samples at 50 μL/well, in duplicate, to the remaining wells, and then add to each of the wells 50 μL of the diluted antibody preparations, before covering the plates with paraffin sheets and incubating at 37°C for 1 h.

7. Using a multichannel pipetor, transfer 50 µL from each well of the polypropylene plates to the respective well of the HDC, C1, 2C-KLH, NC4, or COL2-KLH coated plates. Incubate these plates for 30 min at 4°C and then wash three times with TBS-Tween.

8. Dilute the secondary antibody conjugated to AP in TBS-BSA-Tween, as recommended by the manufacturer or optimized in the specific assay. Add 50 µL/well and incubate for 1 h at 37°C. Wash the plates three times with TBS-Tween and three times with dH$_2$O.

9. Use a two-step ELISA amplification system according to the manufacturer's instructions (Gibco-BRL) or 50 µL/well of AP substrate (COL2-3/4m assay), and after the color development is stopped with 0.3 *M* H$_2$SO$_4$, read the absorbance at either 490 nm (amplification system) or 405 nm (AP substrate).

10. Determine the concentration of the C1, 2C, NC4, COL2, and COL2-3/4m epitopes in each sample from a log/linear plot of concentration (µg/mL) vs corrected absorbance (sample absorbance – mean of nonspecific binding absorbance) for the standards. Use nonlinear regression to establish a sigmoidal dose–response curve with variable slope for determination of the concentrations of the unknowns. Typical standard curves for these immunoassays are shown in **Fig. 3**.

3.2.4. Assay Validation

Assays that are developed for use in clinical sciences must be validated. There are guidelines published by the International Federation of Clinical Chemistry.

The features of any assay that need to be validated are specificity, sensitivity, precision (within run and between run), analytic recovery, and identity of calibrant and unknown sample.

3.2.4.1. ANTIBODY SPECIFICITY

Antibody specificity refers to the ability of an antibody to produce a measurable response for the analyte of interest, whereas crossreactivity measures the response of the antibody to other substances. The polyclonal C1, 2C antibody has selective high affinity for both the immunizing C1, 2C peptide and collagenase (MMP-1 and MMP-13)-cleaved human type II collagen 3/4 α-chain fragments, when compared on a molar basis *(1)*. The antibody demonstrates a lower affinity for similarly cleaved human type I collagen α-chains. There is negligible binding to uncleaved triple-helical and heat-denatured human types I and II collagen, as well as intact or cleaved type III collagen α-chains. The materials required for these procedures are listed in **Subheading 2.1.4.** and **Note 1**.

The NC4 and COL2 antibodies have selective high affinity for both the immunizing peptide and type IX collagen extracted from tissue *(3)*. There was no cross reactivity with collagens types I, II, III, V, VI, and X. Antisera speci-

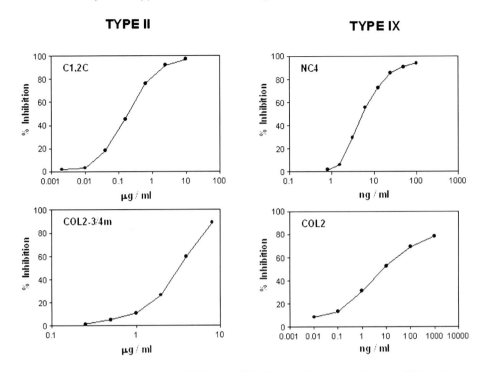

Fig. 3. Standard curves for NC4 and COL2 domain assays for type IX collagen α_1(IX) chain are shown together with those for type II collagen α_1(II) chain intact and cleaved, namely, COL2-3/4m and C1, 2C, respectively.

ficities were also characterized with inhibition ELISA using purified NC4 domain (for NC4 antiserum), pepsin digested type IX collagen (for COL2 antiserum), and collagen types I, II, III, V, VI, and X as competing antigens. Only the corresponding peptides, pepsin-digested type IX collagen (for COL2 antiserum) and purified NC4 domain (for NC4 antiserum), were inhibitory, whereas collagen types I, II, III, V, VI, and X had no effect *(4)*. There was no crossreactivity with collagen types I, II, III, V, VI, and X.

The COL2-3/4m antibody reacts with denatured type II collagen but not denatured types I, III, or X collagen. It crossreacts with the α-3 chain of type XI collagen, as the sequence is identical to that of the $\alpha1$(II)-chain. It does not react with native (triple-helical) type II collagen.

3.2.4.2. Sensitivity

The sensitivity of an assay is the lowest dose at which there is a significant difference in response from zero. This is generally determined by the upper 2 or 3 SD limit in a zero standard study. The minimum detection limit of the C1, 2C assay is 4.9 nM.

3.2.4.3. Precision

Within-run (intra-assay) and between-run (interassay) precision is determined by assaying different samples that cover the range of detectable levels of epitope, in a series of runs. For within-run precision, a single sample is assayed in multiple replicates on the same plate ($n = +20$). The coefficient of variation (% CV) is determined by dividing the SD by the mean of the concentration values obtained and then multiplying by 100. The between-run precision is determined from the same samples assayed on multiple plates ($n = +5$), and the % CV is determined from the SD of the plate means and the overall concentration mean. Values obtained for collagenase-cleaved human type II collagen and culture medium from IL-1–stimulated bovine articular cartilage explants range from CVs of 4.6–8.3% for within-run precision to CVs of 5.4–6.9% for between-run precision for the C1, 2C immunoassay.

3.2.4.4. Analytic Recovery

"Spike recovery" is determined by the addition of known quantities of the purified peptide into fluid samples with different levels of endogenous epitope. Typical results for synovial fluid, urine, and cartilage explant culture medium range from 89 to 110 % recovery for the C1, 2C immunoassay.

Linearity is shown by diluting samples serially and comparing the observed values with those expected. Typical recovery rates of 94–111% have been noted for cleaved type II collagen and culture medium from IL-1–stimulated articular cartilage explants using the C1, 2C immunoassay.

3.2.4.5. Identity of Analyte and Calibrant

The demonstration of parallelism between the dose response curves of the calibrant and the unknown sample proves identity *(4)*. The C1, 2C, NC4, COL2, or CB11B peptides and the sample (cleaved type II collagen for C1, 2C, type IX collagen for COL2, heat-denatured type II collagen for COL2-3/4m, NC4 domain, culture medium, serum, synovial fluid, urine, and so on) are each progressively diluted and assayed separately as described above in **Subheading 3.2.3.** The results for each are plotted on the same graph of concentration (dilution) vs % inhibition, and the curves for each are compared for parallelism *(1–3)*.

3.2.5. Experimental Studies Using the C1, 2C, NC4, COL2, and COL2-3/4m ELISAs

The C1, 2C ELISA can be used to assess the degree of MMP activity, specifically for the collagenases MMP-1, MMP-8, and MMP-13, in terms of cleaved product, in any system in which there is type I and/or II collagen. It can be used to evaluate the effect of MMP inhibitors on the generation of collagenase-cleaved collagen products in vivo and in vitro *(1,5–7)*. To evaluate the levels of collagenase-cleaved collagen *in situ*, tissue is digested with α-chymotrypsin, which releases cleaved and denatured collagens from the extracellular matrix and preserves the recognition of the neoepitope by the C1, 2C antibody *(1,7,8)*.

The NC4 assay can be used to determine the content of the long form of type IX collagen, and the COL2 assay can be used to determine total type IX collagen content in any system in which type IX collagen is present *(4)*. To evaluate the levels of these collagens *in situ*, the tissue is digested with α-chymotrypsin and proteinase K, which releases cleaved and denatured collagens from the extracellular matrix and preserves the recognition of the epitopes.

The COL2-3/4m assay can be used to determine the absolute amount of type II collagen and the proportion of denatured type II collagen in arthritic articular cartilage as well as intervertebral disks *(2,9–11)*.

The protocol for digestion of articular cartilage and extraction of degraded collagen is as follows:

1. Mince articular cartilage and incubate 10–50 mg overnight at 37°C with 500 μL of 1 mg/mL α-chymotrypsin digestion solution (containing protease inhibitors, as described above) in 1.5-mL centrifuge tubes with a V-shaped bottom and a screw-cap lined with an O-ring.
2. Incubate the digest for 20 min at 37°C with 200 μL (160 μg/mL final concentration) of TPCK.
3. For the NC4 and COL2 ELISAs, digest with 500 μL of proteinase K digestion solution containing protease inhibitors. Centrifuge the samples and remove the supernatants for assaying with the respective ELISA, as described in **Subheading 3.2.3.**
4. For the COL2-3/4m assay, using an appropriate pipete, transfer all the α-chymotrypsin cartilage-extract solution (CE) to a new screw-capped 1.5-mL centrifuge tube, taking care to leave all the undigested cartilage residue (CR) in the original tube. Mix the CE and then transfer 300 μL to another screw-capped 1.5-mL centrifuge tube for further digestion of the extract (DE). Store the remaining CE at 4°C.
5. To the CR add 500 μL of 1 mg/mL proteinase K (including proteinase inhibitors, as described in **step 3**). Put the cap on tightly and tap the tube until all the cartilage is submerged in the solution. To the DE add 100 μL of 1 mg/mL proteinase K and put the cap on.
6. Incubate CR and DE overnight in an oven or water bath, at 56°C. Then increase the temperature to 100°C and allow the samples to boil for 10–15 min, to inactivate any remaining proteinase K. *See* **Note 5** for a discussion of problems encountered with digesting cartilage residues.

7. Assay CE, DE, and CR for epitope CB11B, by inhibition ELISA, as described in **Subheading 3.2.3**. Appropriate dilutions of CE, DE, and CR (*see* **Note 6**) should be prepared in Tris-HCl and 50 µL added to duplicate wells already containing antibody in the COL2-3/4m ELISA.

4. Notes

1. If the collagens for the species of interest cannot be purchased, they can be purified from tissues of that species. Type II collagen can be purified from articular cartilage of the species of choice, by pepsin digestion and differential salt precipitation *(12)*, and types I and III collagen can be prepared by pepsin digestion and differential denaturation/renaturation *(13)*.

   a. For cleavage by the collagenases (MMP-1, MMP-8, and/or MMP-13), these lyophilized collagens are dissolved separately in 0.5 M acetic acid and diluted to 2.5 mg/mL in a digestion buffer consisting of 50 mM Tris-HCl, 10 mM CaCl$_2$, 0.5 M NaCl, 0.01% Brij 35, and 0.02% NaN$_3$, pH 7.6.

   b. The proenzymes are activated with 2 mM (final concentration) *p*-aminophenylmercuric acetate (APMA) in the same digestion buffer for 90 min at 37°C.

   c. The activated enzyme solution is added to each of the collagen solutions at molar ratios of from 1:5 to 1:10, the pH is adjusted to 7.5 with NaOH (if necessary), and the samples are incubated at 30°C for 24 h.

   d. The MMPs are inactivated with 20 mM (final concentration) EDTA, and cleavage is confirmed by SDS-PAGE under denaturing conditions using 10%, 1-mm-thick, mini-Protean gels (Bio-Rad).

   e. To confirm immunoreactivity of the cleavage-site neoepitope antibody, the electrophoretically separated collagenase-cleaved α-chain fragments are transferred to a nitrocellulose membrane.

   f. After blocking in PBS-3% BSA, the membrane is incubated overnight with the anti-neoepitope antibody.

   g. After washing with PBS-BSA-Tween, secondary antibody conjugate diluted in PBS-3% BSA-Tween is added for 1 h at 25°C, the membranes are washed three times in PBS-BSA-Tween and three times in dH$_2$0, and substrate solution is added (5-bromo-4-chloro-3-indolyl phosphate and nitroblue tetrazolium) from a kit (Bio-Rad).

   h. After the color has developed for the immunostained bands, and before excess background staining (10–20 min), the substrate is removed, and the membranes are washed with dH$_2$0 before drying on filter paper.

2. Isolation of native type IX collagen and the NC4 domain.

   a. Slices (40 g wet weight) of fetal bovine epiphyseal cartilage can be extracted for 48 h at 4°C with constant stirring in 4 M guanidine HCl in 100 mM sodium acetate, pH 6.0, to remove proteoglycans.

   b. The supernatant can be removed by centrifugation at 2000g for 15 min.

   c. Residual cartilage is washed with 0.5 M acetic acid and then extracted with 1 M NaCl, 0.05 M Tris-HCl, pH 7.4, at 4°C for 48 h *(4)*.

    d. The guanidine HCl and NaCl extractions also contain protease inhibitors 2 mM phenylmethanesulfonyl fluoride (PMSF), 2 mM EDTA-Na$_2$, 5 mM benzamidine, and 10 mM N-ethylmaleimide.

    e. Intact type IX collagen lacking the chondroitin sulfate chain is recovered from the 1 M NaCl salt neutral extract by precipitation with ammonium sulfate at 30% saturation.

    f. The precipitate is redissolved in 0.5 M acetic acid, and native type IX collagen can be enriched in the supernatant after precipitating other molecules with 0.7 M NaCl.

3. The NC4 domain is purified separately *(4)*.

    a. Briefly, proteoglycans are removed from 40g of bovine epiphyseal cartilage slices as described in **step 2**.

    b. After centrifugation at 2000g for 15 min, the residue is resuspended at 4°C in 30 mL of 50 mM Tris-HCl, pH 7.2, 5 mM CaCl$_2$, with inhibitors (as specified above).

    c. After centrifuging and washing the residue by resuspending it in the same buffer several times, 4000 U of collagenase (Clostridiopeptidase A, Sigma) are added, and the sample is incubated at room temperature for 6 h.

    d. After centrifugation at 4000g for 60 min at 4°C, the supernatant is chromatographed on a 3 × 100-cm column of 8% agarose (Bio-Rad A 1.5 m).

    e. The column is equilibrated with 50 mM Tris-HCl, pH 7.6, and 2 M urea.

    f. Two-milliliter fractions are collected and analyzed by PAGE and Western blotting with anti-NC4 antiserum.

    g. Fractions containing the NC4 domain are pooled, dialyzed against 5 mM Tris-HCl, pH 7.6, and 0.2 M urea, and then lyophilized.

4. Checkerboard analysis can be used for titration of both the antigen and antibody to determine the optimum concentration of antigen to coat the microtiter plate wells and the optimum dilution of primary antibody to allow maximum sensitivity and minimal background in the ELISA.

    a. The peptide-carrier conjugate is diluted across the plate from left to right, with the last column of the wells containing no antigen, and allowed to adsorb to the plate.

    b. The primary antibody is then diluted across the plate from top to bottom, thereby obtaining a checkerboard titration of antigen against antibody.

    c. After incubation at room temperature for 1 h, enzyme-conjugated secondary antibody is added, and incubated at 37°C for 1 h, followed by the addition of the enzyme substrate, and the absorbances are read.

    d. A graph is made showing a plot for each antibody dilution of antigen dilution vs optical density (OD), and from this the background of the plate and the nonspecific adsorption of conjugate, as well as the plateau region of maximum antigen binding to the plate (plate saturation), can be determined.

        The anti-collagen antibody (COL2-3/4m) must also be used at an appropriate dilution. If it is too dilute, then the MB value will be too low and inhibition will be difficult to detect. If it is too concentrated, then higher concentrations of epitope will be needed to inhibit its binding to HDC on the ELISA plate. For optimal conditions, the antibody should be bound to HDC at a range of dilutions over a 30-min incubation time at ambient temperature. After washing the plate, bound antibody can be detected using the second antibody/ AP detection system. A plot of log-dilution against OD_{405} will approximate to a straight line. The dilution producing an OD_{405} that is about 40% of maximal OD is optimal for use in the assay. However, note that when the antibody is added to the preculture plate, it is diluted 1:1 with sample (or buffer), so it should be prepared initially at 2X the chosen concentration.

5. Total CB11B in the CE compartment represents the amount of denatured type II collagen. The digestion of CE with proteinase K to generate DE is a means of degrading any native-type II collagen extracted intact by α-chymotrypsin, thus making it available for assay. The amount of CB11B in DE should be equal to or greater than CB11B in CE. Therefore total CB11B epitope in the cartilage = CB11B in DE + CB11B in CR. Calculate type II collagen degradation as:

$$\% \text{ denaturation} = (\text{CB11B in CE/total CB11B}) \times 100$$

6. Digestion of cartilage residues by proteinase K generally results in complete solubilization of the tissue, which is necessary for an accurate estimate of the total collagen content. However, in some instances proteinase K fails to solubilize the tissue. We have found two different reasons for this. The first is if too much cartilage was added to the centrifuge tube. In this case the remaining undigested residue can be transferred to fresh proteinase K. The second is that calcified cartilage is resistant to proteolysis. This problem is most common with cartilage from animals such as rabbits or guinea pigs because the uncalcified tissue layer is very thin. The way to resolve this problem is to increase the concentration of EDTA in the α-chymotrypsin and proteinase K solutions to 400 mM. (The tetrasodium salt of EDTA must be used for this.)

7. The appropriate sample dilutions will vary enormously depending on the type of cartilage, amount of tissue used, and extent of collagen degradation. However, as a general guideline, the CE and DE samples may require no dilution, or they may need to be diluted to about 1:4. The CR samples will always require diluting, often by as much as 1:40 or 1:80. Clearly these values will be even more varied when other tissues are being extracted and assayed for their specific collagens.

Acknowledgments

Financial Support was provided by the Shriners Hospitals for Children, Canadian Institutes of Health Research, National Institutes of Health (to ARP), and the Fonds de la Recherche en Santé du Quebec (to RCB).

References

1. Billinghurst, R. C., Dahlberg, L., Ionescu, M. et al. (1997) Enhanced cleavage of type II collagen by collagenases in osteoarthritic articular cartilage. *J. Clin. Invest.* **99**, 1534–1545.

2. Hollander, A. P., Heathfield, T. F., Webber, C., et al. (1994) Increased damage to type II collagen in osteoarthritic articular cartilage detected by a new immunoassay. *J. Clin. Invest.* **93,** 1722–1732.

3. Nelson F, Dahlberg L, Laverty, S., Reiner et al. (1998) Evidence for altered synthesis of type II collagen in patients with osteoarthritis. *J. Clin. Invest.* **102,** 2115–2125.

4. Mwale, F., Billinghurst, C., Wu, W., et al. (2000) Selective assembly and remodelling of collagens II and IX associated with expression of the chondrocyte hypertrophic phenotype. *Dev. Dyn.* **218,** 648–662.

5. Billinghurst, R. C., Buxton, E. M., Edwards, M. G., McGraw, M. S., and McIlwraith, C. W. (2001) Use of an antineoepitope antibody for identification of type-II collagen degradation in equine articular cartilage. *Am. J. Vet. Res.* **62,** 1031–1039.

6. Dahlberg, L., Billinghurst, R. C., Manner, P., et al. (2000) Selective enhancement of collagenase-mediated cleavage of resident type II collagen in cultured osteoarthritic cartilage and arrest with a synthetic inhibitor that spares collagenase 1 (matrix metalloproteinase 1). *Arthritis Rheum.* **43,** 673–682.

7. Billinghurst, R. C., O'Brien, K., Poole, A. R., and McIlwraith, C. W. (1999) Inhibition of articular cartilage degradation in culture by a novel nonpeptidic matrix metalloproteinase inhibitor. *N. Y. Acad. Sci.* **878,** 594–597.

8. Billinghurst, R. C., Wu, W., Ionescu, M., et al. (2000) Comparison of the degradation of type II collagen and proteoglycan in nasal and articular cartilages by interleukin-1 and the selective inhibition of type II collagen cleavage by collagenase. *Arthritis Rheum.* **43,** 664–672.

9. Laverty, S., O'Kouneff, S., Ionescu, M., et al. (2002) Excessive degradation of type II collagen in articular cartilage in equine osteochondrosis. *J. Orthop. Res.* **20,** 1282–1289.

10. Hollander, A. P., Heathfield, T. F., Liu, J. J., et al. (1996) Enhanced denaturation of the $\alpha 1(II)$ chains of type-II collagen in normal adult human intervertebral discs compared with femoral articular cartilage. *J. Orthop. Res.* **14,** 61–66.

11. Antoniou, J., Steffen, T., Nelson, F., et al. (1996) The human intervertebral disc. Evidence for changes in the biosynthesis and denaturation of the extracellular matrix with growth, maturation, ageing and degeneration. *J. Clin. Invest.* **98,** 996–1003.

12. Squires, G., Okouneff, S., Ionescu, M., and Poole, A. R. (2003) Pathobiology of focal lesion development in aging human articular cartilage reveals molecular matrix changes characteristic of osteoarthritis. *Arthritis Rheum.* **48,** 1261–1270.

13. Miller, E. J. (1971) Isolation and characterization of a collagen from chick cartilage containing three identical achains. *Biochemistry* **10,** 1652–1659.

14. ChandraRajan, J. (1978) Separation of type III collagen from type I collagen and pepsin by differential denaturation and renaturation. *Biochem. Biophys. Res. Commun.* **83,** 180–186.

Table 1
Key Differences Between Apoptosis and Necrosis

Apoptosis	Necrosis
Plasma membrane usually intact early	Plasma membrane disrupted early
No leakage of cell contents	Leakage of cell contents
Minimal inflammation	Inflammation
Cell shrinkage (early)	Cell swelling
Chromatin condensation	Poorly defined clumping of chromatin
Karyorrhexis (nuclear convolution and breakdown)	Karyolysis (nuclear dissolution and disappearance)
Apoptotic bodies (late)	Cell disintegration (late)

and necrosis are listed in **Table 1**. However, it is not always possible to differentiate clearly between apoptosis and necrosis *(2)*. Secondary necrosis or postapoptotic necrosis may occur associated with the late release of lysosomal enzymes, especially in the absence of phagocytosis *(3–5)*. Some toxins can cause apoptosis at low doses and can cause necrosis at high doses *(6)*. Inhibition of apoptosis (by inhibition of caspases) can result in necrosis *(7,8)*. Other forms of cell death such as "dark chondrocytes" or "paralyzed cells," which do not bear all the hallmarks of apoptosis, have been reported *(9)*. In view of the inherent difficulty in accurately detecting apoptosis in chondrocytes, this chapter describes several complementary techniques that may be used in combination.

2. Materials

2.1. Detection of Caspase-3 Processing in Cultured Human Chondrocytes Challenged With Various Death Inducers

1. Primary human chondrocytes.
2. Glucosamine, staurosporine, and sodium nitroprusside (Sigma-Aldrich, St. Louis, MO).
3. Agonistic anti-CD95 antibody, clone CH-11 (Immunotech, Marseille, France).
4. Proteasome inhibitor 1 (PS1; Alexis, Carlsbad, CA).
5. Linbro® 4-well culture plates (ICN, Aurora, OH).
6. Tabletop centrifuge with RTH750 rotor (Sorvall, Newtown, CT).
7. Microcentrifuge (Sorvall).
8. Gel running device for polyacrylamide gel electrophoresis (PAGE) plus blotting apparatus (Novex, San Diego, CA).
9. Nitrocellulose transfer membrane, 0.1 mM pore size (Schleicher & Schuell, Keene, NH).
10. Anti-active caspase-3 antibody (Imgenex, San Diego, CA).

11. Anti-GAPDH (reduced glyceraldehydes-phosphate dehydrogenase) antibody (Ambion, Austin, TX).
12. Goat anti-mouse horseradish peroxidase conjugated antibody (Santa Cruz Biotechnology, Santa Cruz, CA).
13. Supersignal West Pico Enhanced Chemiluminescent Substrate (Pierce, Rockford, IL).
14. Biomax MR Film (Eastman-Kodak, Rochester, NY).
15. Autoradiography cassette (Fisher Scientific, Pittsburgh, PA).

2.2. Quantification of Cell Death in Glucosamine-Stimulated Cultured Chondrocytes by Uptake of Propidium Iodide and Binding of Annexin V

1. Primary human chondrocytes.
2. Propidium iodide (Sigma-Aldrich).
3. Fluorescein-labeled Annexin V Staining Kit (BioVision, Mountain View, CA).
4. Six-well plates (Corning).
5. Centrifuge tubes (Stockwell Scientific, Scottsdale, AZ).
6. Tabletop centrifuge with RTH750 rotor (Sorvall).
7. Microcentrifuge (Sorvall).
8. 5-mL Round-bottomed fluorescence-activated cell sorting (FACS) tubes (Becton Dickinson, Franklin Lakes, NJ).
9. Fluorescence activated cell sorter (Becton-Dickinson).

2.3. In Situ *Detection of Apoptosis by TUNEL*

1. A mechanical compression device (servohydraulic testing machine, cat. no. 8511; Instron, Boston, MA).
2. Fresh (less than 72 h after death) full-thickness human articular cartilage (from tissue banks or autopsies).
3. Glass slides (treated with silane are recommended), cover slips, mounting medium (90% glycerin, 10% phosphate-buffered saline [PBS])
4. 4% Paraformaldehyde buffered at pH 7.4 for fixation.
5. PBS.
6. Xylene.
7. Ethanol: 100, 90, and 80%.
8. 20 µg/mL Proteinase K.
9. Terminal deoxynucleotidyl transferase (TdT; 2.5 U/mL; Roche Diagnostics, Indianapolis, IN).
10. TdT buffer: 30 mM Tris base (pH 7.2), 140 mM sodium cacodylate, 2 mM cobalt chloride (Roche Diagnostics).
11. Fluorescein isothiocyanate (FITC)-dUTP (Roche Diagnostics; also part of the Mebstain kit, MBL, Nagoya, Japan).
12. Termination buffer: 300 mM NaCl, 30 mM sodium citrate (Sigma-Aldrich).
13. Counterstain: propidium iodide, 0.5 µg/mL (Sigma-Aldrich).
14. DNase buffer: 100 µg/mL DNase I, 30 mM Tris base pH 7.2, 140 mM K cacodylate, 4 mM MgCl$_2$, 0.1 mM dithiothreitol (Roche Diagnostics).

3. Methods

3.1. Detection of Caspase-3 Processing in Cultured Human Chondrocytes Challenged With Various Death Inducers

Caspases are zymogens that, in response to a proapoptotic input, are processed into complex-forming large and small fragments either by other caspases or autocatalytically. Activation of caspases occurs in the initiation and/or the execution phase of certain apoptotic programs and represents an early physiologic marker of apoptosis resulting, for example, in the cleavage of substrates such as poly-ADP ribose polymerase (PARP) or lamin *(10)*, or the activation of caspase-activated DNase (CAD) *(11)*. The activation of caspases can be monitored fluorometrically by measuring the cleavage of caspase-specific fluorogenic peptide substrates *(12)*. Although this approach is simple, fast, and quantitative, intercaspase or interprotease reactivity of the substrates may generate experimental artifacts. Monitoring caspase processing by immunoblotting represents a more reliable approach to assess caspase activation. Here we present an immunoblotting technique that allows the detection of caspase-3 processing in cultured human chondrocytes. Cell death is induced by stimulation with staurosporine, sodium nitroprusside (SNP), glucosamine, or agonistic CH-11 antibody with a proteasome inhibitor, PS1 (CH-11/PS1).

3.1.1. Chondrocyte Isolation and Culture and Induction in Cell Death

1. Human chondrocytes were obtained from knee articular cartilage of donors without a recorded history of joint disease. Chondrocytes were isolated from human cartilage using established protocols. The cartilage tissue was processed as described previously *(13)*. The chondrocytes used in this experiment were treated as follows:

    a. After initial medium isolation, the cells were incubated in Dulbecco's modified Eagle's medium (DMEM) supplemented with 25 mM glucose (Gibco), 10% calf serum (Omega Scientific), 10 mM L-glutamine (Gibco), and penicillin/streptomycin (Gibco) and were allowed to attach to the culture flasks.

    b. After incubation the cells were grown to confluence (for approx 3 wk), split once (passage 1), and grown to confluence again.

2. Passage 1 chondrocytes were plated at 1×10^6 cells/well (i.e., confluent) in 4-well plates in DMEM as described above.

3. For stimulation with agonistic CH-11 antibody + proteasome inhibitor PS1 (CH-11/PS1), staurosporine, or SNP, the cells were incubated overnight, and the medium was changed to fresh medium; for stimulation with glucosamine, the cells were cultured overnight and the medium was changed to DMEM supplemented with 5 mM glucose, 10 mM glutamine, penicillin/streptomycin, and 2% calf serum. All cultures were incubated for an additional 24 h.

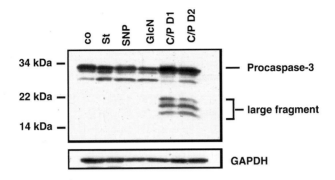

Fig. 1. Immunoblot analysis of caspase-3 processing. The chondrocytes were stimulated with staurosporine (St), SNP, glucosamine (GlcN), or CH-11/PS1 (C/P) to induce cell death. Control chondrocytes (co) were not stimulated. The effects of CH-11/PS1 stimulation on two different donors (D1, D2) are shown. Signals for GAPDH obtained upon reprobing of the blot suggest that similar amounts of protein (approx 25 µg) were loaded in each lane. The large fragment of caspase-3 occurs in three distinct processing forms of approx 22, 20, and 17 kDa.

4. The cells were then stimulated with 20 mM glucosamine, 0.5 mg/mL staurosporine, 1 mM SNP, or CH-11/PS1 (1 mg/mL CH-11 + 20 mM PS1) for 16–24 h (*see* **Note 1.**).
5. The cells were harvested by collecting the supernatants, which contained the floating cells, and by trypsinizing the adherent cells; supernatants and adherent cells were combined and centrifuged for 5 min at 800g using a Sorvall tabletop centrifuge equipped with an RTH750 rotor.
6. The supernatants were carefully and completely aspirated.

3.1.2. Immunoblotting

Whole cell lysates were prepared from approx $1–1.5 \times 10^6$ chondrocytes that were either left unstimulated (control) or stimulated as indicated in **Fig. 1**.

1. The cell pellets from **step 6**, **Subheading 3.1.1.** were lysed with 0.2 mL of ice cold lysis buffer (10 mM Tris, pH 7.6, 158 mM NaCl, 1 mM EDTA, 0.1% sodium dodecyl sulfate [SDS], 1% Triton X-100, leupeptin, aprotinin [1 mg/mL each], and 1 mM phenylmethylsulfonyl fluoride [PMSF; which was added immediately before use]).
2. The lysates were transferred to Eppendorf tubes, and the protein concentration was determined using a protein dye reagent from Bio-Rad according to the protocol supplied.
3. Similar amounts of protein were separated by SDS-PAGE for 2 h using 15% polyacrylamide gels (Novex).

4. The proteins were transferred to nitrocellulose filters by electroblotting for 1.5 h at 20 V (Novex blotting apparatus); the large fragment of active caspase-3 ranges in molecular weight from 17 to 22 kDa (*see* **Note 2.**).

5. The filters were blocked overnight at 4°C in Tris-buffered saline solution supplemented with 0.1% Tween-20 (TBS-T) and 4% calf serum. The membrane was then incubated with antibody against the p17 subunit of caspase-3 (1:1000) for 2 h at room temperature. The membrane was washed three times for 10 min with TBS-T and then further incubated with horseradish peroxidase-conjugated secondary antibody (1:1000) for 1 h. Afterward the membrane was washed three times with TBS-T and was developed using the enhanced chemiluminescent substrate from Pierce.

6. The blot was exposed for 5 min to obtain optimal signals for the large fragment of active caspase-3.

7. The blot was then normalized for protein loading: the membrane was washed twice for 5 min with TBS-T and blocked for 1 h in TBS-T plus 4% calf serum.

8. The blot was incubated with antibody against GAPDH, 1:3000, for 1 h, washed three times with TBS-T, and further incubated with horseradish peroxidase-conjugated secondary antibody (1:3000) for 1 h.

9. The membrane was washed three times, and the blot was developed using the enhanced chemiluminescent substrate from Pierce.

10. The blot was exposed for 2 s to obtain optimal signals for GAPDH.

3.1.3. Interpretation of the Results

Despite induction of substantial cell death, neither glucosamine, SNP, nor staurosporine induced detectable processing of procaspase-3 into its active form (**Fig. 1**). In addition, glucosamine appeared to reduce the expression of procaspase-3 in chondrocytes. Cell death induced by any one of the three stimuli is therefore unlikely to utilize pathways that converge or depend on the activation of caspase-3. In contrast, CH-11/PS1 stimulation causes substantial induction of procaspase-3 processing. This stimulus may therefore serve as a model for the induction of "classic" apoptosis in cultured chondrocytes.

3.2. Quantification of Cell Death in Glucosamine-Stimulated Cultured Chondrocytes by Uptake of Propidium Iodide and Binding of Annexin V

The method is based on the loss of membrane integrity in dead or dying cells, which predisposes them for the uptake of propidium iodide. Apoptosis, as well as necrosis, leads to plasma membrane asymmetry and to externalization of phosphatidylserine residues, which are bound with high affinity by annexin V *(14,15)*. The technique described here is fast and simple and allows for the simultaneous processing of a large number of samples. Unlike methods that are based on the measurement of mitochondrial function, DNA fragmentation, or adhesion assays, this approach directly measures cell death.

Necrosis is associated with early disruption of the cell membrane; therefore, necrotic cells will stain positive with both propidium iodide and annexin V. In the early stages of apoptosis, cells typically have an intact cell membrane. Apoptotic cells will not stain positive with propidium iodide, whereas externalization of phosphatidylserine will be detected by annexin V.

3.2.1. Isolation of Chondrocytes

1. Isolate chondrocytes from human cartilage using established protocols as described above in **Subheading 3.1.1.**
2. Plate chondrocytes at 50,000 cells/well (i.e., subconfluent) in 6-well plates using 3 mL of DMEM supplemented with 25 mM glucose (Gibco), 10 mM glutamine (Gibco), penicillin/streptomycin (Gibco), and 10% calf serum (Omega Scientific).
3. Culture cells overnight and change medium to DMEM supplemented with 5 mM glucose, 10 mM glutamine, penicillin/streptomycin, and 2% calf serum.
4. Incubate for 24 h and stimulate the cells with 5, 10, or 20 mM of glucosamine for another 16–24 h.
5. Collect the supernatants (floating cells); trypsinize (0.5 mL of trypsin solution per well) the adherent cells; add 3 mL of medium to trypsinized cells, and combine supernatants and adherent cells in centrifuge tubes. Centrifuge for 5 min at 800g using a tabletop centrifuge.
6. Resuspend pellets in 1 mL of PBS containing 0.4% calf serum, and transfer the cell suspensions to Eppendorf tubes. The cells may form clumps owing to the loss of membrane integrity; a single-cell suspension can typically be obtained by carefully forcing the cells through an 18-gage needle attached to a 1-mL syringe.
7. Centrifuge at 800g using a microcentrifuge.

3.2.2. Staining of the Cells

1. Resuspend cell pellets in 0.5 mL of Annexin V binding buffer and add 1 µL of Annexin V-FITC supplied with the kit; mix briefly.
2. Incubate for 10 min in the dark.
3. Centrifuge at 800g.
4. Wash cells once with 0.5 mL of PBS containing 0.4% calf serum.
5. Resuspend in 0.5 mL of PBS + 0.4% calf serum and add propidium iodide (final concentration 10 mg/mL); mix briefly.
6. Transfer the cell suspensions to FACS tubes.
7. Immediately analyze the cells by flow cytometry; Annexin V-FITC is detected using the FL-1 channel, and propidium iodide (PI) is detected using the FL-3 channel.
8. Analyze results using CellQuest software (Becton Dickinson).

3.2.3. Interpretation of the Results

At 5 mM, as well as at 10 mM, glucosamine induces only a marginal increase in propidium iodide uptake (compare upper left quadrants in **Fig. 2**). At these

3.3.2. Tissue Preparation

1. Fix the tissue samples overnight in 4% buffered paraformaldehyde and embed in paraffin. The paraformaldehyde fixes the tissue by crosslinking and prevents the loss of DNA during the ethanol treatment.
2. Microtome tissue sections between 2 and 5 μm thick.
3. Deparaffinize the tissue sections by heating in an incubator for 30 min at 60°C (*see* **Note 4**). Then rehydrate with xylene (three times, 3 min each), 100% ethanol (twice, 3 min each), 90% ethanol (once, 3 min), 80% ethanol (once, 3 min), and finally wash in distilled water (four times, 2 min each).

3.3.3. Digestion

1. Incubate in PBS at 37°C for 30 min.
2. Tap off the PBS from the slide and add 250 μL of proteinase K solution on the section (*see* **Notes 5–7**). Incubate again at 37°C for 30 min.
3. Wash slide with distilled water (four times, 2 min each).

3.3.4. DNA Nick-End Labeling

1. Immerse (or pipet) 50 μL TdT buffer.
2. Prepare the TdT solution: 45 μL TdT buffer + 2.5 μL FITC-dUTP + 2.5 μL TdT (*see* **Note 8**).
3. Incubate the section in TdT solution at 37°C for 1 h.
4. Halt the reaction by incubating the section in termination buffer at 37°C for 15 min.
5. Wash in PBS solution (three times, 5 min each).

3.3.5. Counterstain

1. Pipet 50 μL of propidium iodide onto the section and incubate at 4°C for 20 min.
2. Wash with PBS for 3 min.

3.3.6. Controls

1. Digest with DNase buffer (10 min at 20°C, followed by distilled water washes) before DNA nick-end labeling. DNase I produces DNA strand breaks at the 3'-OH end (similar to DNA fragments found in apoptosis).
2. Negative control: do not add TdT to the TdT solution. This will not catalyze the polymerization of nucleotides at the DNA strand break.

3.3.7. Interpretation of the Results

Figure 3 displays the results of TUNEL in cartilage explants subjected to 30% compression. The TUNEL-positive cells are stained green, and the TUNEL-negative cells are counterstained red (propidium iodide). This provides presumptive evidence of apoptosis. Further confirmation is necessary and is provided by electron microscopic examination. Morphologic changes characteristic of apoptosis are shown in **Fig. 4**. These include nuclear condensation, cell shrinkage, and matrix vesicles (*see* **Note 9**).

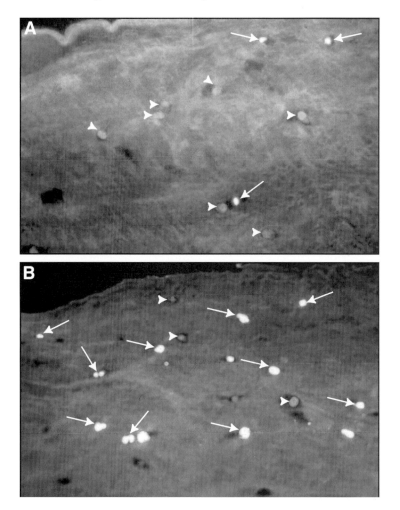

Fig. 3. (A) Control (uninjured) cartilage showing three TUNEL-positive cells (white arrows pointing to bright TUNEL-positive cells). The TUNEL-negative cells were counterstained with propidium iodide (white arrowheads pointing to less bright cells). **(B)** Cartilage subjected to mechanical injury showing widespread TUNEL-positive cells (white arrows). Only a few cells were TUNEL-negative (white arrowheads).

4. Notes

1. For CH-11/PS1, staurosporine, and SNP an incubation period of 16 h was sufficient to induce substantial cell death; for CH-11/PS1 stimulation, incubation for more than 16 h is not recommended as it may result in a reduced cellular content of processed caspase-3. With respect to glucosamine, incubation times may have to be increased to achieve substantial induction of cell death.

Normal chondrocytes

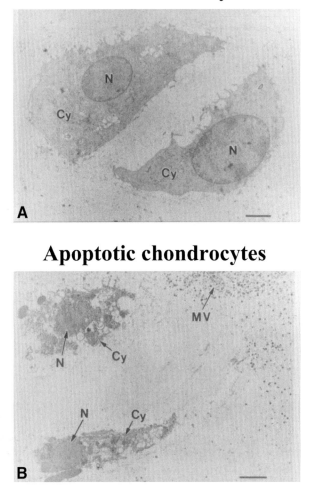

Apoptotic chondrocytes

Fig. 4. Electron microscopic images of chondrocytes. Original magnification 4700×, bar = 2 μm. (**A**) Normal chondrocytes. (**B**) Chondrocytes displaying morphology of apopotosis: cell shrinkage, nuclear condensation, and formation of matrix vesicles. N, nucleus; Cy, cytoplasm; MV, matrix vesicles. Reprinted from ref. *25* with permission from *The Journal of Bone and Joint Surgery*, Inc.

2. The large fragment of active caspase-3 ranges in molecular weight from 17 to 22 kDa. The small size of these fragments requires careful adjustment of the blotting conditions to ensure optimal signal intensity; the use of nitrocellulose membranes with a 0.1 m*M* pore size is recommended since this reduces the effects of "blotting through" the membrane.

3. The Instron servohydraulic machine that was used to injure cartilage is an expensive piece of equipment. Less expensive mechanical compression machines can be used. If access to a precision compression device is not available, manual compression can also be achieved by loading the cartilage explant with a suitable weight that approximates the desired strain. The results may be more variable than those achieved by using precision equipment, but cell death can be induced.

4. A parafilm coverslip can be used to prevent drying during incubation. Fold up one corner of the parafilm to facilitate removal

5. Frozen sections do not need proteinase K digestion.

6. The concentration of proteinase K depends on the type of tissue being stained. It is recommended that proteinase K be titrated against positive controls to reduce the number of false positives and false negatives. Use only nuclease-free proteinase K because the presence of nucleases might lead to false-positive results.

7. Instead of proteinase K, a limited microwave digestion has been recommended *(28)*. Place the slide in a plastic jar containing 200 mL 0.1 *M* citrate buffer, pH 6.0. Microwave at 350 W for 5 min (from the In Situ Cell Death Detection Kit, Roche Diagnostics).

8. Fluorescent labels are easier to visualize and are easier to count automatically through computerized image analysis.

9. Apoptosis and necrosis can have overlapping features. TUNEL has been reported to be positive in necrosis. If it is essential to distinguish between apoptosis and necrosis, additional confirmation using other tools such as morphological analysis and PARP-1 cleavage are necessary.

References

1. Thornberry, N. A. and Lazebnik, Y. (1998) Caspases: enemies within. *Science* **281**, 1312–1316.

2. Trump, B. F., Berezesky, I. K., Chang, S. H., and Phelps, P. C. (1997) The pathways of cell death: oncosis, apoptosis, and necrosis. *Toxicol Pathol.* **25**, 82–88.

3. Thompson, C. B. (1995) Apoptosis in the pathogenesis and treatment of disease. *Science* **267**, 1456–1462.

4. Kroemer, G. (1995) The pharmacology of T cell apoptosis. *Adv Immunol.* **58**, 211–296.

5. Wertz, I. E. and Hanley, M. R. (1996) Diverse molecular provocation of programmed cell death. *Trends Biochem Sci.* **21**, 359–364.

6. Kroemer, G., Petit, P., Zamzami, N., Vayssiere, J. L., and Mignotte, B. (1995) The biochemistry of programmed cell death. *FASEB J.* **9**, 1277–1287.

7. McCarthy, N. J., Whyte, M. K., Gilbert, C. S., and Evan, G. I. (1997) Inhibition of Ced-3/ICE-related proteases does not prevent cell death induced by oncogenes, DNA damage, or the Bcl-2 homologue *Bak. J Cell Biol.* **136**, 215–227.

8. Hirsch, T., Marchetti, P., Susin, S. A., et al. (1997) The apoptosis-necrosis paradox. Apoptogenic proteases activated after mitochondrial permeability transition determine the mode of cell death. *Oncogene* **15**, 1573–1581.

9. Roach, H. I. and Clarke, N. M. (2000) Physiological cell death of chondrocytes in vivo is not confined to apoptosis. New observations on the mammalian growth plate. *J. Bone Joint Surg. Br.* **82,** 601–613.

10. Lazebnik, Y. A., Takahashi, A., Poirier, G. G., Kaufmann, S. H., and Earnshaw, W. C. (1995) Characterization of the execution phase of apoptosis in vitro using extracts from condemned-phase cells. *J. Cell Sci. Suppl.* **19,** 41–49.

11. Enari, M., Sakahira, H., Yokoyama, H., Okawa, K., Iwamatsu, A., and Nagata, S. (1998) A caspase-activated DNase that degrades DNA during apoptosis, and its inhibitor ICAD. *Nature* **391,** 43–50.

12. Gurtu, V., Kain, S. R., and Zhang, G. (1997) Fluorometric and colorimetric detection of caspase activity associated with apoptosis. *Anal. Biochem.* **251,** 98–102.

13. Kuhn, K., Hashimoto, S., and Lotz, M. (1999) Cell density modulates apoptosis in human articular chondrocytes. *J. Cell Physiol.* **180,** 439–447.

14. Waring, P., Lambert, D., Sjaarda, A., Hurne, A., and Beaver, J. (1999) Increased cell surface exposure of phosphatidylserine on propidium iodide negative thymocytes undergoing death by necrosis. *Cell Death Differ.* **6,** 624–637.

15. Lecoeur, H., Prevost, M. C., and Gougeon, M. L. (2001) Oncosis is associated with exposure of phosphatidylserine residues on the outside layer of the plasma membrane: a reconsideration of the specificity of the annexin V/propidium iodide assay. *Cytometry* **44,** 65–72.

16. Gavrieli, Y., Sherman, Y., and Ben Sasson, S. A. (1992) Identification of programmed cell death in situ via specific labeling of nuclear DNA fragmentation. *J. Cell Biol.* **119,** 493–501.

17. Grasl-Kraupp, B., Ruttkay-Nedecky, B., Koudelka, H., Bukowska, K., Bursch, W., and Schulte-Hermann, R. (1995) In situ detection of fragmented DNA (TUNEL assay) fails to discriminate among apoptosis, necrosis, and autolytic cell death: a cautionary note. *Hepatology* **21,** 1465–1468.

18. Charriaut-Marlangue, C. and Ben Ari, Y. (1995) A cautionary note on the use of the TUNEL stain to determine apoptosis. *Neuroreport* **7,** 61–64.

19. Yasuda, M., Umemura, S., Osamura, R. Y., Kenjo, T., and Tsutsumi, Y. (1995) Apoptotic cells in the human endometrium and placental villi: pitfalls in applying the TUNEL method. *Arch Histol. Cytol.* **58,** 185–190.

20. Pelletier, J. P., Jovanovic, D. V., Lascau-Coman, V., et al. (2000) Selective inhibition of inducible nitric oxide synthase reduces progression of experimental osteoarthritis in vivo: possible link with the reduction in chondrocyte apoptosis and caspase 3 level. *Arthritis Rheum.* **43,** 1290–1299.

21. Tew, S. R., Kwan, A. P., Hann, A., Thomson, B. M., and Archer, C. W. (2000) The reactions of articular cartilage to experimental wounding: role of apoptosis. *Arthritis Rheum.* **43,** 215–225.

22. Loening, A. M., James, I. E., Levenston, M. E., et al. (2000) Injurious mechanical compression of bovine articular cartilage induces chondrocyte apoptosis. *Arch Biochem Biophys.* **381,** 205–212.

23. Chen, C. T., Burton-Wurster, N., Borden, C., Hueffer, K., Bloom, S. E., and Lust, G. (2001) Chondrocyte necrosis and apoptosis in impact damaged articular cartilage. *J. Orthop. Res.* **19,** 703–711.

24. D'Lima, D. D., Hashimoto, S., Chen, P. C., Colwell, C. W. Jr., and Lotz, M. K. (2001) Human chondrocyte apoptosis in response to mechanical injury. *Osteoarthritis Cartilage* **9,** 712–719.

25. D'Lima, D. D., Hashimoto, S., Chen, P. C., Lotz, M., and Colwell Jr, C. W. (2001) In vitro and in vivo models of cartilage injury. *J. Bone Joint Surg. Am.* **83-A (Suppl. 2),** 22–24.

26. Colwell, C. W., D'Lima, D. D., Hoenecke, H., et al. (2001) In vivo changes after mechanical injury. *Clin Orthop.* **391(Suppl),** S116–S123.

27. Kim, H. T., Lo, M. Y., and Pillarisetty, R. (2002) Chondrocyte apoptosis following intraarticular fracture in humans. *Osteoarthritis Cartilage* **10,** 747–749.

28. Roach, H. I. and Clarke, N. M. (1999) "Cell paralysis" as an intermediate stage in the programmed cell death of epiphyseal chondrocytes during development. *J. Bone Miner. Res.* **14,** 1367–1378.

Expression, Activity, and Regulation of MAP Kinases in Cultured Chondrocytes

Jang-Soo Chun

Summary

The mitogen-activated protein (MAP) kinase family consists of extracellular signal-regulated protein kinase (ERK), p38 kinase, and c-Jun N-terminal kinase (JNK) and transduces signals from the extracellular environment to the cytoplasm and nucleus. MAP kinase signaling involves a multistep kinase cascade including MAP kinase kinase kinase (MAPKKK), MAP kinase kinase (MAPKK), and MAP kinase. The MAP kinase subtypes are constitutively expressed in articular chondrocytes and they regulate chondrocyte function, including differentiation, apoptosis, inflammatory responses, and activation of matrix metalloproteinases. Therefore, imbalance or destruction of homeostasis regulating MAP kinase activity is related to the pathogenesis of cartilage diseases such as osteoarthritis. This chapter describes methods for measuring and modulating MAP kinase subtype activity in primary cultured articular chondrocytes and cartilage explants.

Key Words: Chondrocyte; cartilage; osteoarthritis; cyclooxygenase; MAP kinase; ERK; JNK; p38; IL-1β; nitric oxide; PGE$_2$; protein kinase C; apoptosis; differentiation; inflammation; matrix metalloproteinase.

1. Introduction

The mitogen-activated protein (MAP) kinase family regulates a variety of cellular responses by conveying information from the extracellular environment to the cytoplasm and nucleus *(1–4)*. These enzymes occupy one level of three-step kinase cascades that have been conserved during evolution in many organisms **(Fig. 1)**. Upon activation by an upstream component such as small G proteins, MAP kinase kinase kinase (MAPKKK), a dual-specificity kinase, phosphorylates and activates MAP kinase kinase (MAPKK), which in turn phosphorylates threonine and tyrosine on MAP kinase, resulting in MAP kinase activation. The mammalian extracellular signal-regulated protein kinase

From: *Methods in Molecular Medicine, Vol. 100: Cartilage and Osteoarthritis, Vol. 1: Cellular and Molecular Tools*
Edited by: M. Sabatini, P. Pastoureau, and F. De Ceuninck © Humana Press Inc., Totowa, NJ

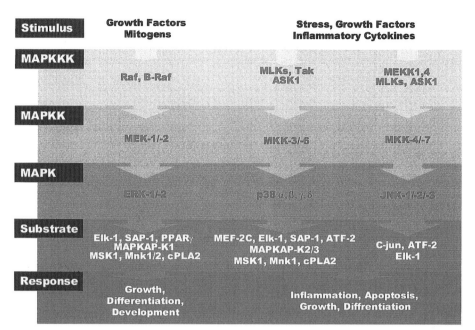

Fig. 1. Mammalian MAP kinase pathways. ASK1, apoptosis signaling-regulating kinase 1; ATF, activated transcription factor; CPLA2, cytosolic phospholipase A2; ELK-1, transcription factor; ERK, extracellular signal-regulated protein kinase; JNK, c-Jun N-terminal kinase; MAPK, mitogen-activated protein kinase; MAPKAP-K1, MAPK-activated protein kinase-1; MEF-2C, mouse embryonic fibroblast-2C; MEKK1,4, MAPK/ERK kinase kinase 1; MKK, MAP kinase kinase; MLK, mixed lineage kinases; Mnk1/2, MAPK-interacting kinase 1/2; MSK1, mitogen and stress-activated protein kinase; PPARγ, peroxisome proliferator-activated receptor γ; SAP-1, shrimp alkaline phosphatase stomach-associated PTP1.

(ERK) consists of ERK-1 (44 kDa) and ERK–2 (42 kDa), the p38 kinase family consists of four members– (p38α, p38β, p38γ, and p38δ), and the c-Jun N-terminal kinase (JNK) family consists of three members, JNK-1 (46 kDa), JNK-2 (54 kDa) and JNK-3 (55 kDa). Among the MAP kinase subtypes, ERK generally regulates growth and differentiation of cells, whereas JNK and p38 kinase subtypes mediate stress responses *(3–5)*.

MAP kinase subtypes are constitutively expressed in most cell types, including chondrocytes, and changes in MAP kinase activity affect a variety of cellular responses. In articular chondrocytes, it has been shown that MAP kinases regulate differentiation, apoptosis, inflammatory responses, and activation of matrix metalloproteinases *(5–10)*. For example, nitric oxide (NO) from the NO donor sodium nitroprusside (SNP) acts via MAP kinases to regulate apoptosis, dedif-

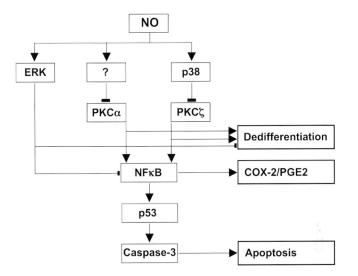

Fig. 2. Signaling pathways involved in nitric oxide (NO)-induced apoptosis, cyclo-oxygenase-2 (COX-2) expression, and dedifferentiation in articular chondrocytes.ERK, eletracellular signal-regulated protein kinase; NFκB; nuclear factor κB; PKC; protein kinase C.

ferentiation, and cyclooxygenases-2 (COX-2) expression in primary articular chondrocytes (**Fig. 2**). However, this regulation can be complex since NO-induced ERK activation induces dedifferentiation and inhibits apoptosis, whereas NO-induced p38 kinase activation induces apoptosis and maintains differentiated phenotypes. In addition to affecting MAP kinase activity, NO inhibits protein kinase C (PKC)α and -ζ activity. Inhibition of PKCα activity is owing to reduced expression, which is independent of MAP kinase signaling, whereas PKCζ activity is blocked as a result of p38 kinase activation. NO-induced activation of p38 kinase also activates nuclear factor (NF)-κB in a manner dependent on MAP kinases and PKC. NO-induced NF-κB activation leads to apoptosis via p53 and COX-2 expression, whereas dedifferentiation is independent of NF-κB signaling.

The primary aim of this chapter is to describe methods for measuring and modulating MAP kinase subtypes, activity in primary cultured chondrocytes.

2. Materials

1. Growth plate chondrocytes from 2-wk-old rabbit knee joint.
2. Recombinant human interleukin (IL)-1β.
3. Dulbecco's modified Eagle's medium (DMEM), fetal bovine-calf serum, streptomycin, and penicillin for cell culture (Gibco-BRL, Gaithersburg, MD).

4. Collagenase type II (381 U/mg solid; Sigma).
5. Antibodies against ERK, p38 kinase, and JNK (New England Biolabs, Beverly, MA).
6. Antibodies against phosphorylated forms of ERK, p38 kinase, and JNK (New England Biolabs).
7. Antibodies against phosphorylated forms of Elk, activating transcription factor-2 (ATF-2), and c-Jun (New England Biolabs).
8. Recombinant ATF-2, Elk, and c-Jun (New England Biolabs).
9. Peroxidase-conjugated secondary antibody (any supplier).
10. Rhodamine- or fluorescein-conjugated secondary antibody (any supplier).
11. Enhanced chemiluminescence reagents (ECL).
12. Protein A/G-sepharose beads (Pierce, Rockford, IL).
13. Lysis buffer A (for Western blot analysis): 50 mM Tris-HCl, pH 7.4, 150 mM NaCl, 1% Nonidet P-40, and 0.1% sodium dodecyl sulfate (SDS), supplemented with protease inhibitors (10 µg/mL leupeptin, 10 µg/mL pepstatin A, 10 µg/mL aprotinin, and 1 mM 4-[2-aminoethyl] benzenesulfonyl fluoride) and phosphatase inhibitors (1 mM NaF and 1 mM Na$_3$VO$_4$). Prepare fresh lysis buffer from concentrated stock solutions of 2 M Tris-HCl, 5 M NaCl, 10% SDS and 1000X protease and phosphatase inhibitors.
14. Lysis buffer B (for immune-complex kinase assay): 20 mM Tris-HCl, pH 7.5, 150 mM NaCl, 1 mM EDTA, 1 mM EGTA, 1% Triton X-100, 2.5 mM sodium pyrophosphate, and 1 mM β-glycerophosphate, plus inhibitors of proteases and phosphatases as in buffer A. Prepare fresh lysis buffer from concentrated stock solutions of 2 M Tris-HCl, 5 M NaCl, 0.5 M EDTA, 80 mM EGTA, 250 mM sodium pyrophosphate, 100 mM β-glycerophosphate, and 1000X protease and phosphatase inhibitors.
15. Kinase assay buffer: 25 mM Tris-HCl, pH 7.5, 5 mM β-glycerophosphate, 2 mM dithiothreitol (DTT), 0.1 mM sodium orthovanadate, and 10 mM MgCl$_2$. Prepare from concentrated stock solutions of 2 M Tris-HCl, 0.5 M MgCl$_2$, 1 M DTT, and 1 M sodium orthovanadate.
16. [γ-^{32}P]ATP.
17. Immunohistochemical staining kit (AEC chromogenic substrate-streptavidin-peroxidase system; DAKO, cat. no. K 0672).
18. Mammalian expression vector for dominant-negative and constitutively active MAP kinase subtypes.
19. LipofectaminePLUS (Gibco-BRL).
20. Standard minigel apparatus.
21. Gel transfer apparatus.
22. Standard fluorescence microscope.
23. Pharmacological inhibitors such as PD98059, SB203580, SB202190, and SP600125 can be obtained from Calbiochem (Darmstadt, Germany), Biomol (Plymouth Meeting, PA), Cell Signaling (Beverly, MA), Promega (Madison, WI), A.G. Scientific (San Diego, CA), Alexis Biochemicals (Montreal, Canada), Sigma (St. Louis, MO), and other supplies.

3. Methods

The methods below detail the culturing of primary articular chondrocytes, measurement of MAP kinase activity, and modulation of MAP kinase activities using genetic tools and pharmacological inhibitors.

3.1. Primary Culture of Articular Chondrocytes

Articular chondrocytes can be obtained from human osteoarthritic joint cartilage of patients undergoing total knee arthroplasty, or from 2-wk-old or 3-mo-old New Zealand white rabbit knee joint articular cartilage. Here we briefly describe procedures for the isolation and culture of growth plate articular chondrocytes (Detailed procedures for primary culture of chondrocytes are provided in Chaps. 1, 14, and 15).

1. Digest enzymatically cartilage slices from 2-wk-old rabbits for 6 h in 0.2% collagenase type II in DMEM, and obtain single cells by collecting the supernatant after brief centrifugation.
2. Resuspend cells in DMEM supplemented with 10% (v/v) fetal calf serum, 50 µg/mL streptomycin, and 50 U/mL penicillin.
3. Plate the cells on culture dishes at a density of 5×10^4 cells/cm^2.
4. Change the medium every 1.5 d after seeding; cells are confluent by d 4 or 5.
5. Confluent primary cultures can be subcultured by plating cells at a density of 5×10^4 cells/cm^2 *(10,11)*.

3.2. Assay of MAP Kinase Activity

Activation of chondrocyte MAP kinase subtypes following exposure to extracellular stimuli such as IL-1β and tumor necrosis factor-α can be determined by detecting phosphorylated (hence activated) MAP kinase subtypes using Western blot analysis. Kinase activity can be directly measured using an *in vitro* immune complex kinase assay. Although there are many commercially available kits, the methods below outline standard procedures for determining MAP kinase activity in primary articular chondrocytes treated with IL-1β (1–5 ng/mL).

3.2.1. Assay of MAP Kinase Phosphorylation by Western Blot Analysis

MAP kinase subtypes are activated by dual phosphorylation on conserved threonine and tyrosine residues. The development of commercially available antibodies that specifically recognize dually phosphorylated MAP kinase subtypes makes it possible to detect activated MAP kinase subtypes by Western blot analysis (*see* **Notes 1** and **2**).

1. Incubate confluent primary chondrocytes (35- or 60-mm dishes) with activating agent (e.g., 5 ng/mL IL-1β) for the desired time.

2. Wash cells twice with ice-cold phosphate-buffered saline (PBS), add ice-cold lysis buffer A (150 or 300 µL for 35- or 60-mm dishes, respectively), harvest cells by scraping, and place suspension in a 1.5-mL microcentrifuge tube.

3. Incubate on ice for 30 min with occasional vortexing, pellet cellular debris by microcentrifugation for 10 min at 4°C (10,000*g*), and collect supernatant (total cell lysate). In general, up to 150 and 300 µg of supernatant protein can be obtained from 80–90% confluent chondrocytes on 35- and 60-mm dishes, respectively.

4. Separate proteins (30 µg/lane) by standard 8% SDS-polyacrylamide gel electrophoresis (SDS-PAGE) using a minigel apparatus, and transfer to a nitrocellulose membrane.

5. After blocking the nitrocellulose sheet with 3% nonfat dry milk in Tris-buffered saline, incubate the membrane with 1 µg/mL of primary antibody (i.e., anti-p-ERK, anti-p-p38 kinase, or anti-p-JNK antibodies) overnight at 4°C.

6. Develop membrane using a peroxidase-conjugated secondary antibody and the ECL system (*see* **Fig. 3**).

3.2.2. Assay of MAP Kinase Activity by In Vitro Kinase Assay

The steps below outline the procedure for immunoprecipitation of MAP kinase subtypes and determination of their activity by immune complex kinase assay (*see* **Notes 3** and **4**).

1. Treat subconfluent primary chondrocytes with stimulating agents (e.g., 5 ng/mL IL-1β) for the desired time. Two 60-mm dishes per treatment will provide a sufficient amount of protein (600 µg) for immunoprecipitation.

2. Wash cells twice with ice-cold PBS, add lysis buffer B, scrape cells from plate, and transfer suspension to a 1.5-mL microcentrifuge tube. Incubate suspension on ice for 30 min with occasional vortexing, pellet cellular debris by microcentrifugation for 10 min at 4°C (10,000*g*), and collect supernatant for immunoprecipitation. Using lysis buffer B, adjust protein concentration and volume to approx 300–600 µg/600 µL.

3. Add 25 µL Protein A/Protein G-sepharose slurry and 1 µg antibody against ERK, p38, kinase or JNK, and rock overnight at 4°C.

4. Pellet immune complexes by microcentrifugation for 2 min at 4°C (10,000*g* or maximum speed in general microfuge).

5. Remove supernatant, wash pellets with lysis buffer B, and resuspend on ice in 20 µL kinase assay buffer.

6. Start kinase reactions by adding 1 µg (1 µL) of recombinant substrate (Elk for ERK, ATF-2 for p38 kinase, and c-Jun for JNK) and 10 µCi (1 µL) [γ-^{32}P]ATP (*see* **Note 3**).

7. Incubate for 30 min at 30°C, then stop the reaction by adding 4X Laemmli's sample buffer, and boil for 3 min.

8. Resolve proteins using 10% SDS-PAGE, and detect phosphorylation of substrate by autoradiography (*see* **Fig. 4**).

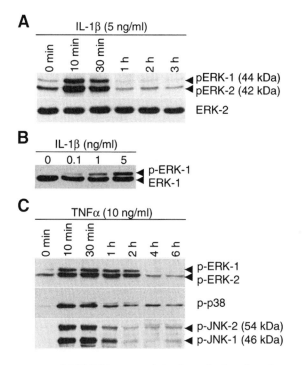

Fig. 3. Measurement of MAP kinase activity in articular chondrocytes using Western blot analysis. (**A**) Primary articular chondrocytes were treated with 5 ng/mL interleukin-1β (IL-1β) for the indicated times. Levels of phosphorylated extracellular singal-regulated protein kinase (ERK)-1 and -2 were determined by Western blotting using antibodies that specifically recognize phosphorylated ERK. The same samples were run in parallel and used to determine ERK-2 as a control. (**B**) Chondrocytes were treated with the indicated concentrations of IL-1β for 30 min. Total cell lysates were separated by 10% SDS-PAGE, and ERK-1 was detected by Western blot analysis. Phosphorylated ERK-1 was identified by its slower mobility. (**C**) Human HTB-94 chondrosarcoma cells were treated with 10 ng/mL of tumor necrosis factor-α (TNF-α) for the indicated time periods. Phosphorylation of ERK, p38 kinase, and c-Jun N-Terminal kinase (JNK) was determined by Western blotting using antibodies that specifically recognize phosphorylated MAP kinase subtypes.

3.2.3. Assay of MAP Kinase Activation by Immunohistochemistry and Immunofluorescence Microscopy

It is often not possible to obtain sufficient amounts of protein from osteoarthritic cartilage for biochemical analysis. The methods below outline the procedure for assaying MAP kinase subtypes in osteoarthritic cartilage or cartilage explants by immunohistochemistry and immunofluorescence microscopy.

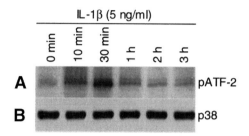

Fig. 4. Measurement of MAP kinase activity in articular chondrocytes using the immune complex kinase assay. Primary articular chondrocytes were treated with 5 ng/mL interleukin-1β (IL-1β) for the indicated times. **(A)** p38α kinase activity was determined by immunoprecipitation and in vitro kinase assay using activated transcription factor-2 (ATF-2) as substrate, followed by SDS-PAGE and autoradiography. **(B)** p38α kinase protein level (p38) was determined by Western blotting using a specific antibody.

3.2.3.1. Immunohistochemical Assay

1. The types of samples suitable for this assay include cartilage explants (~125 mm³) organ cultured in DMEM for 48 h in the absence or presence of 5 ng/mL IL-1β, human osteoarthritic joint cartilage obtained from patients undergoing total knee arthroplasty, and cartilage from experimental rheumatoid arthritic joints of 12-wk-old male DBA/1 mice *(12)*.
2. Fix samples in 4% paraformaldehyde in PBS at 4°C overnight, and then wash with PBS.
3. Dehydrate samples with graded ethanol (once in 30, 50, 70, 80, 90, and 95%, and, then twice in 100%, each for 15 min), embed in paraffin, and cut 4-µm sections using standard protocols.
4. Deparaffinate sections with xylene, and rehydrate with graded ethanol.
5. Incubate sections overnight at 4°C with antibodies (1 µg/mL) against p-ERK, p-p38, kinase or p-JNK.
6. Wash with PBS (three times), and visualize MAP kinase by using a secondary antibody and the AEC substrate-streptavidin-peroxidase kit (DAKO) following the manufacturer's instructions.

3.2.3.2. Immunofluorescence Microscopy

1. Expression and distribution of phosphorylated MAP kinase subtypes can also be determined by indirect immunofluorescence microscopy using cartilage explants, arthritic joint cartilage, and articular chondrocytes in primary culture.
2. To do this, cartilage tissue should be cryosectioned instead of paraffin embedded for better detection of MAP kinase subtypes. Articular chondrocytes should be cultured on round cover slips (12 mm, Bellco Glass, Vineland, NJ).

Normal **OA**

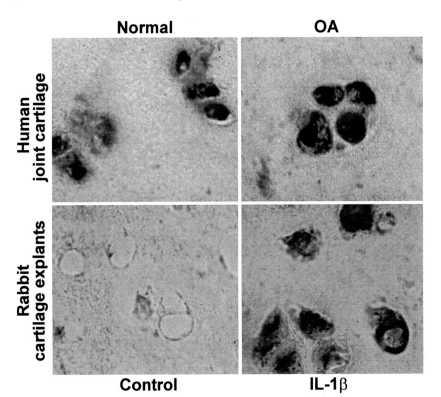

Control **IL-1β**

Fig. 5. Immunohistochemical detection of cyclooxygenase-2 in osteoarthritic (OA) cartilage and cartilage explants treated with IL-1β. Cyclooxygenase-2 protein was detected from undamaged part of (OA) cartilage (normal) and OA human joint cartilage (upper panels) and rabbit cartilage explants untreated (control) or treated with 5 ng/mL interleukin-1β (IL-1β) for 72 h (lower panels). Tissue sections from explants were counterstained with hematoxylin.

3. Fix chondrocytes on cover slips (or cryosections) in 4% paraformaldehyde in PBS containing 10% fetal calf serum at 4°C for 10 min and wash (four times) with PBS.
4. Incubate cover slip for 1 h with primary antibody (1 μg/mL). After washing (four times) with PBS, incubate with rhodamine- or fluorescein-conjugated secondary antibodies (2 μg/mL) for 30 min, and observe under a standard fluorescence microscope (**Fig. 5**).

3.3. Modulation of MAP Kinase Activation

Modulating MAP kinase activity allows for study of the role of MAP kinases in chondrocyte functions. Described in this subheading are pharmacological and genetic tools that can be used to modulate MAP kinase activity.

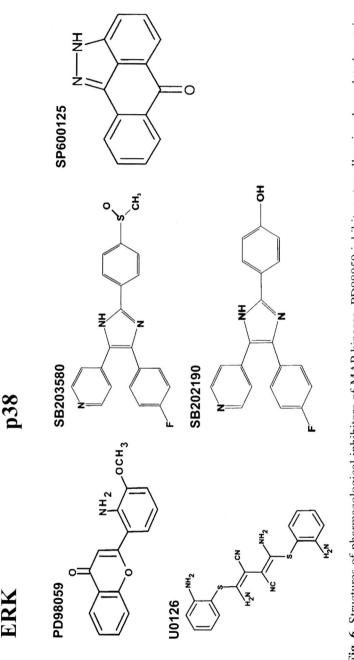

Fig. 6. Structures of pharmacological inhibitors of MAP kinases. PD98059 inhibits extracellular signal-regulated protein kinase (ERK) activation by preventing MEK-1 activation. U0126 is a highly selective inhibitor of MEK-1 and -2. SB203580 and SB202190 inhibit p38α and p38β kinase activity. SP600125 blocks activation of c-Jun N-Terminal kinase (JNK)-1, JNK-2, and JNK-3.

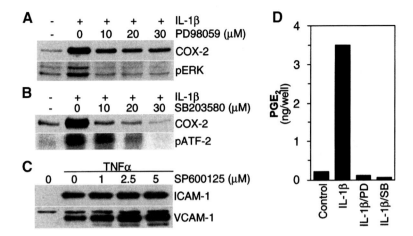

Fig. 7. Inhibition of extracellular signal-regulated protein kinase (ERK), p38 kinase, and JNK by specific chemical inhibitors. **(A,B)**, Primary articular chondrocytes or **(C)** HTB-94 chondrosarcoma cells were treated with the indicated concentrations of **(A)** PD98059 (PD), **(B)** SB203580 (SB), and **(C)**, SP600125 for 1 h and then incubated with 5 ng/mL interleukin-1β (IL-1β) or 10 ng/mL tumor necrosis factor-α (TNF-α) for 12 h. Phosphorylation of ERK and expression of cyclooxygenase-2 (COX-2), vascular cell adhesion molecule (VCAM)-1, and intercellular adhesion molecule-1 (ICAM-1) were determined by Western blot analysis. p38 kinase activity was determined by immune complex kinase assay. **(D)** Prostaglandin E^2 (PGE_2) synthesis was determined by using an assay kit (Amersham Pharmacia Biotech). AFT-2, activated transcription factor-2; PD, PD98059, a MEK-1/2 inhibitor; SB, SB203580, a p38 kinase inhibitor; SP600125, a JNK inhibitor.

3.3.1. ERK Inhibitors

1. *PD98059* (**Fig. 6**) is a flavone compound that binds to the inactive form of MAP kinase kinase (MEK-1), preventing its activation *(13)*. PD98059 appears to stabilize the inactive form of MEK-1, and, unlike inhibitors of other MAP kinases, does not compete for ATP binding sites. PD98059 is 5–10-fold less effective on MEK-2, which is 90% identical in amino acid sequence to MEK-1. It does not block related kinases such as MEK-3, MEK-4, ERK-1, or ERK-2, nor is it known to inhibit other kinases *(13)*. In primary articular chondrocytes, IL-1β activates ERK-1 and -2, and pretreatment with PD98059 prevents ERK activation. Inhibition of ERK with PD98059 partially blocks oxygenase COX-2 expression **(Fig. 7A)** but completely prevents its activity **(Fig. 7D)**.
2. *U0126* is also a highly selective inhibitor of MEK-1 and -2. U0126 shows a significantly higher affinity for MEK-1 compared with PD98059, and PD98059 and U0126 share a common binding site *(14)*.

3.3.2. p38 Kinase Inhibitors

The mammalian p38 kinase family consists of four members, p38α, p38β, p38γ, and p38δ. *SB203580* and *SB202190* (**Fig. 6**) are the most commonly used inhibitors of p38 kinase. They are pyridinyl imidazoles that inhibit p38α and p38β but not other kinases such as p38γ, p38δ, ERK, JNK, or MEK *(15,16)*. These compounds inhibit p38 kinase by binding to the ATP binding site. SB203580 and SB202190 are also effective in treating inflammatory disease such as rheumatoid arthritis. IL-1β-stimulated p38α kinase activity and COX-2 expression and activity were inhibited by *SB203580* pretreatment in primary articular chondrocytes (**Fig. 7B,D**).

3.3.3. JNK Inhibitors

Although the mammalian JNK family consists of three members, JNK-1, JNK-2, and JNK-3, splice variants result in a total of 10 isoforms. *SP600125* (**Fig. 6**) (1,9-pyrazoloanthrone) is a potent, cell-permeable, reversible inhibitor of all JNK family members. SP600125 competes with ATP binding and exhibits over 300-fold higher selectivity for JNK compared with ERK and p38 kinase *(17)*. Recently, a cell-permeable peptide inhibitor of JNK, BC-095 (Kamiya Biomedical, Seattle, WA), has been developed, which blocks interaction of JNK with its substrate, rather than competing with the ATP-binding site *(18)*. In the HTB-94 chondrosarcoma cell line, inhibition of JNK with *SP600125* blocked tumor necrosis factor-α-induced vascular cell adhesion molecule-1 expression (**Fig. 7C**), whereas modulation of other MAP kinase subtypes had no effect.

3.3.4. Genetic Approaches

Although chemical inhibitors are useful for dissecting the roles of MAP kinases in signaling pathways, they inevitably cause undesired side effects. The use of dominant negative or constitutively active mutants of MAP kinase subtypes is an alternative and possibly more physiological way to modulate MAP kinase activities. For example, mutating Lys[71] and Lys[52] to Arg in ERK-1 and -2, respectively, generates dominant negative kinase forms *(19)*. Replacement of Thr[180] and Tyr[182] with Ala and Phe, respectively, creates a dominant-negative p38α kinase, whereas, Lys[55] to Arg substitution generates a dominant-negative JNK-3 *(20)*. MAP kinase subtypes can also be constitutively activated by the expression of mutant upstream kinases. For example, substituting Ser[189] and Thr[193] for Glu in MAP kinase kinase (MKK3) and substituting Ser[207] and Thr[211] for Glu in MKK6 constitutively activate p38 kinase *(21)*.

Infection of primary chondrocytes with adenovirus or retrovirus carrying mutant MAP kinase cDNA resulted in approx 80% of cells overexpressing mutant. Although lipid-based transfection methods are less efficient, still more

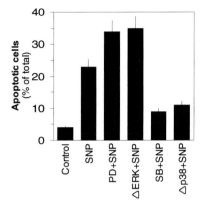

Fig. 8. Modulation of apoptosis by dominant negative mutants of ERK and p38α kinase. Primary culture articular chondrocytes were untreated or treated for 30 min with 20 μ*M* PD98059 (PD) or 20 μ*M* SB203580 (SB). Alternatively, chondrocytes were transfected with dominant-negative extracellular signal-regulated protein kinase (ERK)-2 (ΔERK) or p38α kinase (Δp38) and cultured in complete medium for 24 h. Cells were then treated for 24 h with 1 m*M* sodium nitroprusside (SNP), a nitric oxide (NO) donor that causes apoptosis in chondrocytes. Apoptotic cells were determined by FACS sorting. Treatment with PD98059 or expression of dominant-negative ERK-2 prevented NO-induced ERK activation (data not shown), whereas treatment with SB203580 or expression of dominant-negative p38α kinase blocked NO-induced p38α kinase activation (data not shown).

than 30% of cells can be transfected and MAP kinase activities modulated *(7–12)*. The method below outlines a procedure for transfecting chondrocytes with mammalian expression vectors (*see* **Fig. 8**).

1. Seed chondrocytes at a density of 5×10^4 cells/cm^2 on 35- or 60-mm dishes.
2. When cells are 50–60% confluent (d 3), transfect them with the expression vector using the Lipofectamine reagent (Gibco-BRL) following the procedure recommended by the manufacturer. We found the best transfection efficiency in chondrocytes when using 2 μg vector, 6 μL PLUS reagent, 100 μL dilution medium, 4 μL Lipofectamine reagent, and 0.8 mL serum-free transfection medium in 1 mL transfection volume (35-mm dish).
3. Incubate at 37°C for 4 h, and then replace transfection medium with serum-containing complete culture medium.
4. Culture cells for an additional 36 h prior to assaying the effects of mutant MAP kinase overexpression.

4. Notes

1. Commercially available antibodies against phosphorylated MAP kinase subtypes efficiently recognize human p-ERK, p-p38 kinase, and p-JNK. Of the commercial

antibodies raised against MAP kinases, we found that anti-p-ERK antibodies work well in rabbit cells, but antibodies against p-p38 kinase and p-JNK are not so effective. To detect rabbit p-p38 kinase and p-JNK, it is best to use more lysate (up to 50 µg), higher antibody concentration, and longer exposure time during ECL.

2. ERK phosphorylation (i.e., activation) reduces mobility in SDS-PAGE gels. Therefore, Western blotting using anti-ERK antibody following 10% SDS-PAGE separation of proteins can distinguish phosphorylated and unphosphorylated ERK (*see* **Fig. 3B**). However, it is not so easy to detect shifts in phosphorylated p38 kinase and JNK.

3. An alternative method, avoiding the use of radioisotopes, is to detect phosphorylation of MAP kinase substrates by Western blot analysis. To do this, the in vitro kinase reaction is performed using "cold" ATP. Following electrophoresis and transfer of proteins to nitrocellulose membrane, phosphorylated substrate can be detected by Western blotting using antibodies against phosphorylated ATF-2, Elk, or c-Jun.

4. Here we described, the use of Elk, ATF-2, and c-Jun as substrates in immune complex kinase assays. There are other substrates for each MAP kinase subtype such as myelin basic protein, which can be phosphorylated by each subtype.

Acknowledgments

This work was supported by the National Research Laboratory Program (M1-0104-00-0064) of the Korea Ministry of Science and Technology.

References

1. Johnson, G. L. and Lapadat, R. (2002) Mitogen-activated protein kinase pathways mediated by ERK, JNK, and p38 protein kinases. *Science* **298,** 1911–1912.
2. Schaeffer, H. J. and Weber, M. J. (1999) Mitogen-activated protein kinases: specific messages from ubiquitous messengers. *Mol. Cell. Biol.* **19,** 2435–2444.
3. Garrington, T. P. and Johnson, G. L. (1999) Organization and regulation of mitogen-activated protein kinase signaling pathways. *Curr. Opin. Cell. Biol.* **11,** 211–218.
4. Weston, C. R. and Davis R. J. (2002) The JNK signal transduction pathway. *Curr. Opin. Genet. Dev.* **12,** 14–21.
5. Kim, S.-J., Ju, J.-W., Oh, C.-D., et al.(2002) ERK-1/2 and p38 kinase oppositely regulate nitric oxide-induced apoptosis of chondrocytes in association with p53, caspase-3, and differentiation status. *J. Biol. Chem.* **277,** 1332–1339.
6. Kim, S.-J., Hwang, S.-G., Shin, D.-Y., Kang, S.-S., and Chun, J.-S. (2002) p38 kinase regulates nitric oxide-induced apoptosis of articular chondrocytes by accumulating p53 via NFκ B-dependent transcription and stabilization by serine 15 phosphorylation. *J. Biol. Chem.* **277,** 33,501—33,508.
7. Kim, S.-J., Kim, H.-G., Oh, C.-D., et al.(2002) p38 kinase-dependent and -independent inhibition of protein kinase C-ζ and -α regulates nitric oxide-induced apoptosis and dedifferentiation of articular chondrocytes. *J. Biol. Chem.* **277,** 30,375—30,381.

8. Yoon, Y.-M., Kim, S.-J., Oh, C.-D., et al. (2002) Maintenance of differentiated phenotype of articular chondrocytes by protein kinase C and extracellular signal-regulated protein kinase. *J. Biol. Chem.* **277,** 8412–8420.

9. Kim, S.-J. and Chun, J.-S. (2003) Protein kinase Cα and ζ regulate nitric oxide-induced NFκB activation that mediates cyclooxygenase-2 expression and apoptosis but not dedifferentiation in articular chondrocytes. *Biochem. Biophys. Res. Commun.* **303,** 206–211.

10. Yoon, Y.-M., Kim, S.-J., Oh, C.-D., et al. (2002) Maintenance of differentiated phenotype of articular chondrocytes by protein kinase C and extracellular signal-regulated protein kinase. *J. Biol. Chem.* **277,** 8412–8420.

11. Ryu, J.-H., Kim, S.-J., Kim, S.-H., et al. (2002) β-Catenin regulation of the chondrocyte phenotypes. *Development* **129,** 5541–5550.

12. Kim, S.-J., Lim, D.-S., Kim, S.-H., et al. (2002) β-Catenin regulates expression of cyclooxygenase-2 in articular chondrocytes. *Biochem. Biophys. Res. Commun.* **296,** 221–226.

13. Alessi, D. R., Cuenda, A., Cohen, P., Dudley, D. T., and Saltiel A. R. (1995) PD098059 is a specific inhibitor of the activation of mitogen-activated protein kinase kinase in vitro and in vivo. *J. Biol. Chem.* **270,** 27,489–27,494.

14. Favata, M. F., Horiuchi, K. Y., Manos, E. J., et al. (1998) Identification of a novel inhibitor of mitogen-activated protein kinase kinase. *J. Biol. Chem.* **273,** 18,623–18,632.

15. Jiang, Y., Chen, C., Li, Z., et al. (1996) Characterization of the structure and function of a new mitogen-activated protein kinase (p38β). *J. Biol. Chem.* **271,** 17,920–17,926.

16. Cuenda, A., Rouse, J., Doza, Y. N., et al. (1995) SB 203580 is a specific inhibitor of a MAP kinase homologue which is stimulated by cellular stresses and interleukin-1. *FEBS Lett.* **364,** 229–233.

17. Bennett, B. L., Sasaki, D. T., Murray, B. W., et al. (2001) SP600125, an anthrapyrazolone inhibitor of Jun N-terminal kinase. *Proc. Natl. Acad. Sci. USA* **98,** 13,681–13,686.

18. Bonny, C., Oberson, A., Negri, S., Sauser, C., and Schorderet, D. F. (2001) Cell-permeable peptide inhibitors of JNK: novel blockers of beta-cell death. *Diabetes* **50,** 77–82.

19. Robbins, D. J., Zhen, E., Owaki, H., et al. (1993) Regulation and properties of extracellular signal-regulated protein kinases 1 and 2 in vitro. *J. Biol. Chem.* **268,** 5097–5106.

20. Raingeaud, J., Gupta, S., Rogers, J. S., et al. (1995) Pro-inflammatory cytokines and environmental stress cause p38 mitogen-activated protein kinase activation by dual phosphorylation on tyrosine and threonine. *J. Biol. Chem.* **270,** 7420–7426.

21. Raingeaud, J., Whitmarsh, A. J., Barrett, T., Derijard, B., and Davis, R. J. (1996) MKK3- and MKK6-regulated gene expression is mediated by the p38 mitogen-activated protein kinase signal transduction pathway. *Mol. Cell. Biol.* **16,** 1247–1255.

21

Mechanical Loading of Chondrocytes Embedded in 3D Constructs

In Vitro Methods for Assessment of Morphological and Metabolic Response to Compressive Strain

David A. Lee and Martin M. Knight

Summary

Mechanical loading of chondrocytes in 3D constructs has been used to investigate mechanotransduction and its potential for stimulating tissue-engineered cartilage repair. This chapter describes the preparation of 3D agarose or alginate constructs seeded with isolated chondrocytes and specific test rigs for applying gross compressive strain to individual constructs on a confocal microscope or for longer term compression of constructs cultured within an incubator. Experimental methods are described to quantify the level of cell deformation and the elaboration of extracellular matrix. The chapter thus provides an introduction to the experimental techniques used to examine chondrocyte mechanotransduction and downstream cell function.

Key Words: Agarose; bioreactor; cartilage; cell deformation; cell mechanics; cell proliferation; chondrocyte; confocal microscopy; extracellular matrix; mechanical compression; mechanotransduction; proteoglycan synthesis; sulphate incorporation; thymidine incorporation.

1. Introduction

During normal activity, the articular cartilage of the major load-bearing joints is exposed to a complex array of compressive, tensile, and shear forces. It is well known that this mechanical environment is essential for the health and homeostasis of the tissue. Previous studies have reported that whereas static compression of cartilage causes a downregulation of matrix synthesis, cyclic compression causes a frequency-dependent upregulation *(1,2)*. Consequently it has been suggested that mechanical conditioning may be applied within a

From: *Methods in Molecular Medicine, Vol. 100: Cartilage and Osteoarthritis, Vol. 1: Cellular and Molecular Tools*
Edited by: M. Sabatini, P. Pastoureau, and F. De Ceuninck © Humana Press Inc., Totowa, NJ

tissue engineering context to stimulate in vitro biosynthesis by cells within three-dimensional (3D) scaffolds prior to implantation *(3–5)*. However, the intracellular mechanotransduction pathways through which chondrocytes are able to sense and respond to mechanical loading remain unclear both for chondrocytes in cartilage matrix and for isolated cells in 3D tissue-engineered scaffolds. Potential primary signaling events include cell deformation, fluid flow, hydrostatic pressure, and factors associated with compression of a charged extracellular matrix such as electrical streaming potentials and changes in pH and osmolarity *(6–8)*.

Numerous previous studies have examined chondrocyte mechanotransduction using a well-characterized experimental system consisting of isolated chondrocytes embedded within agarose hydrogel. This in vitro model system maintains chondrocytic phenotype over extended culture periods *(9–11)* while enabling the application of cell deformation through gross compression of the cell-agarose construct *(12,13)*. The model system therefore enables the role of cell deformation in cartilage mechanotransduction to be examined in isolation from factors associated with compression of the charged extracellular matrix *(4,14–17)*. In addition, the model provides insight into mechanotransduction within tissue-engineered constructs, with results indicating important differences between the potential signaling pathways within cartilage and cell-seeded scaffolds *(13)*.

Although compression of cell-agarose constructs will initiate transient changes in hydrostatic pressure and fluid flow, which have both been implicated in mechanotransduction, it is widely believed that cell deformation is the primary mediator. Therefore, before examining the effect of mechanical loading on chondrocyte metabolism, it is important first to identify the effect of loading on cell morphology and deformation. In the vast majority of studies, physiological compressive strain rather than stress is applied to the cell-agarose construct with typical strains in the order of 5 to 20% *(18)*. Various factors have been shown to influence the level of cell deformation and hence the ability of the cells to respond to gross compressive strain. These include the presence and mechanical properties of elaborated extracellular matrix *(19,20)*, the modulus of the scaffold relative to that of the cells and matrix *(21,22)*, and the loading regime and viscoelastic properties of the scaffold *(12)*. Having established the nature of the cell deformation induced by mechanical loading, studies can subsequently examine the metabolic response and the associated intracellular signalling pathways.

This chapter describes the experimental techniques employed for preparing chondrocyte-agarose constructs, quantifying the level of cell deformation, and analyzing the influence of compression on cell proliferation and proteoglycan synthesis using [^{3}H]thymidine and $^{35}SO_4$, incorporation, respectively.

2. Materials

2.1. Isolation of Bovine Chondrocytes

1. Front feet from approx 18-mo-old steers. (Obtain from local slaughterhouse.)
2. 70% (v/v) Industrial methylated spirits (IMS) in water.
3. Dissection kit: metal dissection tray, and sterile scalpels fitted with nos. 20, 11, and 15 blades.
4. Earle's balanced salt solution (EBSS; Sigma, cat. no. E-2888 or equivalent).
5. Culture medium: Dulbecco's minimal essential medium (Sigma, cat. no. D-5921 or equivalent) supplemented with 20% (v/v) fetal calf serum (Sigma, cat. no. F-9665 or equivalent), 2 mM L-glutamine (200 mM stock solution, Sigma, cat. no. G-7513 or equivalent), 20 mM HEPES (1M stock solution, Sigma, cat. no. H-0887 or equivalent), 50 U/mL penicillin plus 50 µg/mL streptomycin (100X concentrated stock solution, Sigma, cat. no. P0906), and 150 µg/mL L-ascorbic acid (Sigma, cat. no. A-0278). Sterilized by filtration through a 0.2-µm-pore size filter. Aliquot and store at –20°C prior to use.
6. Pronase solution: 700 U/mL pronase (Merck, cat. no. 39052 2P) in culture medium.
7. Collagenase solution: 100 U/mL collagenase type XI (Sigma, cat. no. C9407) in culture medium.
8. Trypan blue solution: 0.4% (w/v) trypan blue in 0.81% (w/v) sodium chloride/0.06% (w/v) potassium phosphate (Sigma, cat. no. T-8154 or equivalent).
9. 35-mm-Diameter sterile Petri dishes.
10. 50-mL Capacity sterile polypropylene centrifuges tubes.
11. 70-µm Pore size cell sieve (Falcon, cat. no. 35 2350).
12. Class II safety cabinet.
13. Roller mixer within an incubator or warm room at 37°C.
14. Centrifuge: up to 2000g, compatible with 50-mL centrifuge tubes.
15. Hemacytometer.
16. Inverted microscope with phase contrast facility.

2.2. Preparation of Chondrocyte/Agarose Constructs

1. Culture medium.
2. Isolated chondrocytes.
3. Agarose suspension: 6% (w/v) agarose (type VII, Sigma, cat. no. A4018,) in EBSS, sterilized by autoclaving.
4. Mold for preparing constructs (*see* **Note 1**).
5. Positive displacement pipet and sterile tips (Gilson Microman M250 or equivalent).
6. Water bath, maintained at 37°C.
7. Roller mixer within an incubator or warm room at 37°C.

2.3. Measurement of Cell Deformation in Compressed Cell-Seeded Scaffolds

1. Chondrocyte/agarose constructs seeded with viable cells and prepared as either rectangular blocks or half-cores.

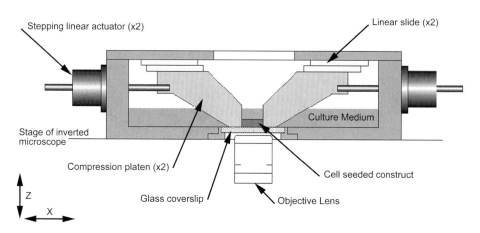

Fig. 1. Schematic diagram of the compression rig that mounts on the stage of an inverted microscope.

2. Microscope-mounted compression rig in which compressive strain may be applied perpendicular to the microscope axis (**Fig. 1**) *(12,19,20,22,23)*.
3. Inverted microscope associated with a confocal microscope system.
4. EBSS buffer solution: EBSS plus 1mM Ca^{2+}, 20 mM HEPES, pH 7.4.
5. Calcein-AM (Molecular Probes) viable cell staining solution prepared in culture medium at 5 µM.
6. 5-mL Universal tube.
7. Pipets.

2.4. Compressive Cell Strain Bioreactor

The equipment comprises the following components, as illustrated in **Fig. 2**:
1. Loading frame to incorporate Hereaus tissue culture incubator (Zwick Testing Machines, Leominster, UK).
2. Servo-hydraulic loading actuator incorporating load cell and Linear Variable Displacement Transducer (Zwick Testing Machines).
3. Hydraulic power supply (Zwick Testing Machines).
4. Digital control unit (Dartec 9610, Zwick Testing Machines).
5. Hereaus B6060 incubator.
6. Custom-designed construct loading assembly and box (Department of Engineering, Queen Mary, University of London, London, UK).

For culture within the bioreactor the following are required:
1. 70% IMS.
2. Culture medium.
3. 24-Well cell culture plate (Costar, cat. no. 3524).

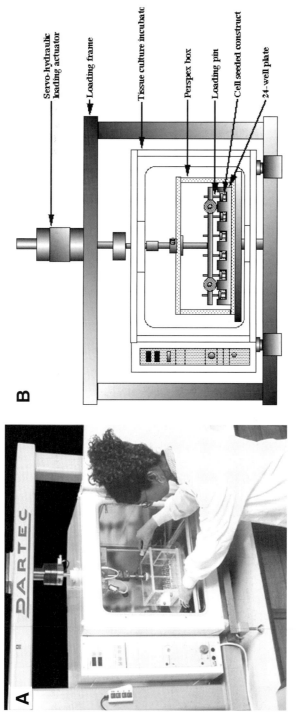
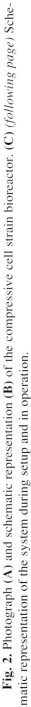

Fig. 2. Photograph (**A**) and schematic representation (**B**) of the compressive cell strain bioreactor. (**C**) (*following page*) Schematic representation of the system during setup and in operation.

Servo-hydraulic loading actuator

Loading frame

Tissue culture incubator

Perspex box

Loading pin

Cell seeded construct

24-well plate

311

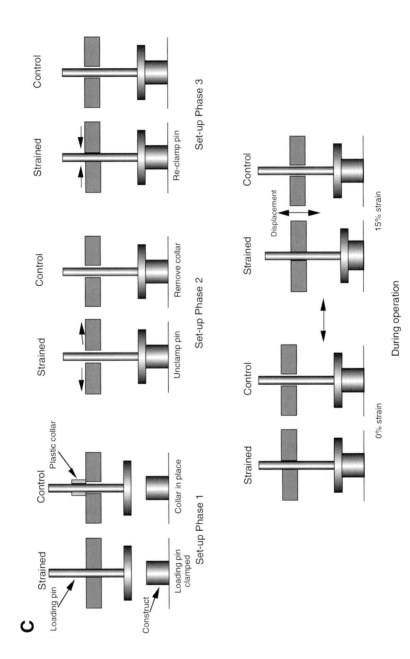

C

Strained | Control
Loading pin | Plastic collar
Construct | Loading pin clamped | Collar in place

Set-up Phase 1

Strained | Control
Unclamp pin | Remove collar

Set-up Phase 2

Strained | Control
Re-clamp pin

Set-up Phase 3

During operation

Strained | Control
0% strain

Strained | Control
Displacement
15% strain

4. Cell seeded constructs.
5. 1-mL Capacity sterile syringe with right-angled needle (*see* **Note 2**).

2.5. Analysis of Proteoglycan Synthesis and Cell Proliferation

2.5.1. Metabolic Labeling

1. Radiolabeled medium: culture medium supplemented with 1 µCi/mL [^{3}H]Thymidine (Amersham Life Sciences, cat. no. TRK61) + 10 µCi/mL ^{35}SO$_4$ (Amersham Life Sciences, cat. no. SJS1).

2.5.2. Digestion of Constructs

1. Papain digest buffer: 150 mM sodium chloride, 55 mM trisodium citrate (BDH, cat. no. 10242), 5 mM EDTA disodium salt, 5 mM L-cysteine hydrochloride (Sigma, cat. no. C7880) in distilled water.
2. Papain suspension (Sigma, cat. no. P3125).
3. Agarase (Sigma, cat. no. A6306).
4. Incubators set at 70°C and 37°C.

2.5.3. ^{35}SO$_4$ and [^{3}H]Thymidine Incorporation for Proteoglycan Synthesis and Cell Proliferation

1. Acetate buffer: 50 mM sodium acetate, pH 5.8, 85 mM magnesium chloride in distilled water.
2. Alcian blue solution: 0.2% (w/v) alcian blue 8GX (Sigma, cat. no. A5268) in acetate buffer.
3. Acetate buffer with 100 mM sodium sulfate (BDH, cat. no. 103984T).
4. Guanidine solution: 4 M guanidine HCl (Sigma, cat. no. G4630), 4.3 M propan-2-ol (Sigma, cat. no. I9516) in distilled water.
5. Trichloroacetic acid (TCA, Sigma, cat. no. 490-10), 10% and 20% (w/v) solutions in distilled water.
6. Vacuum filtration system (Millipore Multiscreen®, or equivalent), including vacuum manifold and multiple punch.
7. Vacuum filtration plates, 0.65-µm-pore size (Millipore Multiscreen, cat. no. MADVN6550).
8. Scintillation cocktail (Emulsifier Safe, Packard or equivalent).
9. Scintillation vials, 4-mL capacity (Packard or equivalent).
10. Liquid scintillation counter (e.g., Wallac 1409, Perkin Elmer, or equivalent).

2.5.4. DNA Analysis

1. Hoechst 33258 solution: 1 µg/mL Hoechst 33258 (Sigma, cat. no. B2883) in 150 mM sodium chloride (BDH, cat. no. 10241), 55 mM trisodium citrate (BDH, cat. no. 10242, Poole, UK), pH 7.0.
2. DNA solutions: Calf thymus DNA (0-100 µg/mL, Sigma, cat. no. D3664) in 150 mM sodium chloride, 55 mM trisodium citrate (BDH, cat. no. 10242), pH 7.0.
3. White microtiter plates (Nunc, cat. no. 437796).
4. Microplate fluorimeter (e.g., BMG FLUOstar Galaxy, BMG Labtechnologies).

3. Methods

3.1. Isolation of Bovine Chondrocytes

1. Clean bovine front feet with water and immerse in 70% IMS for 5 min to sterilize skin.
2. Within the class II safety cabinet, expose the metacarpalphalangeal joint and remove full-depth cartilage slices from the proximal articular surfaces of the joint using a no. 15 blade (*see* **Note 3**). Transfer the slices to a 60-mm Petri dish containing 8 mL of EBSS.
3. Aspirate EBSS, dice the tissue into pieces approx 1 mm^3, and transfer to a 50-mL centrifuge tube containing 10 mL of pronase solution (*see* **Note 4**). Incubate on rollers for 1 h at 37°C.
4. Allow the tissue pieces to settle and remove pronase solution. Add 30 mL of collagenase solution and incubate on rollers for 16 h at 37°C (*see* **Notes 4** and **5**).
5. Allow any remaining tissue pieces to settle and carefully remove the collagenase solution containing isolated cells. Filter the solution through a 70-µm pore sieve into a fresh 50 mL centrifuge tube.
6. Centrifuge at 2000*g* for 5 min to pellet cells. Aspirate the supernatant and resuspend the cells in 10 mL of culture medium using a 10-mL sterile graduated pipet. Repeat this process twice.
7. Add 50 µL of cell suspension to 50 µL trypan blue solution, mix, and add resultant suspension to a hemacytometer. Determine total cell number and cell viability and adjust cell concentration to 2×10^7 cells/mL.

3.2. Preparation of Chondrocyte/Agarose Constructs

1. Assemble the parts of the mold used for preparation of agarose/chondrocyte constructs (*see* **Note 1**).
2. Add the cell suspension, adjusted to 2×10^7 cells/mL to an equal volume of agarose suspension. Mix thoroughly using a positive displacement pipet.
3. Aliquot the agarose/chondrocyte suspension into individual wells of the mold and complete the assembly by adding the second glass slide and clamping the three components of the mold to ensure it is sealed.
4. Incubate for 30 min at 4°C.
5. Carefully dismantle the mold to allow removal of the gelled agarose/chondrocyte constructs.

3.3. Measurement of Cell Deformation in Compressed Cell-Seeded Scaffolds

1. Incubate constructs in Calcein-AM solution for 1 h at 37°C. Allow sufficient staining solution to cover the constructs (*see* **Note 6**).
2. Transfer constructs to EBSS at room temperature to allow complete de-esterization of Calcein-AM.
3. Place an individual construct on the glass coverslip within the compression rig, as shown in **Fig. 1**.

4. Advance the compression platens until they are just touching the construct (*see* **Note 7**).
5. Use the pipet to add EBSS buffer carefully to maintain hydration of the construct throughout testing. Repeat as necessary.
6. Configure the confocal microscope for high-resolution imaging (pixel size ≤ 0.2 μm) with a high-magnification objective lens ($\geq 40\times$). Use a laser excitation of 488 nm with fluorescent emissions detected above 500 nm.
7. To minimize boundary conditions, select individual cells that are at least 30 μm (approx three cell diameters) from each other and from the bottom surface of the construct. Also select cells away from the ends and sides of the construct (*see* **Note 8**).
8. To image an individual cell, adjust the Z focus until the confocal X-Y section image bisects the center of the cell (*see* **Note 9**).
9. In some instances it may be necessary to define the boundary of the cell more clearly. This may be achieved by using a high-pass filter with an intensity threshold. For example, previous studies have used a threshold of 50% of the maximum intensity *(19,24)*.

The subsequent method protocol will depend on whether a paired or non-paired approach is employed.

3.3.1. Analysis Using a Paired Data Approach

This approach relies on the ability to image an individual cell first in the unstrained state and then to follow that cell as gross compression is applied to the construct, enabling the same cell to be imaged again in the compressed state.

1. Select a group of approx 10 individual cells and make a confocal section image through the center of each cell as described above in **steps 6–9**, **Subheading 3.3.**
2. Apply the compressive strain while visualizing the cells using transmitted light microscopy. As the compression is applied, track the individual cells by adjusting the focus and the stage position as necessary. The strain rates should be less than 5%/s (*see* **Note 10**). An example set of images is provided in **Fig. 3**.
3. Image the same sample of individual cells. It is important to be aware of the viscoelastic stress relaxation properties of the scaffold since each cell is imaged at a different time post compression. For scaffolds with an equilibrium modulus significantly greater than that of the cells (i.e., $E_{construct} > 10$ kPa), any relaxation in the scaffold should not influence the level of cell deformation *(22)*.
4. Repeat the test using a new sample on each occasion to avoid artifacts associated with hysteresis and strain history of the scaffold.
5. Calculate the percentage change in cell X and Y diameters measured parallel and perpendicular to the axis of compression (**Fig. 4**).
6. Calculate the percentage change in cell volume ($\pi/6 \cdot X \cdot Y^2$), based on the assumption that the cells deform from a spheroid to an oblate ellipsoid (Y diameter = Z diameter). The paired data approach may also be used to measure the deformation of intracellular organelles such as the nucleus (**Fig. 5**). Specific viable

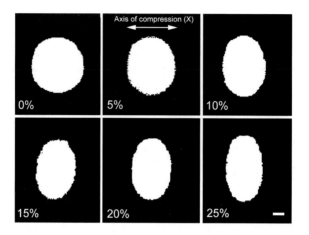

Fig. 3. Confocal section images through the center of an individual cell stained with calcein-AM and visualized within an agarose construct at 0, 5, 10, 15, 20, and 25% compressive strain. An intensity threshold has been applied to each image to clarify the cell boundary to allow measurement of cell diameters. Scale bar = 2 μm.

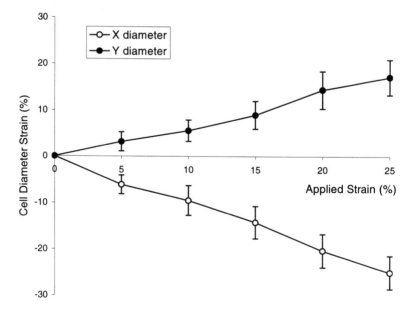

Fig. 4. Percentage change in cell diameter, parallel (*X*) and perpendicular (*Y*) to the axis of compression for freshly isolated chondrocytes compressed in 3% agarose gel. Error bars indicate standard deviation for *n* = 12.

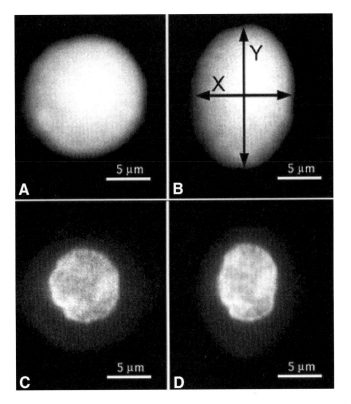

Fig. 5. Confocal images bisecting the center of a single cell (**A,B**) and its nucleus (**C,D**) in unstrained (**A,C**) and 20% compressed (**B,D**) 3% alginate construct. The cells and nuclei have been stained with Calcein-AM and Hoescht, respectively.

fluorescent stains should be used in conjunction with the appropriate excitation and emission settings on the confocal microscope.

3.3.2. Analysis Using a Nonpaired Data Approach

When it is not possible to image the same individual cells in both an unstrained and compressed state, an alternative approach may be used to estimate the level of cell deformation. This so-called nonpaired data or sample population approach uses separate samples of cells imaged in the unstrained and compressed states. However, by using this approach direct, accurate calculation of the percentage change in cell diameter or in cell strains from the sample populations is not possible. This is because of the large variability in unstrained cell diameter associated with cartilage heterogeneity, such that cells isolated from the deep zone are larger than those isolated from the surface zone *(15)*.

Consequently cell deformation is estimated from individual images of cells, using a deformation index (*I*).

1. Image a sample population of cells in the unstrained construct (*see* **Note 11**).
2. Apply a static compressive strain to the construct via the platens (*see* **Note 10**).
3. Allow a period of stress relaxation for the compressive stress in the gel to reach equilibrium (*see* **Note 12**).
4. Image a new sample population of cells.
5. Repeat the test using a new sample on each occasion to avoid artifacts associated with hysteresis and strain history of the scaffold.
6. Calculate the deformation index (*I*) for each cell such that *I* = X/Y, where X and Y are the cell diameters measured parallel and perpendicular to the axis of compression.
7. Freshly isolated chondrocytes in unstrained agarose have been shown to be spherical and to deform at constant volume with rotational symmetry (Y = Z) *(13)*. Therefore, the cell diameter strains in the X and Y axes (ε_X and ε_Y, respectively) may be calculated from the deformation index using the following equations *(22)*:

$$\varepsilon_X = \left| \left(\frac{X_s}{Y_s} \right)^{2/3} - 1 \right| \times 100\% \tag{1}$$

$$\varepsilon_Y = \left| \left(\frac{X_s}{Y_s} \right)^{-1/3} - 1 \right| \times 100\% \tag{2}$$

3.4. Culture of Constructs in Compressive Cell Strain Bioreactor

1. Assemble loading plate, loading pins, and Perspex box, ensuring that the outer pins are held in place with plastic collars and the inner pins are clamped (*see* **Fig. 2B,C**). Sterilize in 70% IMS and allow to dry overnight in a tissue culture hood.
2. Locate constructs at the center of individual wells of a 24-well cell culture plate and locate within the Perspex box.
3. Allow loading pins to drop onto constructs by removing the plastic collars from the outer pins and unclamping the inner pins. Clamp inner pins once in position (*see* **Fig. 2C**).
4. Introduce 1 mL of culture medium into each well through the medium ports associated with the apparatus using a 1-mL syringe and a right-angled needle.
5. Close the box, transfer to the bioreactor, and attach to the loading actuator by means of the central rod. Unlock the central rod to allow free movement.
6. Set the control electronics of the straining apparatus to provide a crosshead movement equivalent to a compressive strain ranging from 0 to 15% in a sinusoidal waveform at a frequency of 1 Hz.

3.5. Analysis of Cell Proliferation and Proteoglycan Synthesis

3.5.1. Radiolabeling and Digestion of Constructs (see **Note 13**)

1. Incubate constructs in 1 mL of radiolabeled medium at 37°C in 5% CO_2 atmosphere for a selected labeling period, typically between 6 and 48 h (*see* **Note 14**).
2. At the end of the labeling period, remove the medium and store at –20°C for analysis (*see* **Subheading 3.5.2.**).
3. Place construct in 1 mL of papain digest buffer and incubate at 70°C until the construct melts (usually 20–30 min).
4. Cool to 37°C and add 10 U/mL agarase and 1 U/mL papain. Incubate at 37°C overnight (*see* **Note 15**).
5. Digested constructs may be stored at –20°C prior to analysis.

3.5.2. $^{35}SO_4$ Incorporation for Proteoglycan Synthesis (see **Note 13**)

1. Add 75 µL of acetate buffer, 25 µL of digested sample or radiolabeled medium, and 150 µL of alcian blue solution, in duplicate, into individual wells of a vacuum filtration plate.
2. Seal the plate and incubate with agitation for 1 h at room temperature.
3. Vacuum aspirate, add 200 µL of acetate buffer with 100 mM sodium sulphate, and incubate at room temperature for 5 min. Repeat this process twice.
4. Vacuum aspirate, carefully blot the underside of the plate to remove excess fluid, and remove the underdrain. Place the plate in an oven, set at 37°C for 1 h.
5. Punch out the filters into individual scintillation vials using the multiple punch and add 500 µL of guanidine solution. Incubate on a rolling mixer for 2 h to resolubilize the precipitate.
6. Add 4 mL of scintillation cocktail and read using a scintillation counter (bound counts in medium or construct).
7. Add 10 µL of recovered radiolabeled medium into individual scintillation vials, add 4 mL of scintillation cocktail, and read using a scintillation counter (free counts in medium).
8. The incorporation of sulfate may be determined as follows:

$$\frac{\text{Sulfate incorpration}}{\left(\mu\text{mol SO}_4 \cdot \text{h}^{-1} \cdot \mu\text{g}^{-1} \text{ DNA}\right)} = \frac{\text{total bound counts in medium and construct} \times 0.81}{\text{total free counts in medium} \times t \times [\text{DNA}]} \quad (3)$$

where t = time of culture in labeled medium in hours and 0.81 = concentration of $^{35}SO_4$ in culture medium in mM.

3.5.3. [^{3}H]Thymidine Incorporation for Cell Proliferation (see **Note 13**)

1. Aliquot 200 µL of 10% TCA into individual wells of a vacuum filtration plate and vacuum aspirate to leave the filters wet.
2. Aliquot 100 µL of 20% TCA, followed by 100 µL of digested sample, in duplicate, into individual wells of the plate in duplicate.

3. Seal the plate and incubate with agitation for 1 h at room temperature.
4. Vacuum aspirate, add 100 µL of 10% TCA solution, and incubate at room temperature for 5 min. Repeat this process twice.
5. Vacuum aspirate, carefully blot the underside of the plate to remove excess fluid and remove the underdrain. Place the plate in an oven, set at 37°C for 1 h.
6. Punch out the filters into individual scintillation vials using the multiple punch and add 500 µL of 0.01 *M* KOH. Incubate on a rolling mixer for 2 h to resolubilize the precipitate.
7. Add 4 mL of scintillation cocktail and read using a scintillation counter.
8. [^{3}H]Thymidine incorporation data are presented as counts per minute (counts/min), normalized to DNA values, i.e., counts/min/µg DNA.

3.5.4. DNA Analysis

1. Aliquot 100 µL of DNA solutions, ranging from 0 to 100 µg/mL, in duplicate, into individual wells of a white microtiter plate.
2. Add 100 µL of digested samples, in duplicate, into individual wells of a white microtiter plate.
3. Add 100 µL of Hoechst 33258 solution into each well (*see* **Note 16**).
4. Read the plate using a microplate fluorimeter with excitation set at 360 nm and emission at 460 nm.
5. Calculate sample DNA concentrations from the standard curve.

4. Notes

1. The molds consist of two glass slides, which act as outer supports for a medical-grade stainless steel central unit, which incorporates a matrix of cylindrical (5-mm diameter × 5mm depth) or rectangular holes (4 × 3 × 3 mm). All three units may be held together using appropriate tape or clamps. For use, the lower glass slide and central unit are clamped together and the resultant wells are filled with the chondrocyte/agarose suspension, taking care to avoid the formation of air bubbles. A positive displacement pipet is ideal for this purpose, and it is recommended that the wells be slightly overfilled at this stage. The top glass slide is carefully located and clamped. Once gelling has occurred, the mold may be disassembled to release cylindrical or rectangular constructs, with dimensions defined by the holes in the central unit. The constructs have plane parallel top and bottom surfaces, which is necessary for mechanical testing. Detailed design drawings may be obtained from David Lee (D.A.Lee@qmul.ac.uk).
2. The right-angled needle is prepared by taking a sterile 21-gage, 50-mm-long length needle and bending it through 90° after partially removing the needle from its sheath.
3. Opening the joint is best performed by making a midline incision using a no. 20 blade, taking care not to enter the joint space. The skin and digital extensor tendons may then be dissected away from the joint capsule. The joint may then be opened with a no. 11 blade, using the distal surface of the metacarpal bone as a guide.

4. The volumes of pronase and collagenase solution are based on the digestion of tissue from one joint. If one is digesting tissue from more than one joint, it is recommended that the tissue be digested in further centrifuge tubes rather than altering the volume of the solutions in each tube. Approximately 1–3 g of tissue can be obtained from a single joint, and this should yield up to 30×10^6 cells.

5. Collagenase batches vary, even when they are purchased from the same supplier. It is highly advisable to test batches prior to use to ensure that all the tissue is digested and that cell viability is maintained. It may be necessary to alter the concentration or incubation times from those stated to achieve optimal cell isolation.

6. These techniques can be combined with a viability assay by incorporating 5 μM Ethidium Homodimer (Molecular Probes) into the staining solution. The use of Calcein-AM ensures that cell deformation is only measured in viable cells.

7. It is useful to visualize the construct and platens using transmitted light microscopy to stop the platens the moment they touch the specimen.

8. At a separation of more than 30 μm between adjacent cells or the construct surface, the mechanical perturbation has been shown to be less than 1% *(25)*.

9. The position of the confocal plane bisecting the center of the cell may be selected from an *X-Z* confocal scan or by taking a confocal *Z* series and selecting the image in which the cell has the largest diameter *(26)*.

10. The magnitude of the compressive strain that can be applied will depend on the mechanical properties of the scaffold material. However, it should be noted that at compressive strains of 25% and above cells show nonreversible membrane blebbing around the equator of the oblate ellipsoid *(26)*.

11. For a sample size of $n = 50$, the mean precision of deformation index measurement in compressed agarose constructs is 0.01 at the 90% confidence interval *(26)*. There is minimal improvement in precision above $n = 50$, although this will depend on the variability within different types of construct.

12. The length of the relaxation period will depend on the modulus and viscoelastic properties of the construct, which may be determined from a stress relaxation test in uniaxial unconfined compression. For constructs with an equilibrium modulus significantly greater than that of the cells (i.e., $E_{construct} > 10$ kPa), it is not necessary to allow a relaxation period *(21,22)*.

13. Safety precautions must be followed when using radiolabeled samples. Gloves must be worn at all times and monitoring should be performed. A GM tube counter will detect $^{35}SO_4$ contamination, but [^{3}H]thymidine contamination can only be detected using a swab test. This involves wiping the area to be tested with a damp swab, which is placed in a scintillation vial containing scintillation cocktail and counted using a scintillation counter. Count per minute values are compared with background levels, determined from an identical swab, added directly to the vial.

14. Labeling periods are dependent on the nature of the study. However, certain points should be considered when conducting radiolabeling experiments with tissue explant or 3D constructs. The radiolabeled molecules must diffuse into the construct prior to incorporation by cells. Accordingly, very short labeling peri-

ods are not recommended as the radiolabeled molecules may not have equilibrated in the construct. Previous studies have demonstrated that [³H]thymidine takes between 4 and 8 h to equilibrate in 3% agarose constructs of 5-mm diameter and 5-mm height *(27)*. It should be noted that an extended labeling period or the use of labeled medium with a high radioactivity may lead to DNA or cellular damage and cause anomalous results. For example, the incorporation of high concentrations of [³H]thymidine into DNA during S-phase may lead to DNA damage, which will activate cellular repair mechanisms involving further DNA synthesis not related to cell proliferation. Further DNA damage is induced, and a cascade of nonproliferative DNA synthesis may occur, resulting in abnormally high [³H]thymidine incorporation values.

15. After extended culture periods, digestion at 37°C may not be sufficient to break up collagenous matrix. In this case, a further incubation period of 1 h at 60°C is recommended. Note that incubation at 60°C will inactivate the agarase, so the 37°C incubation must be included first to digest the agarose.

16. Please note that Hoechst 33258 binds to DNA and may act as a mutagen. Gloves must be worn at all times.

References

1. Sah, R., Kim, Y. J., Doong, J. Y. H., Grodzinsky, A. J., Plaas, A. H. K., and Sandy, J. D. (1989) Biosynthetic response of cartilage explants to dynamic compression. *J. Orthop. Res.* **7,** 619–636.

2. Kim, Y. J., Sah, R. L. Y., Grodzinsky, A. J., Plaas, A. H. K., and Sandy, J. D. (1994) Mechanical regulation of cartilage biosynthetic behaviour: physical stimuli. *Arch. Biochem. Biophys.* **311,** 1–12.

3. Vunjak-Novakovic, G., Martin, I., Obradovic, B., et al. (1999) Bioreactor cultivation conditions modulate the composition and mechanical properties of tissue engineered cartilage. *J. Orthop. Res.* **17,** 130–138.

4. Mauck,R. L., Soltz, M. A., Wang, C. C., et al. (2000) Functional tissue engineering of articular cartilage through dynamic loading of chondrocyte-seeded agarose gels. *J. Biomech. Eng.* **122,** 252–260.

5. Guilak, F., Butler, D. L., and Goldstein, S. A. (2001) Functional tissue engineering: the role of biomechanics in articular cartilage repair. *Clin. Orthop.* **391,** 295–305.

6. Urban, J. P .G. (1994) The chondrocyte: A cell under pressure. *Br. J. Rheumatol* **33,** 901–908.

7. Heath, C. A. and Magari, S. R. (1996) Mechanical factors affecting cartilage regeneration in vitro. *Biotechnol. Bioeng.* **50,** 430–437.

8. Guilak, F., Sah, R., and Setton, L.A. (1997) *Basic Orthopaedic Biomechanics* (Mow, V. C. and Hayes, W. C., eds.), Lippincott-Raven, Philadelphia, PA, pp. 179–207.

9. Benya, P. D. and Shaffer, J. D. (1982) Dedifferentiated chondrocytes reexpress the differentiated collagen phentotype when cultured in agarose gels. *Cell* **30,** 215–224.

10. Aydelotte, M. B., Schumacher, B. L., and Kuettner, K. E. (1990) *Methods in Cartilage Research.* (Maroudas, A. and Kuettner, K. E., eds.), Academic, London, UK, pp. 90–92.

11. Hauselmann, H. J., Fernandes, R. J., Mok, S., et al. (1994) Phenotypic stability of bovine articular chondrocytes after long-term culture in alginate beads. *J. Cell Sci.* **107,** 17–27.

12. Knight, M. M., Ghori, S. A., Lee, D. A., and Bader, D. L. (1998) Measurement of the deformation of isolated chondrocytes in agarose subjected to cyclic compression. *Med. Eng. Phys.* **20,** 684–688.

13. Lee, D. A., Knight, M. M., Bolton, J. F., Idowu, B. D., Kayser, M. V., and Bader, D. L. (2000) Chondrocyte deformation within compressed agarose constructs at the cellular and sub-cellular levels. *J. Biomech.* **33,** 81–95.

14. Lee, D. A., Noguchi, T., Knight, M. M., O'Donnell, L. B., and Bader, D. L. (1997) Differential metabolic response of superficial and deep zone chondrocytes to compressive strain, in *Transactions of the 42nd Annual Meeting of the Orthopaedic Research Society* **22,** abstract.

15. Lee, D. A., Noguchi, T., Knight, M. M., O'Donnell, L., Bentley, G., and Bader, D. L. (1998) Response of chondrocyte subpopulations cultured within unloaded and loaded agarose. *J. Orthop. Res.* **16,** 726–733.

16. Lee, D. A., Noguchi, T., Frean, S. P., Lees, P., and Bader, D. L. (2000) The influence of mechanical loading on isolated chondrocytes seeded in agarose constructs. *Biorheology* **37,** 149–161.

17. Buschmann, M. D., Gluzband, Y. A., Grodzinsky, A. J., and Hunziker, E. B. (1995) Mechanical compression modulates matrix biosynthesis in chondrocyte/agarose culture. *J. Cell Sci.* **108,** 1497–1508.

18. Guilak, F., Ratcliffe, A., and Mow, V. C. (1995) Chondrocyte Deformation and local tissue strain in articular cartilage: A confocal microscopy study. *J. Orthop. Res.* **13,** 410–421.

19. Knight, M. M., Lee, D. A., and Bader, D. L. (1998) The influence of elaborated pericellular matrix on the deformation of isolated articular chondrocytes cultured in agarose. *Biochim. Biophys. Acta* **1405,** 67–77.

20. Knight, M. M., Ross, J. M., Sherwin, A. F., Lee, D. A., Bader, D. L., and Poole, C. A. (2001) Chondrocyte deformation within mechanically and enzymatically extracted chondrons compressed in agarose. *Biochim. Biophys. Acta* **1526,** 141–146.

21. Bader, D. L., Ohashi, T., Knight, M. M., Lee, D. A., and Sato, M. (2002) Deformation properties of articular chondrocytes: a critique of three separate techniques. *Biorheology* **39,** 69–78.

22. Knight, M. M., van de Breevaart Bravenboer, J., Lee, D. A., van Osch, G. J. V. M., Weinans, H., and Bader, D. L. (2002) Cell and nucleus deformation in compressed chondrocyte-alginate constructs: temporal changes and calculation of cell modulus. *Biochim. Biophys. Acta* **1570,** 1–8.

23. Roberts, S. R., Knight, M. M., Lee, D. A., and Bader, D. L. (2001) Mechanical compression influences intracellular Ca2+ signaling in chondrocytes seeded in agarose constructs. *J. Appl. Physiol* **90,** 1385–1391.

24. Knight, M. M., Lee, D. A., and Bader, D. L. (1996) Distribution of chondrocyte deformation in compressed agarose gel using confocal microscopy. *J. Cell. Eng.* **1,** 97–102.
25. Bachrach, N. M., Valhmu W. B., Stazzone, E., Ratcliffe, A., Lai, W. M., and Mow, V.C. (1995) Changes in proteoglycan synthesis of chondrocytes in articular cartilage are associated with the time-dependent changes in their mechanical environment. *J. Biomech.* **28,** 1561–1569.
26. Knight, M. M. (1997) Deformation of isolated articular chondrocytes cultured in agarose constructs. PhD Thesis, University of London, London, UK.
27. Lee, D. A. and Bader, D. L. (1997) Compressive strains at physiological frequencies influence the metabolism of chondrocytes seeded in agarose. *J. Orthop. Res.* **15,** 181–188.

22

In Vitro Physical Stimulation
of Tissue-Engineered and Native Cartilage

Kelvin W. Li, Travis J. Klein, Kanika Chawla,
Gayle E. Nugent, Won C. Bae, and Robert L. Sah

Summary

Because of the limited availability of donor cartilage for resurfacing defects in articular surfaces, there is tremendous interest in the in vitro bioengineering of cartilage replacements for clinical applications. However, attaining mechanical properties in engineered cartilaginous constructs that approach those of native cartilage has not been previously achieved when constructs are cultured under free-swelling conditions. One approach toward stimulating the development of constructs that are mechanically more robust is to expose them to physical environments that are similar, in certain ways, to those encountered by native cartilage. This is a strategy motivated by observations in numerous short-term experiments that certain mechanical signals are potent stimulators of cartilage metabolism. On the other hand, excess mechanical loading can have a deleterious effect on cartilage. Culture conditions that include a physical stimulation component are made possible by the use of specialized bioreactors. This chapter addresses some of the issues involved in using bioreactors as integral components of cartilage tissue engineering and in studying the physical regulation of cartilage. We first consider the generation of cartilaginous constructs in vitro. Next we describe the rationale and design of bioreactors that can impart either mechanical deformation or fluid-induced mechanical signals.

Key Words: Bioreactors; mechanical stress; tissue engineering; cartilage growth; extracellular matrix; compression; perfusion; shear stress.

1. Introduction

One approach to the prevention of end-stage osteoarthritis is to repair articular defects, especially those that are focal in nature, using cartilaginous tissue replacements that are engineered in vitro. Emerging tissue-engineering therapies attempt to reconstitute cartilage structure and function by various processes that typically begin with the in vitro culture of a combination of cells, supporting scaffolding materials, and bioactive molecules (1–5). To date, many of these

From: *Methods in Molecular Medicine, Vol. 100: Cartilage and Osteoarthritis, Vol. 1: Cellular and Molecular Tools*
Edited by: M. Sabatini, P. Pastoureau, and F. De Ceuninck © Humana Press Inc., Totowa, NJ

cell-based tissue-engineering methods have yielded promising but inconsistent results after clinical *(6,7)* or experimental *(8–13)* implantation.

A variety of methods for accelerating the development of biochemical and mechanical properties of growing cartilaginous constructs are under current investigation. One approach has been to subject such constructs to a mechanical environment that is similar to that encountered by native cartilage in vivo. This is accomplished by reproducing select aspects of physiological loading in culture systems collectively known as loading chambers or bioreactors. This strategy is motivated by in vivo and in vitro observations that mechanical signals can be potent regulators of cartilage metabolism.

To the extent that chondrocytes function as the biological "architects" of cartilage in vivo *(14)*, joint loading provides a partial set of instructions. For example, weight-bearing regions of the joint tend to have the highest proteoglycan concentration *(15)*, and the contrast between the articular cartilage in immobilized and weight-bearing limbs of growing dogs suggests that joint loading plays a stimulatory role in local cartilage thickening *(16)*. Immobilized joints in experimental animals also exhibit a reversible decrease in proteoglycan synthesis and content *(17–20)*, whereas moderate exercise stimulates proteoglycan synthesis and accumulation *(18,21)*. Thus, chondrocytes monitor their mechanical environment in vivo and modify the structure and composition of their extracellular matrix over time to meet perceived functional demands *(22)*.

The precise consequences of joint loading can be studied from various perspectives, ranging from the whole joint down to the tissue and molecular length scales (**Fig. 1**). Under physiological joint use, articular cartilage is subjected to a wide range of mechanical loads *(22)*. At the tissue level, the complex mechanical stresses associated with joint loading and articulation can be decomposed into compressive and shear stresses, which are imparted on the successive layers of cartilage (**Fig. 1B**). From the perspective of individual chondrocytes, such loading results in coupled electrical, mechanical, and chemical phenomena that vary in space and time. These phenomena include solid deformation, changes in pH, streaming potentials, fluid-induced shear, hydrostatic pressure, and mass transport of ions and soluble factors *(23–25)* (**Fig. 1C,D**). All these factors represent distinct physical signals that may be important regulators of chondrocyte behavior. Indeed, the role of the matrix in determining the nature of the chondrocyte response has been highlighted in a recent review: "Over the past few years it has been recognized that chondrocytes in cartilage do not respond to load as such but rather to load-induced changes in the matrix" *(26)*. However, because these potential regulatory cues are inherently coupled within intact cartilage matrix, there are significant challenges in identifying which of the biophysical signals play primary roles in triggering specific biological responses by chondrocytes.

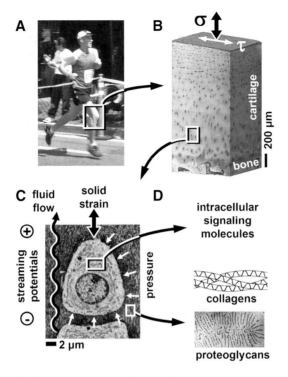

Fig. 1. Mechanical loading of articular cartilage: length scales. (**A**) Normal joint loading and articulation impart (**B**) compression (σ) and shear (τ) to the articular cartilage at joint surfaces. (**C**) The material properties of the extracellular matrix dictate the manner by which loading of cartilage generates discrete biophysical signals to which individual chondrocytes are exposed. (**D**) Embedded chondrocytes may initiate intracellular molecular responses to the induced biophysical signals, leading to cell-mediated alterations in the molecular composition of the matrix. Micrographs and schematics adapted from refs. *115–118*, with permission.

Multiple studies have used in vivo models based on geometrically defined cartilage explants to elucidate the effects of defined mechanical stimuli on cartilage biology. Such explant-based approaches have allowed investigators to confirm and scrutinize in vivo observations that mechanical loading can affect the cellular processes that contribute to matrix remodeling (*see* refs. **27** and **28** for review). In general, *static* compression of cartilage explants, in which a fixed compression level is applied and maintained over time, typically leads to dose-dependent inhibition of matrix synthesis (e.g., refs. *29–33*). On the other hand, the application of *dynamic* compression, which may correspond to the time-varying stresses generated by normal joint activity, can stimulate biosynthesis when certain threshold levels of frequency and amplitude are exceeded *(33–36)*. Under such loading conditions, the stimulated cells appear to be localized to regions predicted to have high fluid flow *(37,38)*. These responses to mechanical compression appear to be reproduced when chondrocytes are isolated from their matrix, cultured in three-dimensional (3D) gels, and then subjected to similar types of compression *(39–41)*, but sometimes only after a significant amount of matrix has accumulated *(39,41)*. Isolated chondrocytes also retain the ability to respond metabolically to different types of mechanical forces, a finding supported by a growing body of research in which they are subjected to distinct components of the *in situ* mechanical environment. In chondrocytes cultured in monolayer, glycosaminoglycan (GAG) biosynthesis was stimulated by cyclic tensile strain *(42)*, fluid-induced shear *(43)*, and extended high-frequency pressurization *(44)*.

In contrast, when compression is applied to cartilage explants at high strain magnitude or strain rate, *injurious* effects can be induced. This type of loading can mimic cartilage impact. The resultant effects have implications for the initiation and progression of cartilage damage and deterioration. Matrix damage in the form of collagen denaturation can occur with a compressive strain magnitude as low as 25% at a relatively low strain rate of 0.1/s in unconfined compression *(45)*, even without chondrocyte death. Cell death, including apoptosis, varies with a number of mechanical loading parameters, including strain magnitude, rate, and duration or number of cycles, with strain magnitude being the major effector. Strain magnitudes as low as 30% can result in cell death, if the strain rate is sufficiently high *(46,47)*. With an increase in applied strain magnitude, chondrocyte viability decreases *(46–50)*, even while the same strain rates are held constant *(46)*. Once injured, cell death can occur either in the short- or the long-term, with cell death sometimes increasing with time after loading *(46,51)*.

Thus, the mechanical signals generated by both normal and injurious joint loading can regulate various cellular processes within chondrocytes in cartilage. The same cellular processes may also underlie the generation of *de novo* extracellular matrix during in vitro tissue engineering procedures, with upregulation of such processes promoting chondrogenesis. The latter observations form the rationale for bioreactor approaches that attempt to exploit *appropriate* mechanical signals for the enhancement of engineered cartilaginous constructs during extended culture periods (weeks to months). The intent of such bioreactors is to apply mechanical stimulation to cartilaginous constructs so that the induced cellular activities result in increased accumulation and assembly of matrix components and concomitant changes in the functional mechanical properties of the tissue. These bioreactors are similar in many respects to chambers that have been used to impart injurious stimuli to cartilage.

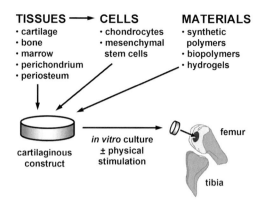

Fig. 2. Tissue engineering strategies to repair an articular cartilage defect in the femoral condyle.

This chapter addresses some of the issues involved in using bioreactors as integral components of current experimental studies of cartilage tissue engineering and physical regulation of chondrocytes and describes some key steps in such studies, namely, sample preparation and mechanical stimulation by solid deformation or fluid-based perfusion. An initial step in cartilage tissue engineering is the fabrication of cartilaginous constructs prior to incubation within a bioreactor.

1.1. Sample Preparation

The cartilage bioengineer is faced with several key design choices on the pathway to fabricating functional cartilaginous constructs (**Fig. 2**). The first of these choices is the selection of an appropriate cell population. The cell types that have been used to generate cartilaginous tissue include chondrocytes *(52)*, perichondrial *(53)* and periosteal cells *(54)*, and other pluripotent cells, including those derived from bone marrow *(55,56)* and fat *(57)*. Once the cell type has been selected, a decision must be made about how to manipulate these cells prior to construct formation. This is a cell-type specific decision, and manipulations can range from direct use of primary cells (as is possible with chondrocytes), to expanding the cell number in monolayer or a 3D gel with or without treatment of growth factors to induce a chondrogenic phenotype (*see* **Note 1**) *(58)*.

After generating a sufficient number of desirable chondrogenic cells, the next step is to decide what type of scaffold, if any, will be used in which to seed the cells and form the initial shape of the construct. A popular class of scaffolds has been biodegradable polymers such as polyglycolic acid (PGA) *(52)*, polylactic acid (PLA) *(59)*, and their co-polymers *(60)*. These materials provide initial mechanical support for the cells, and eventually degrade to leave *de novo* tissue. Other scaffolds use biopolymers such as collagen *(11,61,62)* and hyaluronic acid *(63)*, which are components of the native cartilage matrix. A third class of scaffold materials is hydrogels *(64)*, which have the possible advantage of injection into a defect site. Among the commonly used gels are those polymerized by temperature (agarose) *(65)*, ions (alginate) *(66)*, cross-linking enzymes (fibrin) *(67)*, and light (poly[ethelyne oxide]) and poly[ethylene glycol]) *(68,69)*. Cartilaginous tissue can be formed without scaffolds under certain conditions. These include direct seeding of culture-expanded chondrocytes into a covered defect space *(6)*, micromass culture of chondrogenic cells *(70)*, high-density culture of chondrocytes from immature animals *(71)*, and high-density culture of chondrocytes from adults after preculture in, and recovery from, alginate *(5)*.

When designing construct geometry, it is important to consider bioreactor stimulation, laboratory analysis after in vitro culture, and future clinical application of the engineered cartilage. Having a well-defined geometry, such as a cylindrical disk, can ease the design of bioreactors and allow for simplified models of the solid- and fluid-mechanical environment *(72)*. Additionally, controlling the shape of the developing constructs can allow for more straightforward biochemical and mechanical analysis of the newly formed tissue following culture, without the need for excessive sample manipulation. Although these geometries facilitate tissue formation and subsequent analysis, the application of engineered tissue to cartilage defects may require more complex geometries. If anatomically shaped implants are desired, it is possible to combine 3D imaging techniques such as magnetic resonance imaging (MRI) and sophisticated manufacturing procedures such as 3D printing *(73)* and precision molding *(74)* to generate replacements for very specific defects and possibly even whole joints *(75)*.

Another important choice that significantly affects the growth of the engineered cartilaginous construct is the method of cell seeding. With a preformed scaffold, uniformity and efficiency of seeding are key design goals in the success of tissue generation *(76)*. Static (passive) seeding, in which cells in a dense suspension are allowed to sediment upon (and to a certain extent into) the scaffold, is typically inefficient and results in a high cell density on the periphery of the constructs but a low cell density in the center. Dynamic seeding, either in a well-plate on an orbital shaker or in a spinner flask or rotating bioreactor, enhances both the efficiency and the uniformity of cells seeded into the scaffold *(77)*. If a hydrogel is used, vigorous mixing of the cell/hydrogel suspension, prior to polymerization, facilitates cell dispersion. Also important is minimizing the time needed for polymerization, especially if the curing process has cytotoxic effects. When an exogenous scaffold is omitted (e.g., micromass *[70]* or high-density culture *[5,71]*), the main decisions are the cell seeding density and the amount of time allowed for the cells to form a cohesive mass. With such methods, there is no scaffold to provide volume filling so a very high area density of cells (10^6–10^7 cells/cm^2) is typically formed after cell settling, which is generally an overnight process.

1.2. Mechanical Stimulation In Vitro

The acquisition of mechanical properties in engineered cartilage that approach those of native cartilage does not appear to occur when the tissue is cultured under free-swelling conditions, even for long durations *(78,79)*. After 12 mo, cartilaginous constructs in free-swelling culture attained compressive moduli that were only 10% of those of the native tissue from which the seeded chondrocytes had been derived *(79)*. Although such free-swelling culture conditions provides the investigator with some control over the application of chemical signals (e.g., via addition of growth factors and serum, levels of carbon dioxide, and so on), mechanically proactive culture conditions offer more precise control of the environmental signals, both chemical and mechanical, to which the cells are exposed. Culture conditions that include a mechanical component are made possible by the use of specialized loading chambers, such as bioreactors, in which these aspects of the in vitro culture environment can be regulated.

A number of design criteria are common to all culture approaches that rely on the application of mechanical stimuli. Above all, the loading chambers used must maintain an appropriate environment for tissue culture; thus they must satisfy classical tissue culture criteria *(80)*, including control of ambient temperature and humidity, sufficient exchange of nutrients, gasses, and regulatory factors, sterility, and biocompatibility. Furthermore, bioreactors must be designed to allow the reproducible application of physical stimuli. In this section, we consider details regarding specific modalities of mechanical loading that can be accomplished with the implementation of a bioreactor culture strategy for the tissue engineering of cartilage.

1.2.1. Solid Deformation

During normal ambulation, articular cartilage is subjected to a complex pattern of joint loading that can be decomposed, in general, into time-averaged (static) and time-varying (dynamic) components. Studies indicating that dynamic compression, at certain amplitudes and frequencies, is capable of stimulating the metabolic activities of chondrocytes in cartilage explants in short-term in vitro experiments *(28)* corroborate long-time observations in vivo *(22)* and suggest one modality by which engineered cartilage can be subjected in the long term to the stimulatory influence of physiologic loading (**Fig. 3A**).

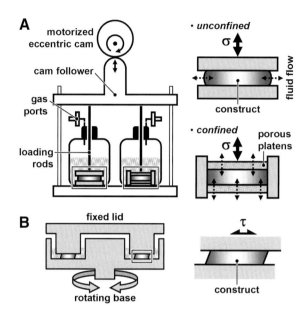

Fig. 3. Various loading configurations for mechanical deformation of cartilaginous constructs. (**A**) Both unconfined and confined compression can be applied using the same incubator-housed actuator apparatus, depending on the sample fixture and platen configuration. (**B**) Tissue shear deformation can be imposed by positioning cartilaginous constructs in contact with culture plate surfaces that rotate relative to each other. Note that for emphasis, the direction of applied shear is shown to be lateral in the figure; in actuality, shear deformation occurs in the direction tangential to the rotation path, which would be into and out of the plane of the page.

In general, accumulation of extracellular matrix *de novo* involves a balance between a number of biological processes, including matrix synthesis, post-translational processing, and extracellular assembly, deposition, and degradation.

Although the stimulatory effects of moderate dynamic compression on overall matrix synthesis have been shown, such loading may reduce the efficiency at which newly synthesized matrix molecules are deposited in cartilage explants, with the induced fluid convection causing an increase in the release of such molecules into medium *(81,82)*, partially counteracting the increased synthesis. Therefore, for long-term accumulation and assembly of cartilaginous matrix, it may be beneficial to introduce periods of load-free, free-swelling culture between controlled duty cycles of dynamic loading, especially since the release of compression exerts stimulatory effects on protein synthesis that can persist for hours *(33,83)*. Bioreactor approaches that include both duty cycles of dynamic compression and periods of load-free culture have been introduced recently *(65,84,85)*. In one such study *(65)*, chondrocytes from 3–5 mo-old bovines were seeded into agarose hydrogels. Once introduced into the bioreactor chamber, cartilaginous constructs underwent 10% dynamic compression at a frequency of 1 Hz for a period of 3 h per day. At the end of 21 d of culture, the loaded constructs exhibited an equilibrium modulus that was approx six times greater than that of their unloaded counterparts and approached 25% of that of native calf cartilage *(86)*, demonstrating the potential value of dynamic loading in the engineering of functional cartilage replacements.

Other modalities of cartilage loading have been investigated as possible regulators of matrix synthesis by the chondrocytes in cartilage explants. Although dynamic compressive loading of a relatively low amplitude has been associated with cartilage stimulation and maintenance *(28)*, excessive loading to the point of impact has been implicated in initiating a cascade of injurious biological processes, such as chondrocyte necrosis and apoptosis and loss of matrix molecules, during subsequent culture of cartilage explants *(46,87,88)*. On the other hand, the application of dynamic shear deformation to cartilage tissue (**Fig. 3B**) stimulated both proteoglycan and protein synthesis *(89)*. The effects of such macroscopic shear deformation did not vary with shear amplitude or frequency. This mode of mechanical loading, in particular, provides novel mechanistic information about the signals to which chondrocytes respond, since under dynamic shear deformation, cartilage undergoes dynamic deformation in the absence of significant induction of fluid flow. Such insights into specific mechanical regulators of cartilage have significant tissue engineering implications: although the role of appropriate mechanical loading in maintaining healthy cartilage is well documented, there are many mechanical strategies for enhancing matrix accumulation in a tissue-engineered construct.

A variety of specialized loading chambers for applying various forms of mechanical loading have been developed for *short-term* studies using cartilage explants (e.g., **ref. 90**). The design of incubator-housed bioreactors for the *long-term* application of mechanical deformation requires some modifications to accommodate both a highly humidified atmosphere and the extended culture periods that necessitate strict standards for sterility and biocompatibility. In general, apparati designed for applying mechanical loads in extended culture must include a culture chamber component that satisfies traditional criteria for tissue culture environments and an actuator component to impart mechanical deformation to samples in a controlled and reproducible manner. The apparatus can be designed to impose either a prescribed displacement or a prescribed load. It may be desirable either to measure or to predict theoretically the other parameter, since prior knowledge of the range in these parameters is critical in determining whether the apparatus has enough stiffness to resist deflection.

It is also important to consider that the nature of physical stimulation may require adjustment over time in culture, as the growing tissue-engineered construct will probably undergo concomitant changes both in geometry and in material properties. These changes in the developing tissue can potentially alter the nature of the physical signals that are transmitted to indwelling cells by the bioreactor and must be considered in any long-term loading protocol design. For instance, a given applied load may be associated with progressively less strain as constructs under dynamic compression acquire increased mechanical stiffness. Also, in the case of tissue shear deformation, slippage between the platen and the tissue sample can also occur at higher strain amplitudes. For these reasons, it may be desirable to monitor aspects of the applied mechanical signals. Such instrumentation can be incorporated into the bioreactor design as part of a feedback control system.

1.2.2. Fluid-Based Perfusion

Perfusion bioreactors, including rotating-wall and direct perfusion bioreactors, represent common forms of bioreactors currently used in cartilage tissue engineering. One of the major design goals of such bioreactors is to promote exchange of nutrients, oxygen, and metabolites between the tissue and culture medium. In addition, the concomitant application of fluid-induced shear stress, compression, hydrostatic pressure, and other factors may provide necessary mechanical signals for enhancing cartilaginous tissue formation. In general, perfusion bioreactors are connected to a medium reservoir that provides a continuous supply of fresh or recycled medium at a controlled flow rate to cartilaginous constructs.

Rotating-wall bioreactors provide a simulated microgravity environment for suspension culture of constructs, while providing laminar flow to enhance mass transfer and to provide mechanical signals (**Fig. 4A**). Although most of the fluid flows around the constructs, and the flow through the constructs is complex, these vessels have been quite successful in stimulating cartilaginous growth and development. Tissue-engineered constructs cultured in rotating-wall bioreactors, for both long (7-mo) and short (6-wk) periods, show increased cell proliferation, accumulation of extracellular matrix, particularly GAG and collagen type II *(91–93)*, and ability to bear compressive load, compared with constructs cultured under free-swelling conditions.

Direct perfusion bioreactors maintain constructs in the path of the fluid flow (**Fig. 4B**) and therefore have the advantage of a more easily defined flow through the constructs. These bioreactors subject constructs to significant physical forces during perfusion culture, including quasi-static compression *(94)* and fluid shear stress, which can directly influence the properties of tissue-engineered constructs *(95)*. Direct perfusion affects matrix metabo-

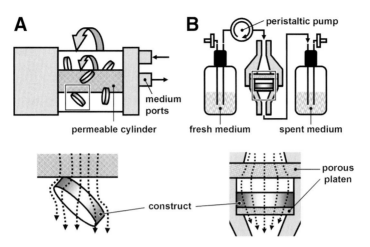

Fig. 4. Culture configurations for perfusion of cartilaginous constructs. **(A)** In rotating wall bioreactors, growing constructs become suspended in the path of the fluid flow induced by the relative motion of the cylindrical walls. The magnified image is a schematic depiction of the fluid path of least resistance, in which fluid flows around the cultured constructs. **(B)** Constructs can also be positioned within perfusion chambers, as shown with accompanying peristaltic pump, media reservoirs, and connecting tubing. In these chambers, the constructs obstruct the path of the fluid flow, and fluid is driven through the cartilaginous constructs.

lism, construct growth, and resultant mechanical properties of constructs. Both intermittent *(96)* and continuous fluid flow *(2,82,95,97,98)* applied at linear velocities of 0.1–100 µm/s to tissue engineered constructs cultured for up to 4 weeks leads to increases in DNA, GAG, and hydroxyproline content compared with static controls *(2,82,97)*. The timing of perfusion stimuli may be important, as application early in culture can inhibit GAG synthesis and accumulation, whereas perfusion later in culture can exhibit the opposite effect *(82)*.

The following sections describe first the generation of cartilaginous constructs in vitro and then the setup of bioreactors that can impart either mechanical deformation or fluid-induced mechanical signals. The intent of some bioreactors is to apply mechanical stimulation over such time that induced cellular activities result in increased accumulation of matrix components and concomitant changes in the functional mechanical properties of cartilaginous constructs. The intent of others is to induce graded levels of cartilage injury.

2. Materials

2.1. Sample Preparation

2.1.1. Cartilage Harvest and Explant Preparation

1. Bovine knee.
2. Table vise.
3. Sterile instruments: scalpel, forceps, squirt bottle, saw blade.
4. Autopsy saw.
5. Sterile phosphate-buffered saline (PBS) at pH 7.4.
6. Penicillin/streptomycin/Fungizone (P/S/F) 100X stock solution, containing 10,000 U penicillin, 10,000 μg streptomycin, and 25 μg amphotericin B per mL (Invitrogen).
7. Sledge microtome (Microm, cat. no. HM440E).
8. Cylindrical punch.

2.1.2. Chondrocyte Isolation

1. Culture medium (DMEM/F12+).
   a. Dulbecco's modified Eagle's medium/Ham's F12 (DMEM/F12).
   b. 0.4 mM L-proline from 100 mM solution, made from powder (Sigma-Aldrich) and filter-sterilized.
   c. 2 mM L-glutamine from 100X stock (Invitrogen).
   d. 0.1 mM nonessential amino acids from 100X stock (Sigma-Aldrich).
   e. P/S/F, diluted 1:100.
2. Fetal bovine serum (FBS; HyClone).
3. Protease type XIV (Sigma-Aldrich).
4. Collagenase P (Roche).
5. Sterile sample cup.
6. Sterile stir bar.
7. 0.22-μm Sterile syringe filter.
8. Cell strainers (40 μm and 70 μm).
9. Trypan blue.
10. Hemacytometer (Neubauer).
11. Centrifuge capable of 750g.

2.1.3. Scaffold Seeding

1. Chondrogenic cells.
2. PLA scaffold (Kensey Nash, DRILAC Cube).
3. Dermal punch.
4. Orbital shaker.

2.1.4. Free-Swelling Construct Culture

1. Ascorbic acid, 25 μg/mL.
2. Multiwell tissue culture plates.
3. DMEM/F12+.

2.2. Mechanical Stimulation In Vitro

2.2.1. Solid Deformation

1. Custom-designed compression or shear bioreactor constructed from biocompatible materials, such as polysulfone or polycarbonate (e.g., **Fig. 3**; *see* **Note 2** for some design considerations).
2. Mechanical actuator capable of imparting desired load or displacement (e.g., linear stepper motors, cam-driven motors, or mechanical testing machines; *see* **Note 3**).
3. Standard incubator for housing bioreactor apparatus to create a culture-like environment (5% CO_2, 95% water-saturated air at 37°C; *see* **Note 4**).
4. Cartilaginous constructs or cartilage explants of defined geometries (e.g., 2–5 mm thick).
5. Medium components.
   a. DMEM/F12+.
   b. FBS.
   c. Ascorbic acid.

2.2.2. Fluid-Based Perfusion

1. Custom-designed perfusion bioreactor constructed from biocompatible materials, such as polysulfone or polycarbonate (e.g., **Fig. 4B**; *see* **Note 5** for some design considerations).
2. Multichannel peristaltic pump (Cole-Parmer Masterflex 9770-50) (*see* **Note 6**).
3. Media reservoir that allows gas exchange.
4. Gas-permeable tubing, such as silicone.
5. Individual polyglycolic acid scaffolds (PGA mesh with 97% porosity and 45-mg/ cm^3 density; Smith & Nephew) of known diameter and thickness to be seeded with cells and placed in individual perfusion bioreactors.
6. Chondrogenic cells in suspension.
7. Medium components.
   a. DMEM/F12+.
   b. FBS.
   c. Ascorbic acid.

3. Methods

3.1. Sample Preparation

The following is an example of steps that may be used to fabricate and mechanically stimulate cartilaginous tissue. First, a method is provided for obtaining geometrically defined cartilage explants that can serve either as control samples for tissue engineering studies, or as samples with which to study the effects of various forms of in vitro stimulation. Then a method to produce cartilaginous constructs, consisting of PLA disks seeded with bovine articular chondrocytes, is provided.

3.1.1. Cartilage Harvest and Explant Preparation (**99**)

1. Obtain an intact bovine knee still surrounded with beef from a local abattoir.
2. Mount the femur in a table vise. Open knee surgically. Use sterile instruments to remove soft tissue and expose the cartilage surfaces of the distal femur. Keep cartilage surfaces irrigated with PBS supplemented with P/S/F.

   If cartilage explants are to be formed, **steps 3–5** are useful. Otherwise, cartilage can be cut off with a scalpel and minced into approx 1-mm³ pieces.
3. Cut osteochondral blocks from the patellofemoral groove and/or femoral condyles using an autopsy saw under copious irrigation with PBS+P/S/F (*see* **Note 7**). Blocks should be rectangular and sized to allow for a relatively flat cartilage surface (~1 ×1 cm²) and should contain approx 1 cm of bone. Store blocks in a sterile sample cup with PBS+P/S/F at 4°C.
4. Mount the blocks on a sledge microtome by gripping the bone such that the cartilage surface is horizontal. Keep blade and cartilage hydrated with PBS+P/S/F.

   a. Incrementally (50–100 μm steps) raise the block until the blade just touches the cartilage surface.
   b. Move the block to the desired thickness (0.2–1.0 mm) and cut the cartilage to obtain slices. Successive cartilage slices can be taken down to the bone (*see* **Note 8**).
5. Trim the slices to fit culture chamber or testing device (*see* **Note 9**).

3.1.2. Chondrocyte Isolation (**100**)

1. Obtain cartilage slices as above, or dissect cartilage off joint directly, mince into pieces, and store them in a sterile sample cup with PBS+P/S/F at 4°C.
2. Digest cartilage enzymatically.

   a. Make medium for enzymatic digestion and cultures.
      i. To DMEM/F12, add sterile L-proline to 0.4 m*M*, L-glutamine to 2 m*M*, nonessential amino acids to 0.1 m*M*, and P/S/F (1:100) to final concentrations of 100 U/mL, 100 μg/mL, and 0.25 μg/mL, respectively. This medium is referred to hereafter as DMEM/F12+.
      ii. Add FBS to DMEM/F12+ (5% final concentration). Make 100 mL for digestion of 3*g* or less of cartilage.
      iii. Dissolve protease type XIV (0.4%) and collagenase P (0.05%) separately in DMEM/F12+ with 5% FBS. Prepare 6 mL of each enzyme solution per gram of cartilage. Use a 0.22-μm syringe filter to sterilize the solutions and keep warm in a 37°C incubator.

   b. Add cartilage to the sample cup with protease solution and incubate for 1 h while stirring using a magnetic stir plate (*see* **Note 10**). Remove medium, and rinse with 50 mL DMEM/F12+ with 5% FBS.
   c. Add collagenase medium to the sample cup with the cartilage slices and incubate for 16 h while stirring (*see* **Note 11**).
   d. Transfer the solution to a sterile 50-mL centrifuge tube through a 70-μm cell strainer. Rinse an additional 25 mL of 4°C PBS through the strainer.

e. Centrifuge at 750*g* for 5 min. Remove and discard the supernatant. Repeat this step an additional two times, each time resuspending the pellet before centrifugation. This removes collagenase activity.

f. Resuspend the cell pellet in DMEM/F12+ with 10% FBS, and filter through a 40-μm cell strainer to obtain a single cell suspension.

g. Measure the volume of the cell suspension, and save 1 drop in a well-plate. Mix 28 μL of the cell suspension with 7 μL of trypan blue. Pipet 10 μL into each side of a hemocytometer. Count the viable (clear) and dead (blue) cells in the main grid of each side.

h. Multiply the average number of live cells by 12,500 to obtain a cell density (cells/mL). Multiply the cell density by the suspension volume to obtain the total number of primary chondrocytes isolated (*see* **Note 1**).

3.1.3. Scaffold Seeding (101)

1. Concentrate the cells to 25 million cells/mL by pelleting the cells and aspirating off the appropriate volume of medium.
2. Create sterile cores of nonwoven PLA mesh using a 3.7-mm-diameter dermal punch on prefabricated polymer cubes. Cut these cores into 3-mm-long segments.
3. Prewet the scaffolds in DMEM/F12+ with 10% FBS for 1 h in a 6-well plate, while revolving at 100 rpm on an orbital shaker.
4. Place PLA scaffolds into individual 50-mL tubes. Seed 80 μL of the cell suspension in each tube. Place the tubes on ice and on an orbital shaker. Shake the tubes at 100 rpm for 1 h to seed the scaffolds efficiently and form cell-laden constructs.

3.1.4. Free-Swelling Construct Culture

1. Place the scaffolds in individual wells of a non-tissue culture-treated 24-well plate. Add 4 mL of medium (DMEM/F12+ with 10% FBS and 25 μg/mL ascorbic acid) to each well.
2. Incubate the plate at 37°C in a humidified incubator for 2 d to allow cells to attach firmly to the scaffold.
3. Collect and freeze a portion of the medium for future analysis.
4. Culture for a given period of time (e.g., 2 wk), with medium changes every other day. Collect and freeze medium for future analysis (*see* **Note 12**).

3.2. Mechanical Stimulation In Vitro

3.2.1. Solid Deformation

Once a bioreactor has been designed for the application of solid deformation, the culture protocol can proceed in a relatively straightforward manner. What follows are the general steps to synthesize cartilaginous constructs under the influence of mechanical deformation (e.g., **refs. 33** and **65**; **Fig. 3**):

1. Prepare cartilaginous constructs or cartilage explants of defined thickness (2–5 mm).
2. Determine the specifics of the loading protocol (*see* **Note 13**).

    a. Configuration (e.g., confined or unconfined compression, or shear loading).
    b. Amplitude (physiological or injurious levels).
    c. Frequency.
    d. Duty cycles and/or periods of load-free culture.
3. Connect bioreactors to mechanical actuators.
4. House the apparatus in a standard incubator (5% CO_2, 37°C).
5. Maintain samples in bioreactors containing 2 mL per million cells of medium, such as DMEM/F12+ supplemented with 10% FBS and 50 µg/mL ascorbate.
6. Maintain free-swelling controls in sterile containers in parallel culture.
7. Change medium three to seven times a week, at regular intervals.

3.2.2. Fluid-Based Perfusion

Varying levels of perfusion can be used to modulate matrix content and can also be used to enhance growth of tissue-engineered cartilage in vitro. Below is an example of one design approach for generating tissue-engineered articular cartilage under conditions of direct perfusion culture using PGA scaffolds seeded with bovine articular cartilage chondrocytes (**Fig. 4B**) *(2)*:

1. Connect bioreactors to media reservoir using gas-permeable tubing such as silicone.
2. Connect bioreactors to a multichannel peristaltic pump with silicone tubing.
3. House apparatus in a standard incubator (5% CO_2, 37°C).
4. Perfusion seeding *(82)*.
    a. Press-fit PGA scaffolds of known diameter and thickness into individual perfusion bioreactors.
    b. Inject chondrocytes in suspension in DMEM/F12+ supplemented with 10% FBS and 25 µg/mL ascorbic acid for a targeted seeding density of 25 million cells/cm^3 scaffold material.
    c. Seed the cells at a flow rate of 2.5 mL/min (corresponding to a linear fluid velocity of ~500 µm/s) for 5 h.
    d. Decrease the flow rate after seeding to 0.05 mL/min (~10 µm/s) and leave the constructs overnight (for 1-d seeding) or longer, making sure to change the medium every 2–3 d.
6. Once the initial growth and seeding is complete, constructs in bioreactors can be subjected to continuous or intermittent flow for the remainder of the culture period (*see* **Note 14**).

3.3. Discussion

In clinical practice, the biological resurfacing of regions of damaged articular cartilage may involve the transplantation of site-matched osteochondral allografts *(102–107)*. Such a transplantation material may immediately withstand the normal mechanical demands placed on joint cartilage, a challenging environment that would disrupt tissue with substantially inferior mechanical properties.

Because of the limited availability of donor tissue, the engineering of mechanically functional cartilage replacements for biological resurfacing has tremendous clinical implications. This chapter has reviewed some of the promising methodologies that are currently being investigated as aids to this ultimate goal of generating tissue-engineered cartilaginous tissue that will become, or remain, functional in the recipient. Some of the same methodologies can be used to study the response of cartilage explants to injurious compression. In summary, the in vitro development of cartilage-like material properties in cartilaginous constructs may require exposure to appropriate mechanical signals that essentially "precondition" the growing tissue in preparation for the mechanical challenges in vivo.

4. Notes

1. Monolayer expansion of cells tends to cause chondrocytes to dedifferentiate into a more fibroblastic phenotype, but further treatment in a three-dimensional gel can induce redifferentiation (*108,109*).
2. Bioreactor design.
   a. Materials such as polysulfone or polycarbonate are convenient choices for bioreactor materials because, in addition to being relatively biocompatible, they can be fabricated by either injection molding or machining, and also can be sterilized in an autoclave.
   b. Particular care must be taken in selecting biocompatible materials for the platens that come into contact with samples and transmit mechanical loads. Such platens can be permeable or impermeable, depending on the specifics of the loading protocol.
3. Mechanical actuator design.
   a. These actuators can be based on cam-driven (*65*) or linear stepper motors (*90*) and may induce deformations directly (displacement control [*90*]) or via spring-loaded rods (load control [*110,111*]).
   b. Alternatively, the chambers may be attached to a mechanical testing machine (*33*).
   c. If load-free cycles are to be inserted between duty cycles, it may be necessary to disengage the culture chambers from the actuators during periods of free-swelling culture.
   d. It may be desirable to monitor aspects of the applied mechanical signals in real time. Such instrumentation can be incorporated into the bioreactor design as part of a feedback control system.
   e. The apparatus (bioreactor and mechanical actuator) should be designed to withstand the humidified environment of a standard incubator (e.g., rust-proof, with motorized parts properly sealed).
4. An alternative to incubator-housing the bioreactor apparatus is to circulate warmed, pH-controlled medium through an external apparatus to create a culture-like environment.

5. Bioreactor design (e.g., **ref. *112***). Perfusion-based bioreactors should be designed so that there is a tight fit between the edge of the construct and the inner wall of the bioreactor. This prevents fluid from flowing around the periphery of the construct and directs flow through the construct itself.

6. Perfusion system design.

   a. A multichannel pump is useful if multiple bioreactors are to be subjected to perfusion in parallel flow paths.

   b. Peristaltic pumps may require the use of an inline damper to reduce pressure fluctuations.

   c. Flow medium can be recirculated, both for reducing the amount of medium needed and also to preserve some of the chemical signals, i.e., growth factors or proteins, secreted by cartilaginous constructs. Fresh medium can also be mixed with spent medium to serve this purpose.

   d. The pump should be capable of generating the hydrostatic pressures that occur as the prescribed fluid flow rate is forced through constructs that typically decrease in permeability during culture.

   e. Monitoring pressure may be useful.

7. Alternatively, osteochondral cores can be taken with surgical harvesting devices such as the Osteochondral Autograft Transfer System (Arthrex).

8. The depth of slices, relative to the articular surface, may be important, as there are zonal variations in the chondrocytes of cartilage *(113)*.

9. A typical configuration is a disk (e.g., 3-mm-diameter × 1-mm-thick), formed by using a dermal punch *(111)*.

10. Loosely cap the enzyme solutions during the digestion to allow for gas exchange.

11. After the collagenase incubation, there should not be any visible pieces of tissue remaining, and the medium should be slightly cloudy.

12. Periodically move constructs to a new well-plate to avoid cell outgrowth on the surface of the plate.

13. Loading protocol.

    a. Configuration: although many of the short-term experimental studies on the effects of compression on cartilage have employed explants loaded in a radially unconfined configuration *(28,33)*, loading in confined compression *(110,114)* has the advantage of rigorously maintaining the radial dimension of a growing construct. Shear-loaded samples are typically not confined radially.

    b. Amplitude: low-amplitude dynamic compression tends to mimic stimulatory effects of physiologic loading, whereas high strain rate impact loading can lead to cartilage injury.

    c. Frequency: higher loading frequencies (>0.01 Hz *[33]*) have stimulatory effects on biosynthesis and may approximate such effects of physiologic loading. However, at high frequency-amplitude combinations, lift-off can occur, when the samples do not "rebound" quickly enough and when there is no platen resting on top.

    d. Duty cycle: periods of free-swelling culture in between duty cycles of loading seem to facilitate stabilization of newly synthesized matrix molecules. This may not be necessary for samples loaded with dynamic tissue shear, since little fluid convection occurs in that loading configuration *(90)*.

14. Spent medium from seeding or growth perfusion culture may be saved for later analysis.

References

1. Freed, L. E., Vunjak-Novakovic, G., and Langer, R. (1993) Cultivation of cell-polymer cartilage implants in bioreactors. *J. Cell. Biochem.* **51,** 257–264.
2. Dunkelman, N. S., Zimber, M. P., LeBaron, R. G., Pavelec, R., Kwan, M., and Purchio, A. F. (1995) Cartilage production by rabbit articular chondrocytes on polyglycolic acid scaffolds in a closed bioreactor system. *Biotechno.l Bioeng.* **46,** 299–305.
3. Wakitani, S., Kimura, T., Hirooka, A., et al. (1989) Repair of rabbit articular surfaces with allograft chondrocytes embedded in collagen gel. *J. Bone Joint. Surg. Br.* **71-B,** 74–80.
4. Kim, W. S., Vacanti, J. P., Cima, L., et al. (1994) Cartilage engineered in predetermined shapes employing cell transplantation on synthetic biodegradable polymers. *Plast. Reconstr. Surg.* **94,** 233–237.
5. Masuda, K., Sah, R. L., Hejna, M. J., and Thonar, E. J.-M. A. (2003) A novel two-step method for the formation of tissue engineered cartilage: the alginate-recovered-chondrocyte (ARC) method. *J. Orthop. Res.* **21,** 139–148.
6. Brittberg, M., Lindahl, A., Nilsson, A., Ohlsson, C., Isaksson, O., and Peterson, L. (1994) Treatment of deep cartilage defects in the knee with autologous chondrocyte transplantation. *N. Engl. J. Med.* **331,** 889–895.
7. Peterson, L., Minas, T., Brittberg, M., Nilsson, A., Sjogren-Jansson, E., and Lindahl, A. (2000) Two- to 9-year outcome after autologous chondrocyte transplantation of the knee. *Clin. Orthop.* **374,** 212–234.
8. Breinan, H. A., Minas, T., Barone, L., et al. (1998) Histological evaluation of the course of healing of canine articular cartilage defects treated with cultured autologous chondrocytes. *Tissue Eng.* **4,** 101–114.
9. Brittberg, M., Nilsson, A., Lindahl, A., Ohlsson, C., and Peterson, L. (1996) Rabbit articular cartilage defects treated with autologous cultured chondrocytes. *Clin. Orthop.* **326,** 270–283.
10. Nehrer, S., Breinan, H. H., Ashkar, S., et al. (1998) Characteristics of articular chondrocytes seeded in collagen matrices in vitro. *Tissue Eng.* **4,** 175–183.
11. Sams, A. E. and Nixon, A. J. (1995) Chondrocyte-laden collagen scaffolds for resurfacing extensive articular cartilage defects. *Osteoarthritis Cartilage* **3,** 47–59.
12. Shortkroff, S., Barone, L., Hsu, H. P., et al. (1996) Healing of chondral and osteochondral defects in a canine model: the role of cultured chondrocytes in regeneration of articular cartilage. *Biomaterials* **17,** 147–154.
13. Wakitani, S., Goto, T., Young, R. G., Mansour, J. M., Goldberg, V. M., and Caplan, A. I. (1998) Repair of large full-thickness articular cartilage defects with allograft articular chondrocytes embedded in a collagen gel. *Tissue. Eng.* **4,** 429–444.

14. Muir, H. (1995) The chondrocyte, architect of cartilage. Biomechanics, structure, function and molecular biology of cartilage matrix macromolecules. *Bioessays* **17**, 1039–1048.

15. Slowman, S. D. and Brandt, K. D. (1986) Composition and glycosaminoglycan metabolism of articular cartilage from habitually loaded and habitually unloaded sites. *Arthritis Rheum.* **29**, 88–94.

16. Kiviranta, I., Jurvelin, J., Tammi, M., Saamanen, A.-M., and Helminen, H. J. (1987) Weight bearing controls glycosaminoglycan concentration and articular cartilage thickness in the knee joints of young beagle dogs. *Arthritis Rheum.* **30**, 801–809.

17. Behrens, F., Kraft, E. L., and Oegema, T. R. (1989) Biochemical changes in articular cartilage after joint immobilization by casting or external fixation. *J. Orthop. Res.* **7**, 335–343.

18. Caterson, B. and Lowther, D. A. (1978) Changes in the metabolism of the proteoglycans from sheep articular cartilage in response to mechanical stress. *Biochim. Biophys. Acta* **540**, 412–422.

19. Jurvelin, J., Kiviranta, I., Saamanen, A.-M., Tammi, M., and Helminen, H. J. (1989) Partial restoration of immobilization-induced softening of canine articular cartilage after remobilization of the knee (stifle) joint. *J. Orthop. Res.* **7**, 352–358.

20. Saamanen, A.-M., Tammi, M., Jurvelin, J., Kiviranta, I., and Helminen, H. J. (1990) Proteoglycan alterations following immobilization and remobilization in the articular cartilage of young canine knee (stifle) joint. *J. Orthop. Res.* **8**, 863–873.

21. Kiviranta, I., Tammi, M., Jurvelin, J., Saamanen, A. M., and Helminen, H. J. (1988) Moderate running exercise augments glycosaminoglycans and thickness of articular cartilage in the knee joint of young beagle dogs. *J. Orthop. Res.* **6**, 188–195.

22. Helminen, H. J., Jurvelin, J., Kiviranta, I., Paukkonen, K., Säämänen, A.-M., and Tammi, M. (1987) Joint loading effects on articular cartilage: a historical review, in *Joint Loading: Biology and Health of Articular Structures* (Helminen, H. J., Kiviranta, I., Tammi, M., Säämänen, A.-M., Paukkonen, K,. and Jurvelin, J., eds.), Wright, Bristol, UK, pp. 1–46.

23. Grodzinsky, A. J. (1983) Electromechanical and physicochemical properties of connective tissue. *CRC Crit. Rev. Bioeng.* **9**, 133–199.

24. Maroudas, A. (1979) Physico-chemical properties of articular cartilage, in *Adult Articular Cartilage* 2nd ed., (Freeman, M. A. R., ed.), Pitman Medical, Tunbridge Wells, England, UK, pp. 215–290.

25. Mow, V. C., Wang, C. C., and Hung, C. T. (1999) The extracellular matrix, interstitial fluid and ions as a mechanical signal transducer in articular cartilage. *Osteoarthritis Cartilage* **7**, 41–58.

26. Urban, J. P. (2000) Present perspectives on cartilage and chondrocyte mechanobiology. *Biorheology* **37**, 185–190.

27. Grodzinsky, A. J., Levenston, M. E., Jin, M., and Frank, E. H. (2000) Cartilage tissue remodeling in response to mechanical forces. *Annu. Rev. Biomed. Eng.* **2**, 691–713.

28. Guilak, F., Sah, R. L., and Setton, L. A. (1997) Physical regulation of cartilage metabolism, in *Basic Orthopaedic Biomechanics* 2nd Ed. (Mow, V. C. and Hayes, W. C., eds.), Raven, New York, NY, pp. 179–207.

29. Burton-Wurster, N., Vernier-Singer, M., Farquhar, T., and Lust, G. (1993) Effect of compressive loading and unloading on the synthesis of total protein, proteoglycan, and fibronectin by canine cartilage explants. *J. Orthop. Res.* **11,** 717–729.

30. Gray, M. L., Pizzanelli, A. M., Grodzinsky, A. J., and Lee, R. C. (1988) Mechanical and physicochemical determinants of the chondrocyte biosynthetic response. *J. Orthop. Res.* **6,** 777–792.

31. Guilak, F., Meyer, B. C., Ratcliffe, A., and Mow, V. C. (1994) The effects of matrix compression on proteoglycan metabolism in articular cartilage explants. *Osteoarthritis Cartilage* **2,** 91–101.

32. Jones, I. L., Klamfeldt, D. D. S., and Sandstrom, T. (1982) The effect of continuous mechanical pressure upon the turnover of articular cartilage proteoglycans in vitro. *Clin. Orthop.* **165,** 283–289.

33. Sah, R. L., Kim, Y. J., Doong, J. H., Grodzinsky, A. J., Plaas, A. H. K., and Sandy, J. D. (1989) Biosynthetic response of cartilage explants to dynamic compression. *J. Orthop. Res.* **7,** 619–636.

34. Copray, J. C. V. M., Jansen, H. W. B., and Duterloo, H. S. (1985) Effect of compressive forces on phosphatase activity in mandibular condylar cartilage of the rat in vitro. *J. Anat.* **140,** 479–489.

35. Palmoski, M. J. and Brandt, K. D. (1984) Effects of static and cyclic compressive loading on articular cartilage plugs in vitro. *Arthritis Rheum.* **27,** 675–681.

36. Parkkinen, J. J., Lammi, M. J., Helminen, H. J., and Tammi, M. (1992) Local stimulation of proteoglycan synthesis in articular cartilage explants by dynamic compression in vitro. *J. Orthop. Res.* **10,** 610–620.

37. Buschmann, M. D., Kim, Y. J., Wong, M., Frank, E., Hunziker, E. B., and Grodzinsky, A. J. (1999) Stimulation of aggrecan synthesis in cartilage explants by cyclic loading is localized to regions of high interstitial fluid flow. *Arch. Biochem. Biophys.* **366,** 1–7.

38. Kim, Y. J., Sah, R. L., Grodzinsky, A. J., Plaas, A. H. K., and Sandy, J. D. (1994) Mechanical regulation of cartilage biosynthetic behavior: physical stimuli. *Arch. Biochem. Biophys.* **311,** 1–12.

39. Buschmann, M. D., Gluzband, Y. A., and Grodzinsky, A. J. (1995) Mechanical compression modulates matrix biosynthesis in chondrocyte/agarose culture. *J. Cell Sci.* **108,** 1497–1508.

40. Lee, D. A. and Bader, D. L. (1997) Compressive strains at physiological frequencies influence the metabolism of chondrocytes seeded in agarose. *J. Orthop. Res.* **15,** 181–188.

41. Ragan, P. M., Chin, V. I., Hung, H. H., et al. (2000) Chondrocyte extracellular matrix synthesis and turnover are influenced by static compression in a new alginate disk culture system. *Arch. Biochem. Biophys.* **383,** 256–264.

42. Fukuda, K., Kumano, F., Asada, S., Saitoh, M., and Tanaka, S. (1997) Cyclic tensile stretch loaded on bovine articular chondrocytes inhibits protein kinase C activity. *Osteoarthritis Cartilage* **5**, A38.

43. Smith, R. L., Donlon, B. S., Gupta, M. K., et al. (1995) Effects of fluid-induced shear on articular chondrocyte morphology and metabolism in vitro. *J. Orthop. Res.* **13**, 824–831.

44. Parkkinen, J. J., Ikonen, J., Lammi, M. J., Laakkonen, J., Tammi, M., and Helminen, H. J. (1993) Effects of cyclic hydrostatic pressure on proteoglycan synthesis in cultured chondrocytes and articular cartilage explants. *Arch. Biochem. Biophys.* **300**, 458–465.

45. Thibault, M., Poole, A. R., and Buschmann, M. D. (2002) Cyclic compression of cartilage/bone explants in vitro leads to physical weakening, mechanical break-down of collagen and release of matrix fragments. *J. Orthop. Res.* **20**, 1265–1273.

46. Loening, A., Levenston, M., James, I., Nuttal, M., et al. (2000) Injurious mechanical compression of bovine articular cartilage induces chondrocyte apoptosis. *Arch. Biochem. Biophys.* **381**, 205–212.

47. D'Lima, D. D., Hashimoto, S., Chen, P. C., Colwell, C. W. Jr., and Lotz, M. K. (2001) Impact of mechanical trauma on matrix and cells. *Clin. Orthop.* **391 (Suppl.)**, S90–S99.

48. Kurz, B., Jin, M., Patwari, P., Cheng, D. M., Lark, M. W., and Grodzinsky, A. J. (2001) Biosynthetic response and mechanical properties of articular cartilage after injurious compression. *J. Orthop. Res.* **19**, 1140–1146.

49. Clements, K. M., Bee, Z. C., Crossingham, G. V., Adams, M. A., and Sharif, M. (2001) How severe must repetitive loading be to kill chondrocytes in articular cartilage? *Osteoarthritis Cartilage* **9**, 499–507.

50. Quinn, T. M., Allen, R. G., Schalet, B. J., Perumbuli, P., and Hunziker, E. B. (2001) Matrix and cell injury due to sub-impact loading of adult bovine articular cartilage explants: effects of strain rate and peak stress. *J. Orthop. Res.* **19**, 242–249.

51. D'Lima, D. D., Hashimoto, S., Chen, P. C., Lotz, M. K., and Colwell, C. W. Jr. (2001) Cartilage injury induces chondrocyte apoptosis. *J. Bone Joint. Surg. Am.* **83-A(Suppl. 2)**, 19–21.

52. Freed, L. E., Grande, D. A., Lingbin, Z., Emmanual, J., Marquis, J. C., and Langer, R. (1994) Joint resurfacing using allograft chondrocytes and synthetic biodegradable polymer scaffolds. *J. Biomed. Mater. Res.* **28**, 891–899.

53. Amiel, D., Chu, C. R., Sah, R. L., and Coutts, R. D. (1998) Tissue engineering of articular cartilage: perichondrial cells in osteochondral repair. *Cells Mat.* **8**, 161–174.

54. Nakahara, H., Goldberg, V. M., and Caplan, A. I. (1991) Culture-expanded human periosteal-derived cells exhibit osteochondral potential in vivo. *J. Orthop. Res.* **9**, 465–476.

55. Wakitani, S., Goto, T., Pineda, S. J., et al. (1994) Mesenchymal cell-based repair of large, full-thickness defects of articular cartilage. *J. Bone Joint. Surg.* **76-A**, 579–592.

56. Johnstone, B. and Yoo, J. U. (1999) Autologous mesenchymal progenitor cells in articular cartilage repair. *Clin. Orthop.* **367S,** 156–162.

57. Zuk, P. A., Zhu, M., Mizuno, H., et al. (2001) Multilineage cells from human adipose tissue: implications for cell-based therapies. *Tissue Eng.* **7,** 211–228.

58. Häuselmann, H. J., Masuda, K., Hunziker, E. B., et al. (1996) Adult human chondrocytes cultured in alginate form a matrix similar to native human articular cartilage. *Am. J. Physiol.* **40,** C742–C752.

59. Chu, C. R., Coutts, R. D., Yoshioka, M., Harwood, F. L., Monosov, A. Z., and Amiel, D. (1995) Articular cartilage repair using allogeneic perichondrocyte seeded biodegradable porous polylactic acid (PLA): a tissue engineering study. *J. Biomed. Mater. Res.* **29,** 1147–1154.

60. Moran, J. M., Pazzano, D., and Bonassar, L. J. (2003) Characterization of polylactic acid-polyglycolic acid composites for cartilage tissue engineering. *Tissue Eng.* **9,** 63–70.

61. Ben-Yishay, A., Grande, D. A., Schwartz, R. E., Menche, D., and Pitman, M. D. (1995) Repair of articular cartilage defects with collagen-chondrocyte allografts. *Tissue Eng.* **1,** 119–133.

62. Lee, C. R., Grodzinsky, A. J., Hsu, H. P., and Spector, M. (2003) Effects of a cultured autologous chondrocyte-seeded type II collagen scaffold on the healing of a chondral defect in a canine model. *J. Orthop. Res.* **21,** 272–281.

63. Solchaga, L. A., Yoo, J. U., Lundberg, M., et al. (2000) Hyasluronan-based polymers in the treatment of osteochondral defects. *J. Orthop. Res.* **18,** 773–780.

64. Lee, K. Y. and Mooney, D. J. (2001) Hydrogels for tissue engineering. *Chem. Rev.* **101,** 1869–1879.

65. Mauck, R. L., Soltz, M. A., Wang, C. C., et al. (2000) Functional tissue engineering of articular cartilage through dynamic loading of chondrocyte-seeded agarose gels. *J. Biomech. Eng.* **122,** 252–260.

66. Guo, J. F., Jourdian, G. W., and MacCallum, D. K. (1989) Culture and growth characteristics of chondrocytes encapsulated in alginate beads. *Connect. Tissue Res.* **19,** 277–297.

67. van Susante, J. L., Buma, P., Schuman, L., Homminga, G. N., van den Berg, W. B., and Veth, R. P. (1999) Resurfacing potential of heterologous chondrocytes suspended in fibrin glue in large full-thickness defects of femoral articular cartilage: an experimental study in the goat. *Biomaterials* **20,** 1167–1175.

68. Bryant, S. J. and Anseth, K. S. (2003) Controlling the spatial distribution of ECM components in degradable PEG hydrogels for tissue engineering cartilage. *J. Biomed. Mater. Res.* **64A,** 70–79.

69. Elisseeff, J., Anseth, K., Sims, D., McIntosh, W., Randolph, M., and Langer, R. (1999) Transdermal photopolymerization for minimally invasive implantation. *Proc. Natl. Acad. Sci. USA* **96,** 3104–3107.

70. Pittenger, M. F., Mackay, A. M., Beck, S. C., et al. (1999) Multilineage potential of adult human mesenchymal stem cells. *Science* **284,** 143–147.

71. Kandel, R. A., Chen, H., Clark, J., and Renlund, R. (1995) Transplantation of cartilagenous tissue generated in vitro into articular joint defects. *Artif. Cells Blood Substit. Immobil. Biotechnol.* **23,** 565–577.

72. Williams, K. A., Saini, S., and Wick, T. M. (2002) Computational fluid dynamics modeling of steady-state momentum and mass transport in a bioreactor for cartilage tissue engineering. *Biotechnol. Prog.* **18,** 951–963.

73. Park, A., Wu, B., and Griffith, L. G. (1998) Integration of surface modification and 3D fabrication techniques to prepare patterned poly(L-lactide) substrates allowing regionally selective cell adhesion. *J. Biomater. Sci. Polym. Ed.* **9,** 89–110.

74. Chang, S. C., Rowley, J. A., Tobias, G., et al. (2001) Injection molding of chondrocyte/alginate constructs in the shape of facial implants. *J. Biomed. Mater. Res.* **55,** 503–511.

75. Khouri, R. K., Koudsi, B., and Reddi, H. (1991) Tissue transformation into bone in vivo. A potential practical application. *JAMA* **266,** 1953–1955.

76. Pei, M., Solchaga, L. A., Seidel, J., et al. (2002) Bioreactors mediate the effectiveness of tissue engineering scaffolds. *FASEB J.* **16,** 1691–1694.

77. Vunjak-Novakovic, G., Obradovic, B., Martin, I., Bursac, P. M., Langer, R., and Freed, L. E. (1998) Dynamic cell seeding of polymer scaffolds for cartilage tissue engineering. *Biotechnol. Prog.* **14,** 193–202.

78. Martin, I., Obradovic, B., Treppo, S., et al. (2000) Modulation of the mechanical properties of tissue engineered cartilage. *Biorheology* **37,** 141–147.

79. Ahsan, T., Chen, A. C., Chin, L., et al. (2003) Effects of long-term growth on tissue engineered cartilage. *Trans. Orthop. Res. Soc.* **28,** 309.

80. Freshney, R. I. (1994) *Culture of Animal Cells: A Manual of Basic Technique* 3rd. Ed., Wiley-Liss, New York, NY.

81. Sah, R. L., Doong, J. Y. H., Grodzinsky, A. J., Plaas, A. H. K., and Sandy, J. D. (1991) Effects of compression on the loss of newly synthesized proteoglycans and proteins from cartilage explants. *Arch. Biochem. Biophys.* **286,** 20–29.

82. Davisson, T. H., Sah, R. L., and Ratcliffe, A. R. (2002) Perfusion increases cell content and matrix synthesis in chondrocyte three-dimensional cultures. *Tissue Eng.* **8,** 807–816.

83. Gray, M. L., Pizzanelli, A. M., Lee, R. C., Grodzinsky, A. J., and Swann, D. A. (1989) Kinetics of the chondrocyte biosynthetic response to compressive load and release. *Biochim. Biophys. Acta* **991,** 415–425.

84. Kisiday, J., Siparsky, P. N., and Grodzinsky, A. J. (2003) Anabolic and catabolic response to dynamic compression in a chondrocyte-seeded self-assembling peptide hydrogel. *Trans. Orthop. Res. Soc.* **28,** 304.

85. Kisiday, J., Jin, M., and Grodzinsky, A. J. (2002) Effects of dynamic compressive loading duty cycle on in vitro conditioning of chondrocyte-seeded peptide and agarose scaffolds. *Trans. Orthop. Res. Soc.* **27,** 216.

86. Williamson, A. K., Chen, A. C., and Sah, R. L. (2001) Compressive properties and function-composition relationships of developing bovine articular cartilage. *J. Orthop. Res.* **19,** 1113–1121.

87. Quinn, T. M., Grodzinsky, A. J., Hunziker, E. B., and Sandy, J. D. (1998) Effects of injurious compression on matrix turnover around individual cells in calf articular cartilage explants. *J. Orthop. Res.* **16**, 490–499.

88. Jeffrey, J. E., Thomson, L. A., and Aspden, R. M. (1997) Matrix loss and synthesis following a single impact load on articular cartilage in vitro. *Biochim. Biophys. Acta* **1334**, 223–232.

89. Jin, M., Frank, E. H., Quinn, T. M., Hunziker, E. B., and Grodzinsky, A. J. (2001) Tissue shear deformation stimulates proteoglycan and protein biosynthesis in bovine cartilage explants. *Arch. Biochem. Biophys.* **395**, 41–48.

90. Frank, E. H., Jin, M., Loening, A. M., Levenston, M. E., and Grodzinsky, A. J. (2000) A versatile shear and compression apparatus for mechanical stimulation of tissue culture explants. *J. Biomech.* **33**, 1523–1527.

91. Vunjak-Novakovic, G., Martin, I., Obradovic, B., et al. (1999) Bioreactor cultivation conditions modulate the composition and mechanical properties of tissue-engineered cartilage. *J. Orthop. Res.* **17**, 130–139.

92. Vunjak-Novakovic, G., Obradovic, B., Martin, I., and Freed, L. E. (2002) Bioreactor studies of native and tissue engineered cartilage. *Biorheology* **39**, 259–268.

93. Obradovic, B., Meldon, J. H., Freed, L. E., and Vunjak-Novakovic, G. (2000) Glycosaminoglycan deposition in engineered cartilage: experiments and mathematical model. *AICHE J.* **46**, 1860–1871.

94. Davisson, T. H., Ratcliffe, A., and Sah, R. L. (2000) Flow-induced physical stimuli during cartilage tissue engineering. *Trans. Orthop. Res. Soc.* **25**, 610.

95. Davisson, T. H., Wu, F. J., Jain, D., Sah, R. L., and Ratcliffe, A. R. (1999) Effect of perfusion on the growth of tissue engineered cartilage. *Trans. Orthop. Res. Soc.* **24**, 811.

96. Sittinger, M., Schultz, O., Keyszer, G., Minuth, W. W., and Burmester, G. R. (1997) Artificial tissues in perfusion culture. *Int. J. Artif. Organs* **20**, 57–62.

97. Pazzano, D., Mercier, K. A., Moran, J. M., et al. (2000) Comparison of chondrogensis in static and perfused bioreactor culture. *Biotechnol. Prog.* **16**, 893–896.

98. Davisson, T. H., Kunig, S., Chen, A. C., Sah, R. L., and Ratcliffe, A. (2002) The effects of perfusion and compression on modulation of tissue engineered cartilage. *Trans. Orthop. Res. Soc.* **277**, 488.

99. Buschmann, M. D., Gluzband, Y. A., Grodzinsky, A. J., Kimura, J. H., and Hunziker, E. B. (1992) Chondrocytes in agarose culture synthesize a mechanically functional extracellular matrix. *J. Orthop. Res.* **10**, 745–758.

100. Mok, S. S., Masuda, K., Häuselmann, H. J., Aydelotte, M. B., and Thonar, E. J. (1994) Aggrecan synthesized by mature bovine chondrocytes suspended in alginate. Identification of two distinct metabolic matrix pools. *J. Biol. Chem.* **269**, 33,021–33,027.

101. Giurea, A., Klein, T. J., Chen, A. C., et al. (2003) Adhesion of perichondrial cells to a polylactic acid scaffold. *J. Orthop. Res.* **21**, 584–589.

102. Bugbee, W. D. and Convery, F. R. (1999) Osteochondral allograft transplantation. *Clin. Sports Med.* **18**, 67–75.

103. Outerbridge, H. K., Outerbridge, A. R., and Outerbridge, R. E. (1995) The use of a lateral patellar autologous graft for the repair of a large osteochondral defect in the knee. *J. Bone Joint Surg. Am.* **77-A,** 65–72.

104. McDermott, A. G., Langer, F., Pritzker, K. P., and Gross, A. E. (1985) Fresh small-fragment osteochondral allografts. Long-term follow-up study on first 100 cases. *Clin. Orthop.* **197,** 96–102.

105. Yamashita, F., Sakakida, K., Suzu, F., and Takai, S. (1985) The transplantation of an autogeneic osteochondral fragment for osteochondritis dissecans of the knee. *Clin. Orthop.* **201,** 43–50.

106. Bobic, V. (1996) Arthroscopic osteochondral autograft transplantation in anterior cruciate ligament reconstruction: a preliminary clinical study. *Knee Surg. Sports Traumatol. Arthrosc.* **3,** 262–264.

107. Matsusue, Y., Yamamuro, T., and Hama, H. (1993) Arthroscopic multiple osteochondral transplantation to the chondral defect in the knee associated with anterior cruciate ligament disruption. *Arthroscopy* **9,** 318–321.

108. Benya, P. D. and Shaffer, J. D. (1982) Dedifferentiated chondrocytes reexpress the differentiated collagen phenotype when cultured in agarose gels. *Cell* **30,** 215–224.

109. Bonaventure, J., Kadhom, N., Cohen-Solal, L., et al. (1994) Re-expression of cartilage-specific genes by dedifferentiated human articular chondrocytes cultured in alginate beads. *Exp. Cell Res.* **212,** 97–104.

110. Chen, A. C. and Sah, R. L. (1998) The effect of static compression on proteoglycan synthesis by chondrocytes transplanted to articular cartilage in vitro. *J. Orthop. Res.* **16,** 542–550.

111. Li, K. W., Williamson, A. K., Wang, A. S., and Sah, R. L. (2001) Growth responses of cartilage to static and dynamic compression. *Clin. Orthop.* **391S,** 34–48.

112. Schreiber, R. E., Ilten-Kirby, B. M., Dunkelman, N. S., et al. (1999) Repair of osteochondral defects with allogeneic tissue engineered cartilage implants. *Clin. Orthop.* **367 (Suppl),** 382–395.

113. Klein, T. K., Schumacher, B. L., Schmidt, T. A., et al. (2003) Tissue engineering of stratified articular cartilage from chondrocyte subpopulations. *Osteoarthritis Cartilage* **11,** 592–602.

114. Davisson, T. H., Kunig, S., Chen, A. C., Sah, R. L., and Ratcliffe, A. (2002) Static and dynamic compression modulate biosynthesis in tissue engineered cartilage. *J. Orthop. Res.* **20,** 842–848.

115. Sah, R. L. (2003) The biomechanical faces of articular cartilage, in *The Many Faces of Osteoarthritis* (Hascall, V. C., Kuettner, K. E., and Krall, A. M., eds.), Birkhauser Verlag, Basel, Switzerland, pp. 506.

116. Bullough, P. G. and Cawston, T. E. (1994) Pathology and biochemistry of osteoarthritis, in *Color Atlas and Text of Osteoarthritis* (Doherty, M., ed.), Times Mirror International, London, UK, pp. 29–60.

117. Hunziker, E. B. (1992) Articular cartilage structure in humans and experimental animals, in *Articular Cartilage and Osteoarthritis* (Kuettner, K. E.,

Schleyerbach, R., Peyron, J. G., and Hascall, V. C., eds.), Raven, New York, NY, pp. 183–199.

118. Rosenberg, L. C. and Buckwalter, J. A. (1986) Cartilage proteoglycans, in *Articular Cartilage Biochemistry* (Kuettner, K., Schleyerbach, R., and Hascall, V. C., eds.), Raven, New York, NY, pp. 39–57.

Index

DATE DUE